*100% research*

# The Scientific Validation of

# Herbal Medicine

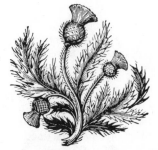

## Daniel B. Mowrey, Ph.D. →

*Speaks 5 languages & plays many musical instruments.*

How to remedy and prevent disease with Herbs, Vitamins, Minerals and other nutrients.

**IMPORTANT!** The information contained in this booklet is intended for educational purposes only. It is not provided in order to diagnose, prescribe, or treat any disease, illness, or injured condition of the body, and the author, publisher, printer(s), and distributor(s) accept no responsibility for such use. Those individuals suffering from any disease, illness, or injury should consult with their physician.

**NOTE:** Many persons, on their first encounter with the information presented in this book, are tempted to throw out their medications and start using nothing but herbs. Please do not do that. Your education in this field is just beginning. In my opinion people should ease into the use of herbs, and ease out of the use of traditional medications only where possible, especially if their health problems are severe. A sudden switch of health regimen can be hazardous.

**NOTE: Throughout the book, I use the word 'treat' to describe the relationship between an herb and its users. The word is not a synonym for 'cure'. It implies only that the herb is used by certain people in an 'attempt to cure'. There is a big difference between treat and cure: While cure involves a successful treatment, treat does not imply success; it only suggests the attempt.**

# FORWARD

It was with great pleasure that I had an opportunity to evaluate the manuscript of Dr. Mowrey's book. The field of herbal products and natural botanical medicines has been fraught with considerable confusion, controversy, and misinformation over the past several years. We have seen consumer interest rise in these natural proucts without knowledge of their positive values, side effects, and hazards from abuse.

It was a breath of fresh air to read through Dr. Mowrey's treatise on The Scientific Validation of Herbal Medicine, which is the first comprehensive manuscript that I have seen which deals with the science, history, pharmacology and clinical applications of herbal materials. The book is highly referenced and illustrates a scientific approach to this complex field. He has weaved a very subtle balance between the clinical anecdote, the history of natural botanicals, and the science which underlies their efficacy. I found the reading to be most enlightening and in a style that flowed and inspired me to read on. We have needed this type of book for some time to clarify issues and separate fact from fiction concerning herbal products.

The birthing of the field of green medicine began when pharmacological evaluations of indigenous aztec medicines yielded agents with important implications in the treatment of modern disease. Since then medicinal plants have provided the foundation of the modern pharmaceutical industry. Certainly, natural products may suffer from a lack of defined dose and potency data, but they benefit from the virtue of containing many specific molecular principles in their natural state possessing a variety of influences upon human physiology, as opposed to the purified synthetic drugs which are based on just a single specific molecular substance derived from the natural product. Dr. Mowrey has described these differences very nicely in this book and I believe this volume (and the forthcoming Volume II) should be of great benefit to any individual who is concerned about natural healing and its clinical applications.


Jeffrey S. Bland, PhD
Director in Nutrition
Analysis Laboratory
Linus Pauling Institute

Dedicated To
Gail & June
Roy & Mable

# PREFACE

The scientific method has been the bedrock of humankind's explosive progress in the medical sciences for the past dozen decades or so (see the Introduction for more details). The use of this method of human inquiry has had profound impact on all cultures that have discovered its power. The material reviewed in this book, unlike the anecdotal material of most books about herbs, rests upon a foundation built with the use of the scientific method.

Here are some preliminary observations about herbal medicine in America that do not necessarily pertain to the rest of the world: The material in this book is not common knowledge. In spite of a resurgence in natural health, ninety percent of the references in this book are from medical journals outside the American continent. Most Americans have a bias against the use of herbal medicines. Medical doctors hesitate to promote the use of herbs. Pharmaceutical companies do not manufacture herbs nor encourage doctors to prescribe them. There is no educational support in the medical community for folk medicine. Why has America ignored the scientific validation of herbal medicine? To understand the uniquely American situation, one needs to examine the development of medical science generally, and the nature of American science specifically.

## Historical Perspectives

A study of the history of herbal research reveals some of the reasons American medicine evolved the way it did, and suggests ways that *sound* herbology and *sound* pharmacology can be united in medical practice.

Historical differences in the development of herbal medicine between Western and Eastern cultures require that the two patterns be discussed separately. We shall see why today, in the East, there is ongoing scientific research in herbs, and why, in the West, especially in America, whole herb materials are seldom if ever investigated.[1]

## The West

At one time in the West, herbs were the subject of intensive scientific investigation. One can find numerous published studies on the effects of herbs on animal and human physiology. As late as the mid 20th century, important herbal research was being undertaken in Europe.

Concomittant with herbal research in this century in the West was the development of powerful synthetic medicines that had the power to virtually wipe out many terrible diseases.[2]

[1]One can observe a slight reversal of this trend in recent research on garlic in the West; hopefully, the trend will continue.

[2]It is hard for those of our generation to understand how it was to live in constant fear of contracting any one of a hundred simple but extremely debilitating, even fatal, diseases. It may have been similar to our fear of nuclear holocast.

As cure after cure was found, great excitement spread through the medical research establishment. Young scientists, especially, were vulnerable to the lure of the exotic new lines of study. Unlike the old vanguard, who recognized the value of the new, but attempted to preserve the fundamental value of botanical medicines and continued to pursue research in them, the young students could not resist the excitement of modern drug research.

The old vanguard died off (or is dying off). Many of the following generation, who had studied medicinal plants while under the tutelage of their masters, left those pursuits at the earliest opportunity in order to join the rush to the exciting sea of synthetic medicines. In time these students have become the masters. Their students have been completely indoctrinated in modern medicine and have never had the chance to develop an interest in herbal research.

Thus, the scientific method spawned a new era in the medicine of the West, especially America. European investigators have used the scientific method as a means to investigate herbal medicines even during the current era of synthetic medicine. And in Asia, the the scientific method did not arrive for decades.

The movement away from the natural and toward the synthetic was not a conscious rejection of medical botany. I don't believe anybody realized how completely the older positions were being abandoned. Nobody in mainstream medical science intended for it to happen that way.[3]

During this period of change, beliefs about the causes of common disease also evolved. As several debilitating diseases were eradicated one by one, western philosophical equivalents of the oriental Yin and Yang were replaced by the notion of *specificity,* which held that each and probably every disease is caused by one and probably only one pathogen. Western scientists were finding these pathogenic organisms and developing specific cures and prophylactics for them (to wit, smallpox, diptheria, tetanus, typhus, cholera, typhoid, tuberculosis).

The abandonment of herbal medicine can be explained partly as the result of not being able to fit a round peg in a square hole. For herbal therapeutics have not changed to fit easily into new conceptions of disease. Herbal medicine continues to view disease as something wrong with the whole body, or at least with whole systems within the body. Terms like alteratives, cholagogues, stimulants, emmenagogues, demulcents, anthelmintics, etc., are still viable in herbal medicine. But this view of disease was abandoned so quickly by the medical researchers that physicians accustomed to the concepts of herbal medicine and unwilling to forsake them soon found they were talking a whole different language than the establishment.[4]

[3]But America did not have a centuries' old heritage of herbal use to contend with. America has always been dedicated to the adventure of exploration and progress, has always by nature been primed to accept the often fallacious premise that new is better.

[4]At best the more potent herbs were examined for their specific active principles and for chemicals that would kill specific germs. This activity still goes on and is called pharmacognosy.

Public attitudes also influenced the course of this 20th century evolution in America. Citizens were no longer content with wholistic ideas. They wanted innoculations, penicillin shots, radical surgery, and other heroic medical methods. Americans, and later, Europeans, entered an era of reckless abandon regarding their health, an era characterized by the adoption of a health creed without parallel in human history: "We shall put our trust in food specialists to insure we receive adequate nutrition; we shall put our trust in medical specialists to prevent most disease and to cure the rest; and, above all, we shall trust in the government to insure that we aren't poisoned, extorted or misled by those in whom we have entrusted health and life itself." Having adopted this creed, the average Westerner was free to eat and drink whatever he chose, whenever he chose, in whatever quantities he chose; furthermore, he could freely choose whichever "experts" he wanted for advise on all other aspects of health. In short, without fear, he freely relinquished all individual responsibility for health.

There are many signs that the public has recently recognized "The Great Error" and is again asserting its "right" of individual responsibility in health care. The one agent-one disease theory is falling on hard times as the number of diseases for which it holds true decreases and the number for which it doesn't pertain stand out as in bold relief. There is an increasing public sentiment that disease is created and nurtured by a general lack of health. Unreasonable trust in the creed has been violated by the reasonable forces of human failing and economic pressure.[5]

This is not to say that the American and European experiment was a failure. And we should not make the mistake of assuming the new climate in health care in any way resembles that of a century ago. It doesn't. What it represents is a whole new paradigm in medicine, a new age. The time has come for ushering in an era of balance between the synthetic and the natural.

We must never return to the way things were before the era of modern medicine. Though it was probably a serious error to abandon centuries of medical experience with natural medicines, it would be an even more grave mistake to overlook the role that proper use of the scientific method can play in making great new advancements in the area of herbal medicine (e.g., see the chapter on NAUSEA).

# Immune Deficiency

The highway of modern medicine and the scenic route of herbal medicine seem to converge at several points. One of these is immune response deficiency. Without recognizing what it was doing, herbal medicine quite naturally enlisted all systems of the body in the fight against disease.

---

[5]Also gaining in popularity is the corollary to the above idea; namely, that careful attention to the general health of the body will help prevent many common diseases. The side effects and dangers of synthesized drugs, as well as the values of herbs, nutritional supplemnts and of whole food substances, are being brought to the public's attention by an increasingly sophisticated press.

Though the treatment may have been aimed at a particular disease, it usually depended on energizing, stimulating or otherwise recruiting the aid of many systems within the organism.[6]

The modern medical approach has, until recently, underplayed the importance of the body's own immune system. In fact, the term itself has entered into popular terminology only in the last few years. The medical establishment now recognizes the immune system as the key to the prevention of cancer and other stubborn diseases.

# Cardiovascular Disease

Another meeting point between the old and new is in the recognition that much cardiovascular disease can be prevented, not simply treated. Many herbal medicines are designed specifically for this purpose (see chapters on HEART and HIGH BLOOD PRESSURE). They bespeak common sense and have been scientifically validated. Modern medicine could easily, and wisely, incorporate the use of herbs such as garlic, hawthorn and echinacea. With the support of more research, other herbal medicines could eventually become a regular part of health, diet and medicine.

We can only eliminate cancer and heart disease in this age by paying more attention to the health of the body and less to treating disease; by devoting more effort to preventing, less to curing. We may then witness a return to medical terminology of terms that describe a substance's effect on whole systems, words that reflect a concern with the ability of the body to withstand the onslaught of environmental pathogens—words like adaptogen, cholagoggue, aperient, etc., words that are the substance of herbal medicine.

# The East

In the East (as in Europe) herbal medicine has a centuries' old heritage. But unlike Europe, and with the possible exception of Japan, countries in the East have generally been slower to adopt the medical advancements of the West.[8]

China incorporates the research methods of the West even as she maintains a strong interest in her native folk methods. And as Americans

---

[6]Thus, if an infection was present, herbal antibiotics were administered *in conjunction with* agents that stimulated blood and lymph flow, mild laxatives, and agents that stimulated phagocytic activity in the white blood cells or leukocytes.

[8]Japan, more than any other Asian country, has adopted the mechanistic philosophy of the West. But over the last 10-15 years a resurgence of interest in wholistic medicine has taken place in Japan, characterized by a revival in Kampo, an ancient Chinese system of medicine first introduced to Japan in the sixth century. But in its new incarnation Kampo has been forced to conform to the reductionistic values of orthodox medicine. Pharmacists and some medical doctors have been pressured by public interest, the press, and the market place to prescribe herbal medicines. The result has been devastating. With complete disregard for the philosophical and empirical bases of Kampo, herbs are prescribed as if they were just other synthetic drugs. Ignored are methods of blending, concepts of prevention, wholistic medical practices, etc., basic to the Kampo system. In essence, the Japanese are exerting great effort to pound the square peg in the round hole with a sledge hammer.

begin to recognize the error in rejecting the totality of their own herbal medical heritage, they increasingly turn toward China as an alternate source of methods and medicines. This is a commendable, but hardly necessary, medical pilgrimage, for a wealth of important folk practices exists right in America's own backyard (e.g., Indian and eclectic medicine). This oversight is partly the ironic result of efforts by American herbalists to indiscriminatly embrace whatever is oriental, exotic or mystic. The medical establishment looks upon such enthusiasm as banal and ridiculous. If Eastern practices are to be accepted in America, careful scientists maintain, they must be selected discriminately and conservatively. And whichever are accepted must be explicable in the language of science. Thus, for example, "wholistic" medicine is acceptable only when it can be explained in terms of the immune response enhancement.[9]

The traditional American approach is to "control"—not "be in tune with", one's inner self. Likewise, it is rather better to control disease, its causes, its symptoms and its cures, than to prepare the body to deal with disease on the body's own wholistic terms, which include physiological, psychological and spiritual forces. Nowhere are the limitations of the philosophy of explore, conquer and control more apparent, even to medical practitioners throughout the West, than in the medical arena. The control of all disease has not been achieved. New disease is continually discovered or created. Iatrogenic disease is rampant.

It is in the shadow of these limitations that I would admonish American medicine to encourage the scientific exploration of alternatives in health maintenance. My goal is to demonstrate that the realm of herbal medicine is a viable and valid alternative or adjunct to orthodox pharmacy.

# Today

The scientific method is a powerful tool, but it has its limits. It cannot provide answers to unasked questions. It cannot sweep away cobwebs of ignorance that are based in professional preconception. It is usually impotent against personal bias, political manipulation, economic suppression and governmental regulation. Yet these very forces have much to say about the relationship between science and medicine in the United States today.

Medical science in America is a unique combination of economic and political factors, which fuse together almost religiously to promote synthesized, highly active chemicals most of which have been around a whole 10 to 15 years. Interesting criteria are used to select which chemicals to promote. Efficacy is, or course, a necessary condition. But it is not sufficient. The chemical must also be potentially profitable. Medicines that cannot be patented (or otherwise made proprietary) are not economically

---

[9]The American way is illustrated in its enthusiastic embrace of bio-feedback following a long history of eschewing the foolishness of Eastern-style meditation. Just the name "Biofeedback" would hook an American to whom the concept of "mind over body" is not inherently attractive, but who can be completely comfortable with the idea of "controlling" biological processes and brain waves through the force of "will".

acceptable. No matter how good a substance is, if a particular pharmaceutical firm does not have the inside tract on patent rights, or if such rights are unobtainable, that firm is not going to invest millions of dollars into development and marketing. If users of a natural, unpatentable, product represent an attractive market share, competitive marketing practices demand that the natural product be discredited, and its users converted to a patented, synthesized product.[10]

One tactic effectively used to discredit natural products is to label them as *unproven*, a strategy that works well among professionals, who by virtue of their training are already predisposed to equate "unproven" with "ineffective", perhaps even "dangerous".[11]

Let me emphasize that the economic and political factors of which I write have slowly produced an entity that is as jealous of profit margins as it is zealous in its self-ordained mission to protect the nation's health. For people educated during this era, there have been no legitimate alternatives. The medical doctor, desiring mainly to engage in an honorable and effective practice, feels tremendous pressure to maintain the status quo.

Asian and to a lesser extent European countries are not reluctant to study medicinal foods such as herbs. Historically, those countries had no political, economic or regulatory reasons for rejecting traditional remedies. Instead, they felt it was very important to scientifically explore natural remedies, accepting or rejecting them as the data came in. When you ask a *priori* questions such as what part of, and how much of a substance is patentable, you sacrifice that same degree of scientific integrity.

Fortunately, even in the United States, herbs still do make economic sense, if not for the large Pharmaceutical companies, at least for a dedicated group of entrepreneurs, who try to provide products for people seeking natural rather than, or in addition to, synthesized health products. It will be a great tragedy and a tremendous blow to the health of our people if big money interests and drug lobbies in the United States succeed in denying the people access to their natural heritage. If herbs continue to be marketed and used in spite of the unproven quackery stigma, there is another method available for ridding them from the marketplace: Admit that herbs work, admit that they have potent properties, and then label them drugs. Let's see how that works.

# Herbs Are Not Drugs

A question of growing importance in the United States is should herbs be classified as drugs because of their biological activity. But the question is not simply one of biology, physiology, or pharmacology. It is, above all else, a political question, the answer to which may have profound effects on the

---

[10]The same holds true for manufacturers of natural products though limited funds makes their efforts largely ineffectual.

[11]In the pharmaceutical business, a substance is not *proven* unless thousands, even millions of dollars have been spent investigating its potential benefits and toxicology. Drugs manufactured by pharmaceutical houses are *proven* substances. Medicinal substances that aren't so manufactured are, by definition, *unproven*, a synonym in the medical community for quackery.

health of the American public.

You can define a drug as anything that enters the body. Water and sunlight are drugs, by this definition. And it is a good definition, the one accepted in most academic circles. However, it is not an acceptable definition in the area of medical politics, for it does not allow discrimination between classes of ingestible agents. The doctor learns the above definition in medical school. He learns the political variants much later. He will eventually learn that there are ingestible chemicals that are to be officially designated as *foods*, and are no longer *drugs*. He learns that there is another group comprised of chemicals which are neither food nor drugs, but *food additives*. With enough experience he can usually correctly guess whether a substance is food, drug or food additive. But, in difficult cases he must rely on the judgments of those with better training than he—political bureaucrats.

So far, herbs are politically designated as foods. But there are forces at work to change all that. Often, drugs and herbs are used for the same purposes. Opponents of herbal medicine argue that herbs should therefore be classified as drugs (not foods)—herbal drugs, not medicinal foods. And were it not for the political implications and consequences, I could almost agree with that. But critics of herbal medicine are not concerned with academic questions of classification and function. Their reasoning is purely political. Classifying herbs as drugs, would prevent your neighborhood health food store from selling them. Only pharmaceutical companies could make them and only doctors could prescribe them. But the doctor wouldn't prescribe them, even if he wanted to, because the pharmaceutical companies wouldn't make them.[12]

## Herbs Are Not Food Additives

A variant of the process has already been successfully used to remove certain herbs from the shelves of stores. If you can't get an herb labeled as a drug, get it labeled a food additive. It can then be controlled by the bureacrats in the F.D.A. For example, sassafras tea has been an established Spring tonic in the United States, since colonial times. But someone found that safrole, one of its constituents, possesses hepatotoxic properties. Protectionists demanded that the herb be banned. Herbal proponents demanded that the herb be left alone. Ban safrole, they said, but don't ban sassafras, for it probably contains other chemicals that neutralize the potential toxic effects of safrole.

It was a sticky problem for two reasons. First sassafras was a food and therefore could not be regulated by the FDA, and second, no study had ever shown the herb to be toxic. In the end, sassafras *tea* was outlawed

[12]Why? The FDA estimates it costs over 7 million dollars to bring a new drug to market. Pharmaceutical companies put that figure closer to 70 million dollars. They say they need two million users of a substance just to break even. Since natural substances cannot be patented, there is even less room for profit in them. Hence, it really doesn't matter how strong the *demand* for a natural substance might be, it would never be economically feasible to go through the expensive process of getting it approved for use by the FDA. No pharmaceutical company would market garlic extract, when the money is in penicillin.

because it was reasoned that when the *food* sassafras was added to the *food* water, the safrole migrated from the sassafras into the water and therefore became a *food additive*, and could therefore be controlled by the FDA. It's reasoning like that that could destroy America's health food industry.

During the entire proceedings, the power of the scientific method, initially utilized to create the controversy, became impotent in resolving the situation. Unasked questions cannot be answered. The question of whether whole sassafras herb or even sassafras tea was toxic to the liver was never experimentally addressed.

In the area of medical politics, substance classification is intrinsically involved with regulations, governmental approval and licensing, the economics of screening tests, and so forth. How a substance is classified, whether as food, drug, or food additive, will determine the nature of its availability to the people.

It is therefore extremely important that herbs (medicinal foods) **never** be classified as drugs (which is meant to include food additives), even if they are used for the same purposes, because they would then, due to strict regulations on drugs imposed by the government, become immediately unavailable to the public, and probably forever remain that way.

Let me emphasize that *medicinal foods are not drugs*, by definition. The only political way to prevent their disappearance *en masse* from the public market is to maintain this definition. If advocates of the "herbs are drugs" fallacy ever win the classification battle, the consequences for personal freedom in diet could be severe, even in areas totally unrelated to herbs. For indeed, eventually the slightest provocation would earmark other foods for control (e.g., fiber, unsaturated oils, etc.). Just as it is now sometimes difficult to distinguish between drugs and medicinal foods, if medicinal foods were called drugs, it would then become difficult to distinguish between regular foods and drugs.[14]

Remember that medicinal foods and regular foods, by their very complex nature, defy the simple chemical classifications that are imposed on synthesized drugs. Extracts and fractions have properties different from the parent source. The total is usually greater than the sum of the parts.

# Where From Here

The political differences between wholistic medicine and pharmaceutical medicine are imposed not by the philosophical divergence of the people, but by the economic realities of the market place. They diverge into a polarized state not because of metaphysical or empirical differences but because of the historical need to acquire market share. Hence, some

[14]Were hawthorn berries to be labeled a drug, what would you do with strawberries? Strawberries contain more toxic chemicals than hawthorn berries. They contain, for example, acetone, acetaldehyde, methyl burrate, ethyl caproate, hexyl acetate, methanol, acrolein, and crotonaldehyde, all of which are poisonous.

cultures, mainly westernized ones, find it more expedient to patent proprietary products, while other cultures, lacking the technology and resources to acquire wealth, gradually incorporate wholistic medicine into modern medicine as expertise in both areas is obtained.

Adherents of both wholistic medicine and pharmaceutical medicine, through the use, respectively, of medicinal foods and drugs, would like to see improvement in the health of humankind.[15]

This book was written for the purpose of dispelling some of the misconceptions about herbs in the minds of most Americans, and in the hope of sparking enthusiasm for the reunion of people and nature's pharmacy, the medicinal plants. It is hoped that this book will help validate this one aspect of the wholistic health movement by presenting a wealth of scientific and ethnopharmacological evidence for the use of medicinal foods, specifically herbs. It is the first effort of its kind of which I am aware, but will hopefully provide the foundation for more, and better, treatments of the scientific foundations of herbal medicine.

[15]The doctor, by reason of political education and indoctrination, will use the drug cholestyramine to help a person reduce cholesterol levels. A wholistic physician may choose garlic or pectin for the same purpose. A ten year study on the effects of cholestyramine in over 3,000 men, and several studies on the effects of garlic or pectin in man and animals, have shown that all three substances reduce serum cholesterol to almost exactly the same extent. The difference between the two approaches is illustrated in the fact, on the one hand, that cholestyramine was so unpleasant to use that a full 27% of the men refused to use it and dropped out of the study. The side effects of garlic, on the other hand, include resistance to infections and fevers, reduced blood pressure if it is high, and better cardiac health. I believe that, given the chance to objectively choose between the drug or the herb, most doctors would choose the herb, or at least some combination of herb and drug.

# INTRODUCTION

Have you ever probed into the validity of therapeutic claims for herbal products? If so, have you discovered that it is extremely difficult to locate reliable and valid information, the kind that inspires confidence in herbal products? Testimonials abound. But you wonder how many result from self-deception (the placebo effect)? There is something about over-confident, over-healthy exuberance that often alienates people who do not share in it. Are you drawn toward the inherent logic of using natural products, yet skeptical of the urge because you haven't found good evidence from legitimate sources? If so, you share those sentiments with thousands of other people. This book is meant to answer some of your questions and erase many of your doubts. It is also designed to educate and enlighten all readers, regardless of interest, background or knowledge.

## The Scientific Method

The validation of herbal medicine has been going on for hundreds of years. But reliable, repeatable verification has been obtained only in modern times, thanks to the advent of the scientific method.[1]

But even with this strong tool, the area of herbal research, especially with blends, has a long way to go. Ideally, herbal blends should be designed around a large body of sound experimental and clinical research.[2]

But such are the realities of pharmacological research that we can only hope for the slow accumulation of good data over decades, even centuries, of work. Meanwhile, whether we like it or not, we must rely on the *ad hoc* compilation of hard facts as they are discovered, soft facts, clinical information, cross cultural verification, anecdotal clues, etc. The relative value of an herb or an herbal blend for human consumption depends on the competent evaluation of the strength of the data supporting its use. In this book you will find data from all the above areas, with a primary emphasis on hard, scientific information.

## Folklore Meets Science

The use of herbs differs in one significant way from the use of other health supplements, such as vitamins and drugs: because herbs have been

---

[1]Most of it comes from countries that have not entirely rejected natural medicine—Japan, Russia, China, and some European nations. The United States, for reasons explored in the Preface, has not been heavily involved in research on natural products.

[2]Ideally, *all* herbal blends would be likewise supported. Furthermore, all interactions *among* the herbs in every blend would ideally have been thoroughly and objectively explored, both experimentally and clinically. Ideally, the interactions among herbal blends and *between* herbal blends and drugs would likewise have been documented. Ideally, all of the above ideals would be accomplished with each and every *form* an herb might take, be it capsule, tea, fresh, dried, or extract.

around for a much longer time, they have a much richer heritage. This is both good and bad. Besides being used in many valuable medicines, herbs have also been subjected to all manner of superstition and magic. Culpeper evolved a whole materia medica based in astrology and the Doctrine of Signatures, the idea that God or Nature designed the appearance of plants to provide clues about their intended purpose. Whether you agree with that philosophy or not, the point is that, for whatever reasons, humankind has maintained an intimate relationship with medicinal plants for centuries. Extremely valuable information has been learned during that time. But it is often difficult to separate myth from fact. Hence the necessity of good research.

The fate of information concerning the medicinal properties of plants has varied throughout history. Before the invention of the printing press, much information was discovered and lost with the passing of individual persons or groups. In the case of South American and African medicine, much still remains unaccessible to modern civilization. Since the advent of the press, a few practitioners have used books to record their experiences in what amounts to an incredibly rich source of clinical data. But most herbalists around the world did not, do not and never will record their knowledge.

Later than books, came Science, characterized by the rigid application of the scientific method. This method is used to determine and publish truth, usually through the systematic elimination of falsehood.[3]

Confronted with an interesting observation, the scientist will postulate a number of explanations.[4] Through carefully controlled experiments, the scientist will attempt to *eliminate* as many explanations as possible, eventually arriving at the one valid, replicable experimental effect. Further experimentation is needed to provide an understanding of the mechanism of action. And then other parameters will be explored. The final results of this process are reviewed by peers and eventually published for the public.

## The World's Herbal Science

A few years ago I committed myself, as one of a very few Americans involved in basic research on the medicinal properties of whole plants, to critically review the scientific literature on herbal medicine, employing translators where necessary, and to finally publish much of this material in a form accessible to all interested parties. The bulk of the material is drawn

---

[3]To the scientist, a statement like "Echinacea cures infections," may or may not be true. He may reject the premise outright, on the basis of some *un*scientific reason, such as political or philosophical bias against herbal medicine. Or, he may accept the statement as a possible *truth.*

[4]If he observes, for example, that 6 out of 10 persons given Echinacea get well in a subjectively brief time, the scientist imagines as many explanations for the effect as he can, only one of which is "The Echinacea did it." He asks, in addition, "Would they have gotten better anyway?" "What about the placebo effect?" "What other medicines were being used?" "How many and what kind of infectious bugs were involved?" "What about the effects of age, sex, physical strength, diet and other medical conditions?"

from medical, pharmaceutical and other professional journals from around the world.[5]

# Science and You

Once you experience the benefits of using herbs, you may find the courage to experiment with proven herbal blends, adapting them to your own needs, exploring new applications and so forth. You are in essence applying the scientific method, and though your findings will lack much of that which defines knowledge as "scientific" or "universal", it will nevertheless still be valid for *you*.

You can do this, even though hundreds of years of folklore experimentation have already witnessed the discovery of many important uses, because the ailments of modern man are in some ways vastly different from those of people just 100 years ago. Cancer, environmental pollution, AIDS, herpes, birth defects, food processing, changes in exercise, diet and work, all of these factors and more have created health problems not shared by our forefathers.

You can discover many new and important uses because you have more versatility in the form in which you can use herbs. The advent of the gelatin capsule, all by itself, is revolutionizing herbal medicine (For example, pungent or acrid substances such as cayenne or ginger root could not be ingested in large quantities before the invention of the gelatin capsule). In addition, the public now has access to high quality tinctures and tablets. Quality control measures have removed the effects of uneven collection, processing and packaging methods that have plagued herbal medicine up until the last 10-12 years. We are poised on the very brink of a new revolution in herbal medicine. As this book may demonstrate, that revolution rests upon a bedrock of scientific evidence.

[5]As the work progressed, I noticed that scientific data often corroborated folklore usage. This finding bolstered my confidence in anecdotal information, especially when I saw radically divergent cultures discovering the same uses for the same or chemically similar plants. Interesting data from folklore and culture (ethnopharmacology) is therefore scattered throughout this book. You may also become more tolerant of medicinal folklore. Purposely included among the major herbs with long lists of solid scientific evidence, are some minor plants that, to me, seem to deserve more attention. Most of these are indigenous to North America and have therefore not been of interest to European or Asian researchers. But each one is potentially as beneficial as any of the more substantially researched herbs.

# TABLE OF CONTENTS

# ACKNOWLEDGEMENTS:

I thank:

For critical analysis of content and style, the fear of whose acrid commentary kept me ever vigilant for inconsistency and embarrassing terminology—Dave Raddatz.

For timely Atta Boy's, Hang In There's and other unearned reinforcments that kept me pecking at the keys, and for daily reassurance that this work wouldn't send me to the poor house—Evan Bybee.

For being a true friend, colleague and the better half of a sporadic but highly effective research partnership—Dennis Clayson.

For incredible patience, understanding, moral support, personal sacrifice, inspiration, strength, unselfishness, and intellectual ability (including editing skills)—my wife, Vickie, and the kids: Tara, Kregg, Korinn, Branna, Erin and Brokk.

Monty Clay, without whom nothing were possible.

# How To Use This Book

Each chapter in this book is devoted to some particular ailment, or physiological system.

*Herbs:* Several herbs are described in each chapter; these may be used separately or, preferrably blended together as indicated. The major herbs, those with the more potent activity, are listed at the beginning of the chapter in **BOLD UPPER CASE**. The other herbs, though potent in other blends, are meant in this case to augment, modulate or otherwise modify the overall activity of the major herbs. In a blend these interactions would be more strongly felt.

*Chapter Titles* The chapters of the book are arranged alphabetically by subject matter. Subjects include **ailments**, such as HAYFEVER/ALLERGY, ARTHRITIS, and NAUSEA; **systems of the body**, such as HEART, NERVES & GLANDS, and WHOLE BODY; **purposes**, such as CHOLESTEROL REGULATION, LAXATIVE, and WEIGHT LOSS; and **miscellaneous** subjects, such as ENVIRONMENTAL POLLUTION. This arrangement, also reflected in the Table of Contents will greatly facilitate finding the topic of interest.

*Purposes:* The main purpose of the major herbs and/or the herbal blend of the chapter is given in this section. It is certain to be closely related to the chapter title and will explain just the major effect the herbs will have regarding the particular chapter topic.

*Other Applications:* This section contains other effects that the particular herbal blend of the chapter may be expected to possess for certain people under certain conditions. These effects are not necessarily substantiated by empirical research, but reflect folklore usage and clinical experience.

*Use:* Here are suggested directions for using the herbs in the chapter in *blend form.* The blend may be used differently for treatment than it is for prevention. It may interact with other blends. Amount used may differ depending on what other herbs are being used. All of these factors are covered in the Use section.

*Contraindications:* When herbs are selected properly, the potential for dangerous side effects, drug interactions and other hazards is very small. However, in this section are listed any precautions that should be taken with certain herbs discussed in the chapter. For example, diuretics have the potential of depleting the body's store of potassium and sometimes require that potassium supplements be taken.

*Text:* The body of the chapter contains information on the individual herbs. This data is grounded as much as possible in sound empirical research. Often, I have also included ethnopharmacological material, interesting folklore anecdotes and pertinent clinical studies.

*References:* The numbers in bold throughout the text correspond to the references listed in this section. The bulk of these references are to studies reported in the world's major medical journals. Over two dozen languages and several hundred different journals are represented. This is, in my opinion, the most important section of every chapter in the book. These references, most of which are presented to the public for the very first time, embody the excitement of herbal medicine and herbal research. I have become attached to them as if to my own children, and it required overcoming intense jealousy to give them away to the public (I could have excluded this section, you know). Ultimately, however, that was my purpose in collecting them all along. And so here they are. . . .

*Index:*   You will notice that most of the herbs appear in more than one chapter. Different information about the herb is listed each time it appears; just exactly what is mentioned would depend on the chapter topic. Therefore, for the convenience of the reader who would like to read everything about a particular herb, the index has been made particularly comprehensive and helpful. The entry for each herb in the index lists each herbal effect and gives the page number where that particular effect is discussed.

The reader will notice another aid for cross-referencing information on a particular herb: At the end of almost every text entry in each chapter is an italicized list of other chapters in which discussions of that particular herb are found. This device is most helpful for the reader who is just browsing but would like to read more about a certain plant.

# ARTHRITIS

## HERBS

**Form:**  Capsule, Tea, Poultice

**CONTENTS: ALFALFA** seed & leaf *(Medicago sativa)*, **CELERY SEED** *(Apium graveolens)*, **Burdock root** *(Arctium lappa)*, **Chaparral** *(Larrea divaricata)*, **Sarsaparilla root** *(Smilax officinalis)*, **Licorice root** *(Glycyrrhiza glabra)*, **Kelp** *(Laminara, Macrocystis, Asocphyllum)*, **Cayenne** *(Capsicum annum)*, **Queen-of-the-Meadow root** *(Eupatorium purpureum)*.

**PURPOSE:**  **To help reduce symptoms such as stiff, inflamed and sore muscles and joints, due to Arthritis, Rheumatism, Lupus, Gout, and Bursitis.**

**Other Applications:**  Atherosclerosis, Blood Cleansing, Acidosis.

**USE:** 1. For General Use: 2 capsules, 4 times per day, with 1/2 glass of liquid (4 capsules, twice per day; or 3 capsules, 3 times per day are satisfactory alternatives).
2. Prevention and during Remission: 2-4 capsules per day.
3. If used in conjunction with the WHOLE BODY TONIC Blend, reduce daily intake by 2 capsules and, for optimum results, increase the ENVIRONMENTAL POLLUTION Blend by two capsules.
4. For an excellent blood purification program, consider using a mixture of this blend with BLOOD PURIFICATION/ DETOXIFICATION and SKIN DISORDERS blends. Three to four capsules of each per day for short periods of time would be appropriate.

1

**Contraindications:**   None. Chaparral, although sometimes called creosote bush, contains **NO** creosote. See Appendix A for discussions of Cayenne and Licorice Root.

There are several kinds of arthritic disorders (including rheumatism, osteo-, lupus, bursitis and gout), all characterized by inflammation and pain in joints, muscles and related connective tissue. Most forms are progressive, i.e., they get worse with time. Early treatment may reverse the damage, leading eventually to healed tissue. Even eroded bone may be replaced. Often, however, when damage is severe, including the loss of critical fluids, and involving muscle atrophy and cartilage destruction, healing can be very difficult, and sometimes impossible. This blend's approach to some stubborn ailments is to help reduce pain and inflammation while cleaning up and strengthening the blood, and while attempting to dissolve troublesome deposits in the joints. Wisely, the blend recognizes both the similarities and the differences in the etiology of complaints under consideration. Though these herbs enjoy a truly distinguished history of intelligent investigation, their usefulness in treating arthritis and rheumatism was not always easily perceived. For example, even though the ancient Arabs recognized Alfalfa as the "Father of all foods" (Al-fal-fa), it was left to the American Indians to become one of the first cultures to discover its medicinal value. Alfalfa grows all over China, but is avoided by the Chinese because they believe it makes a person skinny.

**ALFALFA**'s anti-rheumatic effect is probably due to its extremely high nutritive value, which includes vitamins A, B1, B6, B12, C, D, E and K, niacin, pantothenic acid, biotin, folic acid, minerals, protein, saponins, amino acids, trace elements (calcium, phosphorous, potassium, magnesium, iron, zinc and copper) (**1**). Alfalfa has a proven cholesterol lowering effect (**2**) and it generally helps to improve overall health, vigor and vitality (**3-4**; see also WHOLE BODY). Steroid properties are suggested by its saponin content and by some research that shows an estrogenic effect in ruminants (grazing animals) (**5-7**). Although the treatment of arthritis is difficult at best, it is my opinion that the use of Alfalfa over the long term could significantly help many people deal with the ailment. Alfalfa, as fiber, is also good for cellular detoxification. *See Also ENVIRONMENTAL POLLUTION*

**CELERY SEED** is a traditional diuretic and blood cleanser, well suited for treating rheumatism, especially when combined with

Damiana (**8**). Its inclusion in arthritic blends is a rather modern tradition, but has repeatedly proven itself in clinical trials. The mechanism of action remains obscure, but it is no longer doubted that the herb contains potent active principles. For example, a famous Chinese study showed that it lowered blood pressure in 14 of 16 human patients with chronic high blood pressure (**9**). In Europe, Celery Seed is a common medicinal treatment for gout and rheumatism (**10**). *See Also LIVER DISORDERS*

**BURDOCK ROOT** has been listed for centuries in official Pharmacopoeias of the several countries in which it grows, as an effective blood purifier and pain killer (**11**). This property would partially explain its observed effectiveness in treating rheumatism. American herbalists have testified for the past two hundred years that Burdock can effectively alleviate symptoms of arthritis and other inflammatory diseases (**12-13**). The alterative (blood purifying) nature of Burdock Root enhances the effectiveness of several other blends in this book. *See Also BLOOD PURIFICATION/DETOXIFICATION; DETOXIFY/NURTURE; BONE-FLESH-CARTILAGE*

**CHAPARRAL,** according to the best American Indian folklore, as well as modern science, has good anti-rheumatoid properties. The Indians found it particularly effective (**14**). An Argentine study showed that the primary constituent of Chaparral, NDGA (nordihydroquaiaretic acid), possesses analgesic (pain relieving) and vasodepressant (circulatory depressing) properties (**15**); and in Hungary it was found that NDGA increased ascorbic acid levels in the adrenals (**16**). Stateside studies have further elucidated the physiological properties of Chaparral constituents, confirming antioxidant and anticancer activity (**17**). Such researach has led one researcher to label NDGA as the "Penicillin of hydroquinones," (**18**). On a cellular level, NDGA stimulates mitochondrial respiration (process by which cells utilize foods for energy) (**19**), a fact that may eventually provide the key to its effectiveness in treating arthritic conditions. *See Also SKIN; BONE-FLESH-CARTILAGE; DETOXIFY/NURTURE*

**SARSAPARILLA** was independently discovered in the United States, Honduras, Mexico and China, as well as other countries around the world, to be an effective treatment for rheumatism (**20-21**). Mode of action is not yet fully elucidated, but may stem from its high content of saponins. The saponins make Sarsaparilla a good candidate for a whole body tonic. *See Also INFERTILITY; DETOXIFY/NURTURE; WHOLE BODY; BLOOD PURIFICATION/DETOXIFICATION*

**LICORICE ROOT** and its derivatives, especially glycyrrhetic acid, have been found to possess substantial anti-arthritic activity (**22-24**). The herb's anti-inflammatory properties no doubt account for its profound effect upon the course of arthritis and rheumatism in many people, although certain enzyme systems have also been implicated (**25**). The anti-inflammatory property of Licorice Root was first observed scientifically in treating dermatological problems (**26-28**). Then, in 1958, an English team subjected the herb's derivatives to four established tests for anti-inflammatory properties. The test results were positive on all counts (**29**). Since that time, several studies have been done to verify and extend those initial findings (e.g., **30-36**). In the search for a mode of action, researchers discovered that glycyrrhizin inhibits the anti-granulomatous action of cortisone (**37**) and has a high affinity for glandular receptors that are specific for adrenocortical hormones (**38**). The anti-inflammatory effect is therefore probably related to a release of corticoids from the adrenals (**39**), for in all studies the effect depended on an intact adrenal gland (**40**). The advantage in using Licorice Root is that it has none of the side effects associated with the use of glucocorticoid-type drugs such as cortisone and hydrocortisone. Yet Licorice Root and/or its derivatives can be every bit as effective as hydrocortisone (**30**). See Appendix A for a discussion of Licorice Root toxicity, and why it doesn't pertain to its use in blends such as this. In summary, the above findings suggest a pervasive general effect as well as a cellular locus of action for Licorice Root. *See Also RESPIRATORY AILMENTS; SKIN; FEMALE TONIC; BLOOD PURIFICATION/DETOXIFICATION; CIRCULATION; FATIGUE; WEIGHT LOSS; ENVIRONMENTAL POLLUTION; FEVERS & INFECTIONS; THYROID; WHOLE BODY; DETOXIFY/NURTURE; MENTAL ALERTNESS/SENILITY*

**QUEEN-OF-THE-MEADOW** herb has been established clinically as an effective treatment for rheumatic and gouty conditions due to uric acid deposits in the joints (**41**). Because of its stimulating effect on glands and organs that clear the body of toxins and waste (**42**), it is also helpful in most forms of inflammatory distress. Queen-of-the-Meadow is primarily a diuretic. *See Also DIURETIC*

**KELP** and **CAYENNE** provide nutritive support as well as improve good circulatory stimulation. They measurably enhance the overall effectiveness and usefulness of the blend. The trace mineral content of Kelp is among the highest of any source known, a fortunate circumstance for arthritic patients who use it.

# OTHER NUTRIENTS

*Arthritis and related conditions have been shown to respond very nicely to various nutritional interventions. Individual needs may depart substantially from the recommendations below.*

## VITAMINS

(Daily requirements unless otherwise noted)

Vitamin A *25,000 I.U.*
Vitamin B Complex
Vitamin B1 *25-100 mg*
Vitamin B2 *25-100 mg*
Vitamin B6 *25-100 mg*
Vitamin B12 *4 mcg*
Vitamin C *3,000-4,000 mg*
Vitamin D *2,500 I.U.*
Vitamin E *600-800 I.U.*
Folic Acid
Niacinamide *10 mg*
Pantothenic Acid *300 mg*

## MINERALS

Calcium/Magnesium
Iodine
Phosphorous
Potassium
Sulfur
Manganese

## MISCELLANEOUS

Lecithin
GLA
Essential Fatty Acid
Cod Liver Oil
HCl
Liver

# REFERENCES

1. Leung, A.Y. **Encyclopedia of Common Natural Ingredients.** New York, 1980.
2. Malinow, M.R., McLaughlin, P., Papworth, M.S., Stafford, C., Kohler, G.O., Livingston, A.L., and Cheeke, P.R. "Effect of alfalfa saponins on intestinal cholesterol absorption in rats." **The American Journal of Clinical Nutrition,** 30 (Dec 1977), 2061-2067.
3. Ellingwood, F. **American Materia Medica, Therapeutics and Pharmacognosy.** Eclectic Medical Publications, Portland, Oregon, 1983.
4. Der Marderosian, A. "Medicinal teas—boon or bane?" **Drug Therapy,** 7(2), 178-188, 1977.
5. Schaible, P.J. **Poultry, Feeds and Nutrition,** AVI, Westport, Conn., 1970, p. 358.
6. Keeler, R.F. "Toxins and teratogens of higher plants." **Lloydia,** 38(1), 56-86, 1975.
7. Bickoff, E.M., Livingston, A.L. & Booth, A.N. "Tricin from alfalfa—isolation and physiological activity." **Journal of Pharmaceutical Sciences**, 53(11), 1411-1412, 1964.
8. List, P.H. & Hoerhammer, L. **Hagers Handbuch der Pharmazeutischen Praxis.** Volumes 2-5, Springer-Verlag, Berlin.
9. Grieve, M. **A Modern Herbal.** 2 vols. Hafner, New York, 1967.
10. Kiangsu Institute of Modern Medicine. **Encyclopedia of Chinese Drugs.** 2 Vols. Shanghai, Peoples Republic of China, 1977.
11. Bentlov, U. "The Great Burdock." **The Herbalist,** June, 1978, 32-33.
12. Felter, H. W. **The Eclectic Materia Medica, Pharmacology and Therapeutics.** Eclectic Medical Publications, Portland, Oregon, 1983 (first published 1922).
13. Millspaugh, C. F. **American Medicinal Plants.** Dover Publications, Inc. New York, 1974 (first published 1892).
14. Train, P., Henricks, J.R., & Archer, W.A. "Medicinal Uses of Plants by Indian Tribes of Nevada." U.S. Dept. Of Agriculture, Washington, D.C., 1941, 96.
15. Bergel, M. "Nordihydroquaiaretic acid in therapy." **Semana Medical,** (Buenos Aires), II, 123-131, 1955.
16. Sporn, A. & Schobesch, O. "Toxicity of nordihyroguaiaretic acid." **Igiena,** (Bucharest), 15(12), 725-726, 1966.
17. Waller, C. W. & Gisvold, O. N. "A phytochemical investigation of Larrea Divaricata Cav." **Journal Of the American Pharmaceutical Association**, 34, 78-81, 1945.

18. Burk, D. & Woods, M. "Hydrogen peroxide catalase, glutathione peroxidase, quinones, nordihydroquaiaretic acid, and phosphopyridine nucleotides in relation to x-ray action on cancer cells." **Radiation Research Supplement,** 3, 212-246, 1963.

19. Scharff, M. & Wilson, R.H. "Nordihydroguaiaretic acid effects on the metabolism of mung beam mitochondria." **Plant & cell Physiology,** 16, 865-869, 1975.

20. Leung, A.Y. **Encyclopedia of Common Natural Ingredients.** New York, 1980.

21. Kiangsu Institute of Modern Medicine. **Encyclopedia of Chinese Drugs.** 2 Vols. Shanghai, Peoples Republic of China, 1977.

22. Tangri, K.K., Seth, P.K, Parmar, S.S. & Bhargava, K.P. "Biochemical study of anti-inflammatory and anti-arthritic properties of glycyrrhetic acid." **Biochemical Pharmacology,** 14(8), 1277-1281, 1965.

23. Nikitina, S.S. "Data on the mechanism of anti-inflammatory action by glycyrrhizic acid." **Farmakologiia i Toksikologiia,** 29(1), 67-70, 1966.

24. Gujral, M.L., Sareen, K., Phukan, D.P. & Amma, M.K.P. "Anti-arthritic activity of glycyrrhizin in adrenalectomized rats." **Indian Journal of Medical Science,** 15(8), 625-629, 1961.

25. Parmar, S.S., Tangri, K.K., Seth, P.K. & Bhargava, K.P. "Biochemical basis for anti-inflammatory effects of glycyrrhetic acid and its derivatives." **International Congress of Biochemistry,** 6(5), 410, 1967.

26. Adamson, A.C. & Tillman, W.G. "Hydrocortisone." **British Medical Journal,** 2, 1501, 1955.

27. Colin-Jones, E. & Somers, G.F. "Glycyrrhetinic acid, a non-steroidal anti-inflammatory agent in dermatology." **Presse Medicale,** 238, 206, 1957.

28. Evans, Q. "Glycyrrhetinic acid." **British Medical Journal,** 2, 1239, 1956.

29. Kumagi, A., Yano, S., & Otomo, M. "The corticoid-like action of glycyrrhizin and the mechanism of its action." **Endocrinologia Japonica,** 4, 17-27, 1961.

30. Finney, S.H., & Somers, G.F. "The anti-inflammatory activity of glycyrrhetinic acid and derivatives." **Journal of Pharmacology and Pharmacodynamics,** 10(10), 613-620, 1958.

31. Miyake, T. **Allergy,** 10, 131, 1961.

32. Cappelletti, E.M., Trevisan, R. & Caniato, R. "External anti-heomatic and anti-neuralgic herbal remedies in the traditional

medicine of north-eastern Italy." **Journal of Ethnopharmacology,** 6(2), 161-190, 1982.

33. Kumagi, A., Yano, S., Takeuchi, K., Nischino, K., Asanuma, Y., Nanaboshi, M. & Yamamura, Y. "An inhibitory effect o glycyrrhizin on the anti-granulomatous action of cortisone." **Endocrinology,** 74, 145-148, 1964.

34. Armanini, D., Karbowiak, I., & Funder, J.W. "Affinity of liquorice derivatives for mineralcorticoid and glucocorticoid receptors." **Clinical Endocrinology,** (Oxf), 19(5), 609-612, 1983.

35. Finney, R.S.H., Somers, B.F. & Wilkinson, J.H. "The pharmacological properties of glycyrrhetinic acid—a new anti-inflammatory drug." **Journal of Pharmacy and Pharmacology,** 10, 687-695, 1958.

36. Nasyrov, K.M. & Lazareva, D.N. "Study of anti-inflammatory activity of glycyrrhizin acid derivatives." **Farmakologiia i Toksikologiia,** 43(4), 399-404, 1980.

37. Finney, R.S.H. & Tarnoky, A.L. "The pharmacological properties of glycyrrhetinic acid hydrogen succinate." **Journal of Pharmacy and Pharmacology,** 12(1), 49-58, 1960.

38. Meier, R., Schuler, W. & Dessaulles, P. "Zur frage des mechanismus der hemmung des bindegewebswachstums durch cortisone." **Experientia,** 6(12), 469-471, 1950.

39. Tamura, Y. "Study of effects of glycyrrhetinic acid and its derivatives on delta 4-5 alpha and 5 beta-reductase by rat liver preparations." **Folia Endocrinologia Japonica,** 51(7), 589-600, 1975.

40. Gibson, M.R. "Glycyrrhiza in old and new perspective." **Lloydia,** 41(4), 348-354, 1978.

41. Hutchens, A.R. **Indian Herbalogy of North America.** Merco, Ontario, Canada, 1969.

42. Felter, H. W. **The Eclectic Materia Medica, Pharmacology and Therapeutics.** Eclectic Medical Publications, Portland, Oregon, 1983 (first published 1922).

# HIGH BLOOD PRESSURE

## HERBS

**Form:** Capsule.

**CONTENTS: GARLIC** *(Allium sativum),* **VALERIAN** root *(Valeriana officinalis),* **Black Cohosh root** *(Cimicifuga racemosa),* **Cayenne** *(Capsicum annum),* & **Kelp** *(Laminara, Macrocystis, Ascophyllum).*

**PURPOSE:** **To help the body reduce high blood pressure (Hypertension); To help relieve any condition that may be aggravated by nervous anxiety; To lower serum cholesterol.**

**Other Applications:** Hives, Shingles, Erysipelas, Insomnia.

**USE:** 1. Anxiety attacks: 4 capsules, 3 times per day
2. Prevention: 3-5 capsules per day
3. High blood pressure: 2-3 capsules, 3-4 times per day
4. To assist the body in maintaining proper blood cholesterol levels: 4 capsules daily, in conjunction with the CHOLESTEROL REGULATION Blend.
5. To supplement the HEART Blend: See the HEART Blend for details.
6. To supplement the NERVOUS TENSION Blend: 2-4 capsules per day.

**Contraindications:** None. For a discussion of Cayenne, see Appendix A.

This blend takes a different approach to treating high blood pressure than the HEART blend. Rather than assuming an underlying cardiac problem, it assumes your hypertension is due to high serum cholesterol levels, and perhaps mild arteriosclerosis, plus the aggravation of those problems by emotional stress and nervous anxiety. Hypertension is a hybrid of physiological, emotional and mental factors. Physiologically, it is often aggravated by athero- and arteriosclerosis, obesity and drug abuse (including cigarettes, alcohol and caffeine). Emotionally and mentally, hypertension normally occurs in persons with stressful lifestyles, characterized by worry, hurry and flurry. This blend seeks to reduce blood cholesterol levels, hypertension and anxiety. It relies heavily on Garlic to accomplish those purposes. Garlic, another of those herbal prodigies, holds the promise of extraordinary therapeutic benefits, possessing nearly two dozen major medicinal properties. Only the hypocholesterolemic (ability to lower cholesterol levels), and hypotensive effects concern us here. Hypotensive and vasodilatory activities have also been found in extracts of Black Cohosh. The whole herb, I have found, likewise provides this effect. The hypotensive and sedative properties of Valerian root have also received serious attention in university and medical research labs. People suffering from hypertension, nervous anxiety and the stress of modern living will find this blend a valuable adjunct to their lifestyles—and their health.

**GARLIC** contains several volatile sulphur compounds (like allicin) which are the probable active constituents (**1**). Animal and human basic research has irrefutably established Garlic's ability to lower blood serum cholesterol levels (**2-7**). Dozens of such studies have been carried out in universities and hospitals, located in such places as India, Libia, Japan, England, Poland, Russia, Czechoslovakia, Canada, Finland, Spain, Pakistan, Egypt, Germany, Romania, and elsewhere (but not Transylvania). The typical study compares diets high in fat with and without Garlic. Garlic diets consistently produce the lowest cholesterol levels (**8**). In the 1940s, one investigator found that 40 of 100 patients with high blood pressure experienced a reduction of 20 mmHg or more after about a week of garlic treatment (**9**). In another study, a water extract of garlic was given to hypercholesterolemic patients for two months during which time the patients experienced a 28.5% reduction in cholesterol—the dose was equivalent to about 10 grams of garlic per day (**10**). Summarizing the results of six studies on the effects of Garlic in rabbits fed high cholesterol diets, the herb produced lower blood cholesterol levels (10-80%) than those of the control groups, with

15-50% fewer incidence of atherosclerotic lesions or other signs of atherosclerosis (**11-16**). The extent of the protection in these studies depended on such factors as length of study and dosage levels. Extrapolating from the data, it can be concluded that regular Garlic ingestion could have dramatic beneficial effects of the course of heart disease due to atherosclerosis. It is thought that allicin blocks the biosynthesis of cholesterol (by reacting with sulfhydryl group systems and combining with coenzyme A). In another study, humans were selected on the basis of being vegetarian; however, they were divided into two groups on the further criterion of whether or not they ate Garlic and/or onion on a regular basis. The two groups were carefully matched as to age, sex and social class (the study took place in India). As expected, there was little difference between groups in serum cholesterol levels (since meat was not a part of either diet). However, there were significant differences in other factors which influence the course of atherosclerosis. For example, those who used Garlic and onion had much lower serum-triglycerides, beta lipoproteins, phospholipids and plasma fibrinogen levels (**17**). The mode of action of Garlic is still unclear, but it definitely involves a simple restriction in rise of blood cholesterol and blood lipid, or it may involve increasing the fibrinolytic activity of plasma.

Another important property of Garlic, its hypotensive activity, is similar to the action of the HEART blend. Rabbits and humans who have been given Garlic show a rapid and prolonged decrease in blood pressure (**18**). It seems that dietary Garlic helps to expand vessel walls (**9**). This action has been attributed to the presence of methyl allyl trisulfide in Garlic. Another chemical in Garlic, ajoene, affects the health of the blood and blood vessels in yet another way that has important implications in preventing high blood pressure and heart disease: it inhibits the tendency of blood cells to stick together (platelet aggregation). This property, which results in a reduced tendency by the blood to clot, and restrict the flow of blood, has been demonstrated in both animal and human studies (**19-21**). *See Also FEVERS & INFECTIONS; PARASITES*

**BLACK COHOSH** has been one the favorite herbs of Americans for at least two centuries. Some pharmacological investigation conducted on this plant has confirmed its hypotensive effect. In one study, a fluid extract produced a distinct fall in blood pressure, with no effect on respiration (**22**). Another study demonstrated a hypotensive effect on animals and a vasodilatory effect on humans (**23**). These findings, from America, China and Europe, confirm the validity of Black Cohosh's reputation as a sedative and hypotensive. In Europe, where much research has been done on Black Cohosh, it is believed that the herb, through its resinous constituents, exhibits hypotensive properties by inhibiting the vasomotor centers in the central nervous system (**24**). *See Also FEMALE TONIC; NERVOUS TENSION*

**CAYENNE** will also lower blood cholesterol levels, thereby helping to reduce blood pressure (**25-26**). In one study (**27**), separate groups of rats were fed diets high in cholesterol with or without ground Cayenne or capsaicin, the active constituent of Cayenne, for seven weeks. Both Cayenne and capsaicin prevented rise in liver cholesterol levels, and increased fecal excretions of free cholesterol. These findings show that Cayenne prevents even the absorption of cholesterol. Interestingly, it was also found that Cayenne was more effective than capsaicin on all counts, indicating, as so often happens in pharmaceutical science, that the use of isolated constituents may ignore the beneficial effects of principles left behind in the dross. Cayenne, according to another study, also reduces the blood pressure in an even more direct manner: a number of years ago, a team of researchers discovered that capsaicin acts in a reflexive manner to reduce systemic blood pressure, a kind of coronary chemoreflex (**28**). *See Also CIRCULATION; BLOOD PURIFICATION/DETOXIFICATION; FATIGUE*

**VALERIAN ROOT** is one of the most studied plants. The herb has been investigated in animals and humans alike in hundreds of investigations, in several countries, particularly Germany and Russia. The results are always the same: Valerian root and/or its major constituents, the valepotriates, have marked sedative, anticonvulsive, hypotensive, tranquilizing, neurotropic, and anti-aggressive properties (**29-33**). These effects result from a selective neurotropic action of the root on higher brain centers, as is shown in EEG (electroencepholograph) monitorings of brain waves. The herb's main functional effect is to suppress and regulate the autonomic nervous system. As a result, it has been found effective in treating psychosomatic diseases that involve dysregulation of the autonomic nervous system. Many forms of restlessness and tension also yield to the effects of Valerian root. Interestingly, in Germany, Valerian preparations have been used for about 10 years to treat childhood behavioral disorders (**34**). Unlike other medications for hyperactivity, Valerian root has no side effects, even at rather high doses. In fact, in these children, the preparation enhanced motor coordination and maintained reaction time, while calming anxiety and fears, curing restlessness and curbing aggression. *See Also NERVOUS TENSION; IN-SOMNIA*

**KELP**'s considerable hypotensive activity is discussed in the HEART chapter.

## OTHER NUTRIENTS

*High blood pressure can be markedly affected, for good or bad, by dietary habits. Avoiding high dietary salt, sugar, food additives and saturated fat will greatly help. Individual requirements may vary widely. Use the following recommendations as guidelines only.*

### VITAMINS

*(Daily requirements unless otherwise noted)*

Vitamin B Complex-High Potency
Vitamin B6 *25 mg*
Vitamin C *1,000-3,000 mg*
Vitamin E *200-600 I.U.*
Choline *1,000 mg*
Inositol *1,000 mg*
Niacinamide *100 mg*
Bioflavanoids *100-300 mg*

### MINERALS

Calcium/Magnesium
Potassium
Phosphorous

### MISCELLANEOUS

GLA
Essential Fatty Acid
Cod Liver Oil
Brewer's Yeast
Lecithin
Wheat Germ
Liver

# REFERENCES

1. Bordia, A., Bansal, H.C., Arara, S.K. & Singh, S.V. "Effect of the essential oils of garlic and onion on alimentary hyperlipemia." **Atherosclerosis,** 21, 15-19, 1975.
2. Sial, A.Y. & Ahmed, S.I. "Study of the hypotensive action of garlic extract in experimental animals." **Journal of the Pakistan Medical Association,** 32(10), 237-239, 1982.
3. Kamanna, V.S. & Chandrasekhara, N. "Effect of garlic on serum lipoproteins and lipoprotein cholesterol levels in albino rats rendered hypercholesteremic by feeding cholesterol." **Lipids,** 17(7), 483-488, 1982.
4. Bordia, A. "Effect of garlic on blood lipids in patients with coronary heart disease." **American Journal of Clinical Nutrition,** 34(10), 2100-3, 1981.
5. Petkov, V. "Plants and hypotensive, antiatheromatous and coronarydilating action." **American Journal of Chinese Medicine,** 7(3), 197-236, 1979.
6. Kritchevsky, D. "Effect of garlic oil on experimental atherosclerosis in rabbits." **Artery,** 1(4), 319-323, 1975.
7. Korotkov, V.M. "The action of garlic juice on blood pressure." **Vrachebnoe Deloebnoe,** 6, 123, 1966.
8. Bordia, A. & Bansal, H.C. "Essential oil of garlic in prevention of atherosclerosis." **The Lancet,** II, 1491, 1973.
9. Piotrowski, G. "L'ail en therapeutique." **Praxis,** 37, 488-492, 1948.
10. Augusti, K.T. & Mathew, P.T. "Lipid lowering effect of allicin on long term feeding to normal rats." **Experientia.** 30(5), 468-470, 1973.
11. Bordia, A., Arora, S.K., Kothori, L.K., et.al. "The protective action of essential oils of onion and garlic in cholesterol-fed rabbits." **Atherosclerosis,** 22, 103-109, 1975.
12. Jain, R.C. "Onion and garlic in experimental cholesterol atherosclerosis in rabbits. I. Effect on serum lipids and development of atherosclerosis." **Artery,** 1(2), 115-125, 1975.
13. Jain, R.C. & Konar, D.B. "Onion and garlic in experimental cholesterol atherosclerosis in rabbits. II. Effect on serum proteins and development of atherosclerosis." **Artery,** 2(6), 531-539, 1976.
14. Jain, R.C. "Onion and garlic in experimental cholesterol induced atherosclerosis." **Indian Journal of Medical Research,** 64(10), 1509-1515, 1976.

15. Temple, K.H. "Effect of garlic on experimental cholesterol ather- osclerosis in rabbits." **Medizin und Erhaerung,** 3(9), 197-199, 1962.
16. Bordia, A., Verma, S.K., Vyas, A.K., et.al. "Effect of essential oil of onion and garlic on experimental atherosclerosis in rabbits." **Atherosclerosis,** 26, 379-386, 1977.
17. Sainani, G.S., Desai, D.B. & More, K.N. "Onion, garlic and atherosclerosis." **The Lancet,** Sept 11, 575-576, 1976.
18. Korotkov, V.M. "The action of garlic juice on blood pressure." **Vrachebnoe Delo,** 6, 123, 1966.
19. Srivastava, K.C. "Effects of aqueous extracts of onion, garlic and ginger on platelet aggregation and metabolism of arachido- nic acid in blood vascular system: In vitro study." **Prostaglan- dins Leukotrienes and Medicine,** 13, 227-235, 1984.
20. Bordia, A. "Effect of garlic on human platelet aggregation, in vitro." **Atherosclerosis,** 30, 355-361, 1978.
21. Makheia, A.N., Vanderhoek, J.Y. & Bailey, J.M. "Inhibition of platelet aggregation and thromboxane synthesis by onion and garlic." **The Lancet,** 1, 781, 1979.
22. Macht, D.I. & Cook, H.M. "A pharmacological note on cimicifu- ga." **Journal of the American Pharmaceutical Association,** 21(4), 324-330, 1932. (It was on the basis of many negative findings in this study, that research on the herb was abandoned and it fell into disrepute in traditional medicine in the U.S.A.)
23. Genazzani, E. & Sorrentino, L. "Vascular action of acteina: ac- tive constituent of actaea racemosa L." **Nature,** 194(4828), 544- 545, 1962.
24. List, P.H. & Hoerhammer, L. **Hagers Handbuch der Phar- mazeutischen Praxis.** Volumes 2-5, Springer-Verlag, Berlin.
25. Srinivasan, M.R., Sambaiah, K. Satyanarayana, M.N. & Rao, M.V.L. "Influence of red pepper and capsaicin on growth, blood constituents and nitrogen balance in rats." **Nutrition Reports International,** 21(3), 455-467, 1980.
26. Sambaiah, D., Satyanarayana, M.N. & Rao, M.V.L. "Effect of red pepper (chilles) and capsaicin on fat absorption and liver fat in rats." **Nutrition Reports International,** 18(5), 521-529, 1978.
27. Sambaiah, K. & Satyanarayana, M.N. "Hypocholesterolemic effect of red pepper & capsaicin." **Indian Journal of Ex- perimental Biology,** 18 (8), 898-899, 1980.
28. Toh, C.C., Lee, T.S. & Kiang, A.K. "The pharmacological actions of capsaicin and analogues." **British Journal of Pharmacolo- gy,** 10, 175-182, 1955.

29. Gstirner, F. & Kleinbauer, E. "Zur pharmakologischen Pruefung der Baldrianwurzel." (Toward the pharmacological examination of Valerian root). **Pharmazie,** 13(7), 416-419, 1958.
30. Hauschild, F. "Die problematik der sedativen baldrianwirkung." **Pharmazie,** 13(7), 420-422, 1958.
31. Kempinskas, V. "K voprosu o deystivii valer'yany". (On the action of valerian). **Farmakologiia i Toksikologiia,** 27(3), 305-309, 1964.
32. Zburzhinsky, V.K. "Issledovania sedatibnovo deistvia valer-yany." (An investigation into the sedative effect of valerian) **Farmakologiia i Toksikologiia,** 27(3), 301-305, 1964.
33. Boeters, U. "Behandlung vegetativer regulationsstoerungen mit valepotriaten (Valmane)." (Treament of sympathetic regulation disorders with valepotriates (Valmane). **Muenchener Medizinishe Wochenschrift,** 111(37), 1873-1876, 1969.
34. Klich, R. "Verhaltensstoerungen im kindesalter und deren therapie." (Behavioral disorders of childhood and their treatment). **Medizinische Welt,** 26(25), 1251-1254, 1975.

# BLOOD PURIFICATION AND DETOXIFICATION

## HERBS

**Form:**　Capsule, Tea

**CONTENTS:** **DANDELION root** *(Taraxacum officinale),* **YELLOW DOCK root** *(Rumex crispus),* **Sarsaparilla root** *(Smilax officinalis),* **Echinacea** *(Echinacea augustifolia),* **Licorice root** *(Glycyrrhiza glabra),* **Cayenne** *(Capsicum annum),* & **Kelp** *(Laminaria, Macrocystis, Ascophyllum).*

**PURPOSE:**　**To assist in the purification and detoxification of the blood. To be used by itself or to support several other blends.**

**Other Applications:**　Acne, obesity, gout, moles, viral warts, body odor, venereal disease, general toxicity, skin sores and swellings, skin cancer, endocrine and exocrine gland disorders.

**USE:**　1. Detoxification, purification & cleansing programs: 3-4 capsules, 2-3 times per day, with meals.
2. To support the problems discussed under ARTHRITIS, SKIN DISORDERS, and FEVERS & INFECTIONS. 1 capsule, 3 times per day with meals.
3. Routine Maintenance: 2-4 capsules daily with meals.
4. To help treat liver problems (see LIVER DISORDERS): 2 capsules, four times per day, never on empty stomach.

**Contraindications:**　None. For discussion of Licorice root and Cayenne, see Appendix A.

It is difficult to overestimate the importance of maintaining a healthy supply of blood. The blood must supply oxygen to each of the other sixty trillion cells of the body, transport nutrients, hormones and waste, warm and cool the body, heal itself, ward off invading micro-organisms, seal off wounds in the vessels, and so on. These vital functions sometimes become overtaxed due to the accumulation of bacteria and toxic waste products that result from acute and chronic cellular disease. Under such conditions, the blood may benefit from a boost, supplied by you, that detoxifies, purifies, heals and stimulates the production of plasma, leukocytes and hemoglobin. The therapeutic rationale behind this blend is that many ailments and diseases are either the result of impurities and toxins in the blood or that they can at least be benefited by a pure and vital blood supply. Either way, the blood is seen as a target for effective medicinal intervention. This idea has been around for a long time, though it occurs only rarely in modern medical practice. The old herbalist term for agents that clean up the blood is "alterative," a term that implies that the properties of the blood are gradually being changed from unhealthy to healthy. However, that may be an oversimplification of what is actually transpiring. In reality, toxins and wastes are being filtered out, microbial poisons are being killed, vital salts are being adjusted and balanced, nutrients are being furnished, and important plasma substances are being strengthened and enhanced. You may use this blend for the ailments listed under **Other Applications,** or whenever your symptoms include ugly sores, easy bruising, mucous diseased gums, exhaustion, anemia, cancer, venereal disease, and related conditions.

**DANDELION ROOT** acts primarily by purifying the blood, i.e., by straining and filtering toxins and wastes from the bloodstream. A complete discussion of Dandelion's effects on liver function is presented in the chapters on DIABETES and LIVER DISORDERS. Since a healthy liver is required to provide effective blood detoxification, it is important to note here two studies that demonstrated a liver-healing property in Dandelion. The first showed that in human patients, the herb uniformly remedied chronic liver congestion (**1**). In another study, in England, Dandelion was used in medical practice to successfully treat hepatitis, swelling of the liver, jaundice and dyspepsia with deficient bile secretion (**2**). Although not an herb of major use by the early American eclectics, these physicians did feel it was effective in treating cases of autointoxication (**3**). *See Also NERVES & GLANDS; SKIN DISORDERS; DIABETES; LIVER DISORDERS*

**YELLOW DOCK** also primarily affects liver function and the health of related organs, increasing their ability to strain and purify the blood. In addition, the herb has antibacterial properties (**4**). Formerly, Yellow Dock was a primary treatment for scurvy and anemia (probably because of its high iron content). It is still a favorite alterative (blood purifier) of peoples in many countries. The eclectics used it often when they felt that some particular skin disease incident was caused by blood-borne toxins (see the chapter on SKIN DISORDERS). To this day the herb is an important ingredient in alterative preparations in European countries (e.g., Germany, Russia, France, England and Switzerland), North American countries, China and India. In a search for an explanation for its alterative effect, research has thus far turned up only high thiamine content as a possiblity (**5**). *See Also NERVES & GLANDS; SKIN DISORDERS*

**SARSAPARILLA** root actually attacks microbial substances in the blood stream, neutralizing them (**6**). This effect is primarily due to antibiotic principles (such as special saponins) contained in the plant (**7-8**). The plant is also a strong diuretic, and thereby contributes to this blend by stimulating the excretion of wastes such as uric acid and excess chloride. The urea content of blood is dramatically lowered by this action. To a lesser degree the plant is a diaphoretic—by promoting sweating still more toxins are removed from the lymph and circulatory systems. Psoriasis is especially vulnerable to the effects of Sarsaparilla. *See Also INFERTILITY; ARTHRITIS; WHOLE BODY; DETOXIFY/NURTURE*

**LICORICE** root acts in an extremely complex manner to adjust the concentrations of vital blood salts, thereby stimulating and sustaining proper adrenal function (**9**). Licorice root protects the blood supply and enhances its purity by protecting the body's blood detoxification plant—the liver, from serious diseases, such as cirrhosis (**10**) and hepatitis (**11-13**). Licorice root should be included in blends such as this one that contain a goodly portion of saponin-containing plants since it protects cell membranes from hemolysis (the rupture of red blood cells) that often occurs from the ingestion of plant saponins (**14**).

**CAYENNE** is primarily a kind of catalyst in the blood purification process. It stimulates the vital organs to greater activity, promotes cardiovascular activity, while lowering overall blood pressure (**15-16**). But additionally, it acts directly as a diaphoretic, stimulating excretion of wastes in the sweat (**17**). *See Also CIRCULATION; HIGH BLOOD PRESSURE; FATIGUE; INFLUENZA*

**KELP** is a general nutritive tonic to the blood, supplying essential vitamins and mineral salts (**18**). Kelp is an important adjunct to any cleansing program since it can bind radioactive strontium, barium, cadmium and zinc, some of our most dangerous pollutants, in the gastrointestinal tract, thus preventing their absorption into the body (**19**). From studies carried out to discover why seaweeds dramatically inhibit the formation of human breast cancer (see chapter DE-GENERATIVE DISORDERS for details), it has been postulated that Kelp may activate the body's immune system (**20**). If proven true, this may explain some of Kelp's remarkable alterative properties. Incidentally, several studies have determined that arsenic in Kelp is physiologically inert (**21**). Kelp is neither carcinogenic nor toxic.

**BURDOCK** root comes about as close to a good old fashioned alterative or blood cleanser as anything in this blend. Thus, it produces gradual beneficial changes in the body by improving general nutrition and by gradually altering the health of the blood. It is both diuretic and diaphoretic, meaning it promotes the excretion of wastes in both the urine and sweat. Burdock has also been shown to enhance liver and bile functions (**22**). Bacteriostatic principles have been isolated from Burdock (**23**), and it has been found to inhibit tumor growth (**24**). Though the mechanism of action for these properties is not clear, it is very possible that they and the blood cleansing property are closely related. Clinically, Burdock and Yellow Dock are very similar in action.

In 1978, a major American medical journal printed an article entitled "Burdock root tea poisoning," that reported a case of a 26-year-old woman who was experiencing toxic symptoms after ingesting what she thought was Burdock root tea (**25**). The authors determined that the symptoms were consistent with atropine poisoning. Analysis of the plant revealed the presence of atropine, a fact that should have been a clue to the investigators that the herb was, in fact, not Burdock root, but the article never indicates that anything other than Burdock root was being analyzed (heavily contaminated Burdock root would have been another alternative, but the authors didn't clarify the situation). I called the main investigator and asked about it. He admitted that they did not verify the identity of the plant; in fact, they doubted it was Burdock! That doubt was not expressed in the paper. The bottom line, cutting through the misleading aspects of the paper and the irresponsible editorial style of the journal, is that one should be careful about where one buys herbal products. Burdock root is perfectly safe, as long as it truly is Burdock root. *See Also DETOXIFY/NURTURE; SKIN DISORDERS; BONE-FLESH-CARTILAGE*

**ECHINACEA** is also a classical alterative. A physician during the previous century reported over 100 blood counts made in cases of infectious disease, mainly tuberculosis. He found that Echinacea increased the phagocytic activity of leukocytes (the ability of white blood cells to fight, destroy and eat toxic organisms that invade the body). It increased and stabilized the red blood cell count and stimulated the elimination of waste products. In more technical terms, it stabilized the relative percentage of neutrophils to other leukocytes in the blood, and normalized both hyperleukocytosis (excess of leukocytes) and leukopenia (deficiency in leukocytes) (**26**). These studies were undertaken because Echinacea was one of the most popular medicinal foods of that century. Actually, the therapeutic use of Echinacea can be traced to the North American Indians who used it to heal wounds, for insect and snake bites, to combat infections, both externally and internally. Modern research has validated, explained and extended the observations of the previous century. Enchinacea has been shown to increase the healing rate of bacterial skin infections by a direct stimulation of phagocytosis (**27**). Leukocyte production in radiology patients has been promoted by the herb. In rabbits, the number of circulating granulocytes has been increased by Echinacea (**28**). Finally, Echinacea extracts (injected i.v.) dramatically increased blood properdin levels (**29**). Properdin helps neutralize bacterial and viral blood toxins. These findings suggest that Echinacea significantly stimulates the body's own blood cleansing system. *See Also SKIN DISORDERS; FEVERS & INFECTIONS*

## OTHER NUTRIENTS

*The ability of the blood to perform its many functions depends on a continual and adequate supply of nutrients. The following recommendations are meant as guidelines; individual requirements may differ significantly.*

### VITAMINS

(Daily requirements unless otherwise noted)

Vitamin A *10,000 I.U.* (25,000 I.U. for short intervals)

Vitamin B Complex
Vitamin B-2 *25-50 mg*
Vitamin B-6 *25-50 mg*
Vitamin B-12 *25 mcg*
Vitamin C *500-1,000 mg*
Vitamin D *200-400 I.U.*
Vitamin E *200-600 I.U.*
Niacinamide *100 mg*
Pantothenic Acid *50-100 mg*
Choline *500-1000 mg*
Inositol *500-600 mg*
PABA *10 mg*
Folic acid *400 mcg*

**MINERALS**

Potassium
Calcium/Magnesium

# REFERENCES

1. Leclerc, H. **Phytotherapie (Paris),** 1927, cited by Ripperger, W. "Pflanzliche laxantien und cholagogue wirkungen." **Medizinische Welt,** 9, 1463, 1935.
2. Kroeber, L. "Pharmacology of inulin drugs and their therapeutic use. II. Cichorium intybus; taraxacum officinale." **Pharmazie,** 5, 122-127, 1950.
3. Felter, H. W. **The Eclectic Materia Medica, Pharmacology and Therapeutics.** Eclectic Medical Publications, Portland, Oregon, 1983 (first published 1922).
4. List, P.H. & Hoerhammer, L. **Hagers Handbuch der Pharmazeutischen Praxis.** Volumes 2-5, Springer-Verlag, Berlin.
5. Watt, J.M. & Breyer-Brandwijk, M.G. **The Medicinal and Poisonous Plants of Southern and Eastern Africa.** E. & S. Livingstone, LTd., Edinburgh & London, England, 1962.
6. Tschesche, R. "Advances in the chemistry of antibiotic substances from higher plants." in Wagner, H. & Horhammer, L. **Pharmacognosy and Phytochemistry.** Springer Verlag, N.Y. 1971, pp. 274-276.
7. D'Amico. "Richerche sulla presenza di sostanze ad azione antibiotica nelle piante superiori." **Fitoterapia,** 21(1), 1950, 77-79.
8. Fitzpatrick, F.K. "Plant substances active against Myobacterium

tuberculosis." **Antibiotics and Chemotherapy,** 4(5), 1954, 528-536.

9. Kumagi, A, Asanuman, U., Yano, S., Takevchik, Morimoto, Y., Vemura, T. & Yamamura, Y. "Effect of glycyrrhizin on the suppressive action of cortisone on the pituitary adrenal axis." **Endocrinologia Japonica,** 13, 235-244, 1966.

10. Zhao, M., Han, D., Ma, X., Zhao, Y., Yin, L. & Li, C. "The preventive and therapeutic actions of glycyrrhizin, glycyrrhetic acid and crude saikosides on experimental cirrhosis in rats." **Yao Hsueh Hsueh Pao,** 18(5), 325-331, 1983.

11. Fujisawa, K., Watanabe, Y. * Kimura, K. "Therapeutic approach to chronic active hepatitis with glycyrrhizin." **Asian Medical Journal,** 23, 745-756, 1980.

12. Iwamura, K. "Ergebnisse der therapie mit dem midikament strong neo-minophagen C der chronischaggressiven hepatitis in Japan." **Therapiewoche,** 30, 5431-5445, 1980.

13. Yamamoto, S., Maekawa, Y, Imamura, M & Hisajima, T. "Therapeutic effects of stronger neo-minophagen C on chronic hepatitis." **Clinical Medicine and Pediatrics,** 13, 73-75, 1958.

14. Nakagawa, K & Masukichiro, A. "Effect of glycyrrhizin on hepatic lysosomal systems." **Japanese Journal of Pharmacology,** 31, 849-851, 1981.

15. de Lille, J. & Ramirez, E. "Pharmacodynamic action of the active principles of chillie (capsicum annuum L)." **Anales Inst. Biol.,** 6, 23-37, 1935.

16. Toh, C.C., Lee, T.S. & Kiang, A.K. "The pharmacological actions of capsaicin and its analogues." **British Journal of Pharmacology,** 10, 175-182, 1955.

17. Lee, T.S. **Journal of Physiology,** 124, 528, 1954.

18. Yamamoto, T. & Ishibashi, M. "The content of trace elements in seaweeds." in **Proceedings of the Seventh International Seaweed Symposium,** Wiley & Sons, N.Y., 511-514, 1972.

19. Tanaka, Y., Hurlburt, A.J., Argeloff, L., Skoryna, S.C. & Stara, J.F. "Application of algal polysaccharides as in vivo binders of metal pollutants." in **Proceedings of the Seventh International Seaweed Symposium,** Wiley & Sons, N.Y., 602-607, 1972.

20. Taylor, W.A., Sheldon, D., & Spicer, J.W. "Adjuvant and suppressive effects of grass conjuvac and other alginate conjugates on IgG and IgE antibody responses in mice." **Immunology,** 44, 41-50, 1981.

21. Fukui, S. Hirayama, T., Nohara, M & Sakagami, Y. "The chemical forms of arsenic in some seafoods and in urine after ingestion

of these foods." **Shokihin Eiseigaku Zasshi,** 22(6), 513-519, 1981.

22. Chabrol, E. & Charonnat, R. "Therapeutic agents in bile secretion." **Ann. Med.,** 37, 131-142, 1935.
23. Foldeak, S. & Dombradi, G.A. "Tumor-growth inhibiting substances of plant origin. I. Isolation of the active principle of arctium lappa." **Acta Univ. Szeged., Phys. Chem.,** 10, 91-93, 1964.
24. Schulte, K.E., Ruecker, G. & Perlick, J. "polyacetylene compounds in Echinacea purpurea and e. augustifolia." **Arzneimittel Forschungen,** 17(7), 825-829, 1967.
25. Bryson, P.D., Watanabe, A.S., Rumack, B.H. & Murphy, R.C. "Burdock root tea poisoning." **Journal of the American Medical Association,** 239(20), 2157, 1978.
26. Ellingwood, F. **American Materia Medica, Therapeutics and Pharmacognosy.** Eclectic Medical Publications, Portland, Oregon, 1983.
27. Quadripur, S.A. **Therapie der Gegenwart,** 115, 1072, 1976.
28. Chone, B. "Geziete steuerung der leukozytentinetik durch echinacin." **Arzneimittel-Forschung,** 11, 611-615, 1965.
29. Busing, K.H., "The effect of extracts of Echinacea purpurea on the properdin levels of rabbits." **Zhurnal Immunitatsforschung,** 115, 169-176, 1958.

# LOW BLOOD SUGAR

## HERBS

CONTENTS: **LICORICE** root *(Glycyrrhiza glabra)*, **GOTU KOLA** *(Hydrocotyle asiatica)*, **Siberian Ginseng** *(Eleutherococcus senticosus)*, & **Ginger** *(Zingiber officinale)*.

PURPOSE: **To counter the effects of low blood sugar and to support glucose metabolism.**

Other Applications: Fatigue, Exhaustion, Addison's Disease (adrenal exhaustion).

USE: 1. Anywhere from 4 to 8 capsules per day can be recommended depending on the severity of symptoms.
2. To supplement the FATIGUE Blend: 4 capsules per day.
3. To supplement the MENTAL ALERTNESS/SENILITY Blend: 3-4 capsules per day.

**Contraindications:** Some forms of low blood sugar involve very low serum potassium levels. Please have your physician check your potassium. If it is low, be sure to supplement the use of this blend with potassium tablets. For a discussion of Licorice root, see Appendix A.

Low blood sugar may result from any one of several conditions: 1) Overproduction of insulin; 2) Damage to liver cells; 3) Insufficient secretion of adrenocortical hormones; and 4) Pituitary gland abnormalities. This blend is designed to remedy cause 3 above. Since the effects of stress are felt mainly by the adrenals, it is probable that most cases of hypoglycemia are of this type. You can help the body remedy the first cause by not ingesting refined sugar; cause two by using the blend for LIVER DISORDERS along with this blend; and cause four by prolonged use of the WHOLE BODY TONIC blend with good nutritional planning. Prolonged hypoglycemia that resists the measures presented here should be treated by a competent physician. This product, due to Licorice root, should increase circulating glucocorticoids, (adrenal hormones) in the liver and should also mimic their action somewhat itself. "Functional" hypoglycemia, due to severe muscular exertion, poor nutrition and other stressors, characterized by a general rundown feeling, headache, numbness, chilliness, dizziness and weakness, will yield nicely to the tonic effects of this blend. Gotu Kola and Ginseng build up the body's resistance to stress, and Ginger root strengthens and maintains the G.I. tract so that it can better assimilate nutrients from this and other sources. The WHOLE BODY TONIC blend, and potassium supplements should probably be taken in conjunction with this product.

**LICORICE ROOT**'s role in treating hypoglycemia is to increase the effectiveness of glucocorticoids (adrenal hormones) circulating in the liver, and to mimic the action of these hormones itself (**1-2**). This mechanism would work in cases of low blood sugar brought on by adrenal stress. In a classical example, a person subjects himself to vigorous physical work, poor nutrition and other extremely stressful circumstances. Even in the short run, that person may feel rundown and experience headache, numbness, chilliness, dizziness and weakness. Often the adrenals simply cannot keep up with the demands on the body. Licorice root can help to reverse the symptoms, but long term health maintenance demands better overall nutrition ,at the very least. Complete adrenal exhaustion is known as Addison's disease. In this condition none of the three major classes of adrenal-cortical hormones are being produced. These include the glucocor-ticoids (cortisol, corticosterone), mineralcorticoids (aldosterone), and sex hormones (androgen, estrogen). Some rather severe problems develop. Licorice root constituents have been shown to help the body overcome adrenal failure, which could lead to Addison's disease (**3-4**). Their effectiveness derives from their ability to maintain the proper electrolyte balance in tissues (normally the role of aldosterone), and from their ability to prevent the enzymatic destruction of whatever glucocorticoids and mineralcorticoids happen to be present in the cells (**3-8**), thus allowing these hormones to circulate and be active longer. Furthermore the use of Licorice root alone or in conjunction with drugs used to treat adrenal insufficiency, prevents the destruction (through atrophy) of the adrenal glands that usually occurs when drugs alone are used. Cortisone and other drugs, by interrupting the normal feedback mechanisms that signal the adrenals to begin producing hormones, make the gland "lazy", i.e., the body keeps telling the adrenal gland that there are plenty of hormones in the blood, so the gland quits making them, shrivels up and self-destructs. Licorice root prevents the drug-induced atrophy from happening; instead it helps the adrenal gland recover normal function. There is another interesting case study that sheds light on how licorice root (in conjunction with Ginseng) might help counteract the effects of stress. In this case, a woman was diagnosed as having a severe pituitary deficiency following a tough pregnancy and tougher delivery. Normal treatment would have been ACTH (the pituitary hormone that stimulates the adrenal glands) and corticosterone (to replace steroids not being secreted by adrenal glands). Instead, Licorice root and Ginseng were administered. The woman improved quickly, gaining weight, increasing in energy and blood pressure. The researchers attributed most of the outcome to Licorice root but acknowledged the role of Ginseng in stimulating the pituitary-adrenocortical system (**8**). Even though the best controls were not implemented in this study, the results do conform to predicitions. *See Also DETOXIFY/NURTURE; FEMALE TONIC; WHOLE BODY; FEVERS & INFECTIONS; INFERTILITY; ARTHRITIS; SKIN DISORDERS; BLOOD PURIFICATION/DETOXIFICATION; CIRCULATION; WEIGHT LOSS; ENVIRONMENTAL POLLUTION; MENTAL ALERTNESS/SENILITY*

**GOTU KOLA** is used to build up good adrenal health. See the chapters on FATIGUE, WHOLE BODY TONIC, and MENTAL ALERTNESS/SENILITY for discussions of this herb.

**SIBERIAN GINSENG**, through the interplay of its many active constituents, including the panaxosides, ginsengosides, essential oils, carbohydrates, organic acids, amino acids, peptides, vitamins, minerals, trace elements, enzymes and sterols, is often able to *normalize* physiological imbalances (**10**). In this case, research has shown that it can raise abnormally low blood sugar levels (**11-12**) and that it can lower abnormally high blood sugar levels (**12-13**). These results suggest that Ginseng increases the conversion rate of sugars into the necessary substrates for the formation of fatty acids in the liver. In my opinion, Ginseng's effect on blood sugar levels is an indirect result of its effect on the total organism. Since a person suffering from hyperglycemia or hypoglycemia presents a complex picture of physiological symptoms, including deficiencies and excesses, any agent that improves general cellular health will have a positive effect on both conditions. This is exactly what Ginseng does. It stimulates RNA synthesis (**14**), produces changes in the polysome content, i.e., the content of the bodies in liver cells that are responsible for the production of glucose from lactic acid (**15**), increases the amount of endoplasmic reticulum, i.e., in those cellular structures responsible for metabolic function (**16**), and stimulates protein synthesis (**17**). Whether blood sugar would be produced or used up during that process would depend on substrate requirements of the cell. If too much blood sugar was around, it would be utilized by the liver in protein and fat synthesis. If very little sugar were available, the liver would use other metabolic pathways that would result in increased glycogen synthesis and glucose production. The liver utilizes energy at the most basic level. Changes in RNA content, ATPase (an important enzyme) activity and increases in endoplasmic reticulum after prolonged ingestion of Ginseng suggest that the plant simply increases the efficiency of the body's own natural metabolic processes. *See Also INFERTILITY; FATIGUE; WHOLE BODY TONIC; MENTAL ALERTNESS/SENILITY*

**GINGER ROOT** probably does not have a direct effect on blood sugar levels. Nevertheless, it is an important herb for hypoglycemics to use. It works indirectly to increase the availability of dietary nutrients for digestion and metabolism. Whenever the hypoglycemic condition is attended and/or made worse by improper digestion and assimilation of foods, Ginger root will markedly facilitate the utilization of energy stores (**18-19**). Functional hypoglycemia, that rundown feeling, is especially well-served by this treatment. *See Also CIRCULATION; NERVOUS TENSION; FATIGUE; DIGESTION; NAUSEA; STOMACH/INTESTINAL*

## OTHER NUTRIENTS

*Eating properly and ingesting adequate supplementary vitamins and other nutrients each day will go far toward preventing hypoglycemic episodes. Individual requirements may depart substantially from the following recommendations.*

### VITAMINS

*(Daily requirements unless otherwise noted)*

Vitamin B Complex
Vitamin B1 *25-50 mg*
Vitamin B2 *25-50 mg*

Vitamin B6 *25-50 mg*
Vitamin B12 *25-50 mg*
Pantothenic acid *100-200 mg*
Vitamin C *2,000-5,000 mg*
Vitamin E *600-800 I.U.*

## MINERALS

Calcium/Magnesium
Phosphorous
Chromium
Potassium

## MISCELLANEOUS

HCl
Brewer's yeast

## REFERENCES

1. Tamura, Y. "Study of effects of glycyrrhetinic acid and its derivatives on 4-5 alpha and beta -reductase by rat liver preparations." **Folia Endocrinologia Japonica,** 8, 164-188, 1975.
2. Kumagai, A, Asanuman, U., Yano, S., Takevchik, Morimoto, Y., Vemura, T., & Yamamura, Y. "Effect of glycyrrhizin on the suppressive action of cortisone on the pituitary adrenal axis." **Endocrinologia Japonica,** 13, 235-244, 1966.
3. Borst, J.G.G., Ten Holt, S.P., de Vries, L.A., & Molhuysen, J.A. "Synergistic action of liquirice and cortisone in Addison's and Simmond's disease." **Lancet,** 1, 657-663, 1953.
4. Pelser, H.E., Willerbrands, A.F., Frenkel, M., van der Heide, & Groen, J. "Comparative study of the use of glycyrrhizinic and glycyrrhetinic acids in Addison's Disease." **Metabolism,** 2, 322-334, 1953.
5. Card, J., Strong, J.A., Tompsett, M.W., Taylor, N.R.W. & Wilson, J.M.G. "Effects of liquorice and its derivatives on salt and water metabolism." **Lancet,** 1, 663-668, 1953.
6. Groen, J. Pelser, H.E., Frenkel, M., Wilderbrands, A.F. & Kamminga, C.E. "Extracts of glycyrrhizinic acid on the electrolyte metabolism in Addison's disease." **Journal of Clinical Investigations,** 31, 87-91, 1952.
7. Armanini, D., Karbowiak, I. & Fulder, J.W. "Affinity of liquorice derivatives for mineralcorticoid and glucocorticoid receptors." **Clinical Endocrinology,** (Oxf), 19(5), 609-612, 1983.

8. Tamura, Y., Nishikawa, K., Yamada, M, Yamamotoa, M. & Kumagi, A. "Effects of glycyrrhetinic acid and its derivatives on delta-four-5-alpha and 5-beta reductase in rat liver." **Arzneimit-tel-Forschung,** 29(4), 647-649, 1979.

9. Cheng-chia, L. & Ching-ch'u, T. "Successful treatment of post-partum hypopituitarism with decoction of radix glycyrrhizae and radix ginseng." **Chinese Medical Journal,** 11, 156, 1973.

10. Yugens, I.L. & Kirilov, O.I., "The effect of eleutherococcus on stress." **24th Session of the Committee to Study Ginseng and Other Medicinal Plants of the Far East,** Vlad., 96 pages.

11. Solodkov, A.S., "Changes in some biochemical indices of human blood under the effect of eleutherococcus." **24th Session of the Committee to Study Ginseng and Other Medicinal Plants of the Far East,** Vlad., 96 pages.

12. Jiang, J., Zhang, Z., Zhang, L. & Huang, M. "Effects of general saponin of panax notoginseng and sanchinoside C-1 on blood sugar in experimental animals." **Acta Pharmaceutica Sinica (Yao Hsueh Hsueh Pao),** 17(3), 222-225, 1982.

13. Bedzdetko, G.N. "Experimental investigations of a liquid extract of eleutherococcus as an antidiabetic agent." **24th Session of the Committee to Study Ginseng and Other Medicinal Plants of the Far East,** Vladivostok, 96 pages.

14. Dardymov, I.V., "Basic pharmacological properties of eleutherococcus roots." **24th Session of the Committee to Study Ginseng and Other Medicinal Plants of the Far East,** Vladivostok, 96 pages.

15. Kirilov, O.E. "Investigations on the mechanism of eleutherococcus adaptogenic action and the problem of the pharmacological control of stress." **24th Session of the Committee to Study Ginseng and Other Medicinal Plants of the Far East,** Vladivostok, 96 pages.

16. Bezdetko, G.N., Brekhman, I.I., Dardymov, I.V., Zilber, M.L. & Rogozkin, V.A. "Effect of eleutherococcus glucosides on RNA polymerase activity in nuclei from skeletal muscles and liver after physical strain." **Vop. Med. Khim.,** 19(3), 245-248, 1973.

17. Belonosov, I.S., et. al. "Some results of the studying the effect of eleutherococcus on metabolism." **24th Session of the Committee to Study Ginseng and Other Medicinal Plants of the Far East,** Vladivostok, 96 pages.

18. Thompson, E.H., Wolk, I.D. & Allen, C.E. "Ginger rhizome: a new source of proteolytic enzyme." **Journal of Food Science,** 38(4), 652-655, 1973.

19. Glatzel, H. "Treatment of dyspetic disorders with spice extracts." **Hippokrates,** 40(23), 916-919, 1969.

# BONE-FLESH-CARTILAGE
# SUPPLEMENT

**HERBS**

**Form:** Capsule, Poultice, Compress, Mouthwash

**CONTENTS: HORSETAIL** *(Equisetum arvense)*, **CHA-PARRAL** *(Larrea divaricata)*, **Plantain** *(Plantago ovata)*, **Parsley** *(Petroselinum sativum)*, **Burdock** *(Arctium lappa)*, **Marshmallow** *(Althea officinalis)*, **Slippery Elm** *(Ulmus vulva)*.

**PURPOSE:** **To provide nutritive support for bones, skin and related tissue, and to promote the healing of those parts of the body.**

**Other Applications:** Arthritis, Bursitis, Rheumatism.

**USE:** 1. Internal: 4-8 capsules per day. Use more if severe injury or other conditions warrant.
2. External: 4 capsules for small areas. 8 capsules for larger areas. Apply as poultice or compress.

**Contraindications:** None. Chaparral contains no creosote.

Since bones, skin and related tissue make up the greatest mass of our bodies, it is very important to keep them in good health. This is done best by eating foods that supply the nutrients needed for growth, strength and resistance to disease. It is also important that damaged bones and tissue heal properly with a minimum of permanent damage such as scar tissue, mineral deposits, destroyed nerves, and deformation. In general, the diet must supply adequate amounts of calcium, magnesium, phosphorous, Vitamins A, D, and

31

B complex. The use of herbs can supply some of those nutrients, but herbs also supply active principles that heal, soothe and remedy in a more direct fashion. This blend is probably as effective in external applications as it is when taken internally. Several herbs in the blend contain large quantities of more or less inert mucilage. The mucilage will clean up and sanitize wounds, absorb toxins around sores and wounds on all exposed surfaces, both inside and outside the body, including mucous membranes. One scientist, speaking of Plantain, writes, "The efficiency of the drug would appear to be entirely due to large quantities of mucilage.... It ...passes through the small intestine unchanged and during its passage it lines the mucous membrane acting as a demulcent (a soothing agent) and a lubricant. Further, the mucilage is not acted on by the intestinal bacteria in the large gut. Its presence there in fact would appear to have an inhibiting action on the growth of the organisms....The mucilage...has a remarkable power of absorbing bacterial and other toxins." The same thing could have been written about Slippery Elm, and Marshmallow, all very high in mucilage and very similar in action to Plantain, both internally and externally.

**HORSETAIL** or **SHAVEGRASS** has been shown to possess hemolytic (blood clotting) (**1**) and antibiotic (**2**) activities, properties that contribute to the healing process. Externally, Horsetail can be applied as a poultice to accelerate the healing of stubborn wounds. This remedy was practiced by the American Indians on this continent and by the Chinese in Asia. Horsetail also supplies calcium, the primary mineral required for the healing of bones. Horsetail is rich in several other minerals that the body uses to rebuild injured tissue.

**CHAPARRAL** has substantial clinical and experimental support as a treatment for skin cancer (see DETOXIFY/NURTURE for details). In addition, at the Brooks hospital in Boston, a team of scientists found that the antioxidant nature of NDGA (nordihydroquaiaretic acid), the primary constituent of Chaparral, significantly inhibited the formation of dental caries (73-74% by one measure, 80-83% by another) (**3**). This research implies that a good rinsing of the mouth with Chaparral tea (or this blend) a couple of times per day might reduce bacterial or viral damage to teeth. There is also research that indicates that Chaparral helps reduce the painful symptoms of rheumatism (**4**), reduces inflammation by increasing ascorbic acid (Vitamin C) levels in the adrenals (**5**) and inhibits several strains of bacteria, molds and other pathogens(**6-8**). These data, together with those discussed in other chapters, clearly indicate that Chaparral plays an important role in healing skin and bone tissue, and in preventing pathogenic damage. *See Also SKIN DISORDERS; ARTHRITIS; DETOXIFY/NURTURE*

**PARSLEY** serves two functions in this blend. First it imparts a measure of essential oil that invigorates the body, its blood supply and its tissues. Secondly, it supplies a good deal of nutrients. Its protein content (needed in the mending of bones) is over 20% (**9**), and it contains vitamins A, C, B-complex and K (**10**). Added benefits from ingesting Parsley are its hypotensive or relaxing action (**11**) and its mild antibacterial action (**12**). *See Also DIURETIC; DIABETES; PROSTATE*

**BURDOCK,** due to its high inulin (not be confused with insulin) content (up to 50% in root), is classified as a blood purifier. That is why it is in this blend. The skin and bones need a pure supply of blood in order to heal properly. Nutrients need to be brought to sites of injury, and wastes need to be drawn off. The blood performs these tasks much more efficiently under the influence of herbs such as Burdock. The heart also benefits from the presence of inulin, since this substance is a source of the sugar fructose which is converted by the liver more rapidly into glycogen than other sugars (**1**). Burdock is high in the healing B vitamins and vitamin C. It possesses activity against tumor growth (**13**), and is a natural antibiotic (**14**). *See Also BLOOD PURIFICATION/DETOXIFICATION; DETOXIFY/NURTURE; SKIN DISORDERS*

**MARSHMALLOW** is demulcent and mucilaginous, containing up to 35% mucilage. It soothes mucous membranes, and has been used externally for hundreds of years as a wound healer. Marshmallow ointments and cremes are used on chapped hands and lips. Mainly, it is used internally to treat inflammation and mucosal afflictions of the genito-urinary tract, including cystitis, incontinence, painful urination, gonorrhea, enteritis, diarrhea, dysentery and cholera. It is also used to soothe a respiratory tract irritated by bronchitis, asthma, whooping cough, etc. It is used as a mouthwash and gargle and for helping infants cut new teeth (**1, 15-16**). Incidentally, the above listed uses were known as long ago as the days of Dioscorides and Pliny (**17**). The root of Marshmallow was the original main ingredient in the white spongy marshmallow confection, but it is no longer used for that purpose.

**SLIPPERY ELM** is also demulcent due to its high mucilage content (up to 50%). It is the American equivalent of Marshmallow, the two having been used for almost exactly the same purposes. The presence of Slippery Elm bark may have been one reason why the cultivation and use of Marshmallow in the Colonies, and later the States, never caught on as it did in Europe. Likewise, the Europeans have never found much application for Slippery Elm. As early as 1633, we find records of Slippery Elm use in Europe, as a poultice for wounds and as a remedy for broken bones (**18**), but it never became a truly popular herb among the English settlers until they noticed its use by the Indians. In 1859, a physician wrote "Slippery Elm, the inner bark of which is one of the most useful medical agents we have...is so important an article that it may be had at almost any drug store now...." (**19**). At any rate, medical botanists have never given up the practice of using Slippery Elm bark for just about any condition involving injured or infected tissue or bone. *See Also HEMORRHOIDS/ASTRINGENT; RESPIRATORY AILMENTS*

**PLANTAIN** provides a mucilaginous substance that contains healing properties that other mucilaginous plants do not possess. Evidence for this comes from a report of a rather loosely performed experiment in which several people, having contracted poison ivy dermatitis, were immediately treated with Plantain leaf. The itching immediately subsided and did not return (**20**). It is surprising that this knowledge is not better known. Plantain is also reportedly effective on ringworm. Our early American Physicians used Plantain for any skin infection or inflammation (**21**). One early physician even wrote that Plantain leaves placed upon the feet will ease the pain and fatigue one might experience on long walks (like around shopping malls?). No one currently recommends Plantain to heal bones, but I wonder if we are overlooking something that was once common knowledge. Read these words from Shakespeare's **Romeo and Juliet:**

Romeo: Your plantain leaf is excellent for that.
Juliet: For what I pray thee?
Romeo: For your broken shin.

## OTHER NUTRIENTS

*The importance of nutrients in the repair and growth of tissue is well-known. The following guidelines must be adapted to your individual needs and requirements.*

## VITAMINS

*(Daily requirement unless otherwise noted)*

Vitamin A *25,000 I.U.*
Vitamin B Complex
Vitamin B1 *50 mg*
Vitamin B2 *50 mg*
Vitamin B6 *50 mg*
Vitamin B12 *30-900 mcg*
Vitamin C *500-1,000 mg*
Vitamin D *800-3,000 I.U.*
Vitamin E *600-800 I.U.*
Pantothenic acid *150 mg*

## MINERALS

Calcium/Magnesium
phosphorous
Copper

## MISCELLANEOUS

HCl

# REFERENCES

1. List, P.H. & Hoerhammer, L. **Hagers Handbuch der Pharmazeutischen Praxis.** Volumes 2-5, Springer-Verlag, Berlin.
2. Sommer, L., Mintzer, L. & Rindasu, G. "Antimicrobial activity of the volatile oil extracted from equisetum arvense." **Farmacia Bucharest.,** 10, 535-541, 1962.
3. Lisanti, V.F. & Eichel, B. "Antioxidant inhibition of experimental induced caries." **Journal of Dental Research,** 42, 1030-1035, 1963.
4. Bergel, M. "Dihydroquaiaretic acid in therapy." **Semana Med** (Buenous Aires), II, 123-131, 1955.
5. Sporn, A. & Schobesch, O. "Toxicity of nordihydroquaiaretic acid." **Igiena,** (Bucharest), 15(12), 725-726, 1966.
6. Herrman, K. "Lignans and their practical importance." **Pharmazie,** 12, 147-155, 1957.
7. Epstein, S.S., Sporoschetz, I.B. & Hunter, S.H. "Toxicity of antioxidants to tetrhymena pyriformis." **Journal of Protozoology,** 14(2), 238-244, 1967.

8. Hirose, K., Ose, Y. & Kitamura, J. "Antibacterial property of antioxidants." **Gifu Yakka Daigaku Kiyo,** 6, 66, 1956.

9. Murphy, E.W., Marsh, A.C. & Willis, B.W. "Nutrient content of spices and herbs." **Journal of the American Dietetic Association,** 72, 174-176, 1978.

10. Watt, B.K. & Merrill, A.L. **Composition of Foods—Raw,** Processed, Prepared, Rev., USDA Agricultural Handbook No. 8, 1963.

11. Petkov, V. "Plants with hypotensive, antiatheromatous and coronarodilatating action." **American Journal of Chines Medicine,** 7(3), 197-236, 1979.

12. Abdullin, K.K. "Bactericidal effect of essential oils." **Uch. Zap. Kazansk. Vet. Inst.,** 84, 75-79, 1962.

13. Foldeak, S. & Dombradi, G.A. "Tumor-growth inhibiting substances of plant origin. I. Isolation of the active principle of arctium lappa." **Acta Physiology and Chemistry (Szeged),** 10, 91-93, 1964.

14. Schulte, K.E., Ruecker, G. & Boehme, R. "Polyacetylene compounds in burdock roots." **Arzneimittel-Forschung,** 17(7), 829-833, 1967.

15. Schauenberg, P. & Paris, F. **Guide des plantes medicinales,** Delachaux et Niestle, S.A., Neuchatel, Switzerland, 1969.

16. Wren, R.W. **Potter's New Cyclopedia of Botanical Drugs and Preparations,** 7th ed. Health Science Press, Rustington, England, 1970.

17. Barton, B.H. & Castle, R. **The British Flora Medica,** Chatto & Windus, London, 1877.

18. Gerarde, John. **The Herball or General History of Plants,** Dover edition, 1975 (1st printed 1633, London).

19. Gunn, J.D. **New Domestic Physician or Home Book of Health,** Moore, Wilstach, Keys. Cincinnati, 1st ed., 1857, 2nd ed 1859, 3rd ed 1961.

20. Duckett, S. "Plantain leaf for poison ivy." **Lancet,** 303(10), 583, 1980.

21. Ellingwood, F. **American Materia Medica, Therapeutics and Pharmacognosy.** Eclectic Medical Publications, Portland, Oregon, 1983.

# CHOLESTEROL REGULATION

## HERBS

**Form:** Capsule.

**CONTENTS: APPLE PECTIN, Hawthorn berries** *(Crataegus oxyacantha)*, **Plantain** *(Plantago ovata)*, **Fenugreek** *(Trigonella Foenum-graecum)*, **Black Cohosh root** *(Cimicifuga racemosa)*, & **Cayenne** *(Capsicum annum)*.

**PURPOSE: To help the body lower high serum cholesterol and to help prevent the deposition of dietary cholesterol on arterial walls.**

**Other Applications:** To reduce the risk of heart disease, colon cancer, food poisoning and atherosclerosis; A dieting aid.

**USE:** 1. To reduce or reverse cholesterol build up: 1-2 capsules per meal.
2. To help relieve acute conditions: 4-6 capsules per day (for three month period).
3. As a dieting aid: 1 capsule per meal (Use with WEIGHT LOSS blend).
4. Use in conjunction with the HEART blend to reduce the risk of developing Heart Problems.
5. Use in conjunction with the HIGH BLOOD PRESSURE blend to reduce the contribution of cholesterol to this problem.

6. For enhanced effectiveness of above applications, use Vitamin C (1000 mg daily) (**1**) and polyunsaturated oils (Evening Primrose, Walnut, Eicosapentanoic acid (EPA), corn, cod liver, GLA).

**Contraindications:**   None. Insulin-requiring diabetics should inform their physicians if using this blend for an extended period (see discussion under Pectin below). Hawthorn may potentiate the action of digitalis. Advise your physician if you are using both.

Cholesterol is a waxy, white substance that is classified as a fat. About 1000 milligrams are manufactured each day by the liver, from the fats, proteins and carbohydrates we eat. It is used in all tissues, not just the bloodstream, and is essential to life. Among other functions, it provides the building blocks for several hormones, makes up the major portion of the fatty insulation layer of nerves and is an important structural unit in the outer membrane of cells. However, cholesterol may build up in the bloodstream, accumulating on the arterial walls, slowly inhibiting the flow of blood, until the flow becomes very difficult or stops completely (atherosclerosis); eventually a stroke or heart attack will probably occur. In addition to the cholesterol made by the liver, Americans consume about 400-500 mg of it directly from their diets every day. This cholesterol is only found in animal products (meat, eggs, poultry, fish, dairy products), almost never in vegetable sources.

By now, everyone has heard of low-density lipoproteins, very-low-density lipoproteins and high-density lipoproteins. HDL's are the good guys; VLDL'S and LDL's are the bad guys. They are all made by the liver. However, VLDL's and LDL's, like so many miniature oil tankers, deliver the cholesterol into the body's systems, and HDL's clear it out of the system. Furthermore, LDL and HDL are made from different kinds of fat. LDL is composed primarily of saturated fats such as butter, bacon fat, beef fat and vegetable oils like coconut and palm oil, and saturated fats made by the liver. HDL is made up mainly of polyunsaturated fats which cannot be manufactured by the body, but must be consumed, such as corn, safflower, soybean and sesame oil. By consuming polyunsaturated (essential) oils and eliminating saturated fat, we reduce the number of oil trucks carrying the cholesterol to the system and increase the amount of HDL, with the net result of keeping serum cholesterol levels within normal limits.

Herbs, especially mucilaginous fibers such as Pectin, can help reduce cholesterol levels, prevent heart disease and atherosclerosis, and remedy many already serious conditions. This blend provides a high concentration of herbs with known cholesterol-lowering action, i.e., Pectin, Plantain and Fenugreek in a base of other herbs which, in homeopathic doses, help tone the entire circulatory system, providing nutrition, strength and vitality.

**PECTIN,** as found in citrus fruits, apples, potatoes, green beans and strawberries, serves the natural purpose in plants of binding adjacent cell walls. In 1957 a group of researchers revealed that dietary Pectin (in rats) increased the excretion of lipids, cholesterol and bile acids (**2**). From this inauspicious beginning reports began to mount which verified those data, and extended them to include humans. By 1977, the effect had been thoroughly documented and established. For example, in one 3 week study in humans, plasma cholesterol fell about 13% or more as long as Apple Pectin was administered (about 15 grams/day). When the Pectin was removed, cholesterol levels rose (**3**). Contrast that with a recently ended 10 year study, involving almost 4000 men with high blood cholesterol levels, which investigated the effects of a drug called cholestyramine. It reduced heart attacks and heart disease by reducing blood cholesterol 13.4%, very similar to the results achieved with pectin. But the drug had to be taken six times per day at a cost of $150 per month, achieved success only when accompanied by a diet change, and caused such unpleasant side effects that 27% of the subjects dropped out of the experiment rather than continue taking it. Yet this is what most doctors will recommend ahead of Pectin and other dietary fibers.

It is believed that Pectins operate by binding with bile acids, thereby decreasing cholesterol and fat absorption (**4**). Pectin also increases the excretion of neutral bile acids (**5**) because its ionic charge imparts a high affinity for solubilized biliary salts (**6**). Pectin-salt complexes are excreted as waste, resulting in a reduction of the available biliary salts which would normally be used by the body to make the absorption of cholesterol possible. This, in turn, may indirectly lower cholesterol levels even further because the body will now use up even more endogenous (non-dietary) cholesterol to produce more biliary acids. The results of most experiments indicate that mucilaginous fibers such as Pectin, Plantain and Fenugreek are much better in decreasing serum cholesterol levels than are particulate fibers such as are found in wheat bran (**7-11**). It is important to note that Pectin reduces lymphatic cholesterol absorption best when the diet contains cholesterol (**12**). It is therefore wise to use this blend if your diet contains animal or dairy products. Pectin is also effective when used for producing regressions in, and preventing, gallstones (**13**).

As a bonus benefit for using Pectin, you can expect all nutrients including sugars and carbohydrates to be absorbed by Pectin and released in the intestinal tract over a longer period of time, thereby increasing energy efficiency and producing a much slower rise in blood sugar levels. In fact, there is evidence accumulating that the regular use of Pectin may lessen the severity of diabetes (**14-16**). Along these lines, it has been suggested that fiber-depleted diets actually help cause diabetes mellitus (**17**). One group of researchers found that adding Pectin (and guar) to meals significantly reduced glucose and insulin levels in nondiabetic as well as non-insulin-requiring diabetic patients following meals. Insulin-requiring patients experienced a lowering of glucose levels (**18**). In a similar study, it was found that insulin-requiring diabetic patients, when placed on a long term Pectin-rich diet, experienced a continuing effect of low-ered plasma glucose (**19**). These patients eventually required much less insulin. This study should serve to warn anybody using insulin that the use of this blend could lead to permanent changes in insulin requirements. To prevent the possibility of insulin over-dose, such individuals should make their physician aware of the dietary change. Additional information on Pectin and other fibers can be found under ENVIRONMENTAL POLLUTION.

**HAWTHORN BERRY** and **CAYENNE,** in the carefully measured amounts found in this blend, will slowly eat away cholesterol deposits and provide relief from concurrent hypertension. Cayenne helps regulate cholesterol and lipid levels. In a series of studies carried out in India, it was found that dietary Cayenne, or equivalent amounts of its main constituent, capsaicin, when fed along with dietary cholesterol prevented significantly the expected rise in liver and serum cholesterol levels and brought about enhanced fecal excretion of both free cholesterol and bile acids (**20-22**). Tests a few years ago in my lab showed that serum cholesterol levels in rats maintained on a carefully controlled diet that contained 2 grams/day powdered Hawthorn berries fell anywhere from 10% to 18% over a 2 month period (**23**). Whatever their effect on cholesterol, the main reason for including these herbs in this blend is to provide nutritive support to the heart and circulatory system that you are trying to rescue from the ravages of atherosclerosis. For a more complete discussion of the physiological action of these herbs, see the HEART blend and Appendix A.

**FENUGREEK SEED** is not normally considered by members of American society as an agent for reducing serum cholesterol. However, European research indicates that we have been amiss in overlooking this important medicinal food. And, like Pectin, Fenugreek seeds may be an important remedy for diabetes. In France, several researchers added Fenugreek seeds to the diet of normal dogs or dogs that had been experimentally treated to become diabetic and suffer high blood cholesterol levels. After several days the Fenugreek diet had significantly reduced blood glucose and plasma cholesterol levels in both the normal and diabetic dogs **(24)**. Other studies have confirmed these findings **(25-28)**. In searching for a mode of action, we note first that Fenugreek seeds contain a certain portion of mucilaginous fiber with high viscosity. The herb may affect cholesterol levels in the same fashion as Pectin (see above for details). Fenugreek also contains the glycosidal saponins diosgenin and tigogenin. The saponin-containing plant fibers could inhibit the intestinal absorption of cholesterol much as Alfalfa saponins do, i.e., by adsorbing bile acids and increasing the loss of bile acids by fecal excretion, which then leads to an increased conversion of cholesterol into bile acids by the liver (See ENVIRONMENTAL POLLUTION for additional details). Another possible mechanism has been suggested **(29)** by a researcher who studied the influence of vegetable protein amino acids on serum cholesterol: amino acid patterns affect the ability of vegetable protein to lower cholesterol levels. In his experiments, soybean protein was effective. The amino acid pattern of Fenugreek protein, as it turns out, is very similar to that of soybean **(30)**, but it will require further study to determine if the Fenugreek-Soybean comparison is valid. *See Also FEMALE TONIC; STOMACH/INTESTINAL*

**PLANTAIN SEED** contains mucilage in its outer epidermis and swells when it gets wet. This property makes these seeds a natural candidate for the control of cholesterol levels. The powdered mucilaginous portion has been used for years as a bulking agent in the treatment of constipation and to control appetite **(31)**. More recently it has been used to treat obesity **(32)**. Of more direct interest, however, Plantain has been shown by scientists in Italy, Russia and other countries to reduce the intestinal absorption of lipids **(33-35)**. The consensus of opinion is that the seeds and leaves act by reducing the intestinal absorption of bile acids, as suggested by the significant reduction in plasma bilirubin levels observed in patients being treated. In a larger sense, one cannot discount the possible effect on cholesterol levels that would be derived from lower fatty food intake as a result of the appetite suppressant property of the herb. *See Also WEIGHT LOSS; BONE-FLESH-CARTILAGE; RESPIRATORY AIL-MENTS; VAGINAL YEAST INFECTION*

**BLACK COHOSH** is included here, like Hawthorn and Cayenne, for its tonic action on the heart and circulation. It has been experimentally proven to reduce hypertension (**36**). This action appears to occur through vasodilation of peripheral veins (**37**), as well as through a direct central effect supported by inhibition of vasomotor centers. We do not yet know the whole story on Black Cohosh. The plant exhibits a variety of physiological properties that are only vaguely related to each other, such as antiinflammatory (**38**), hypoglycemic (**39**) and estrogenic (**40-41**) activity. Further research must be done to clarify the behavior of this herb. *See Also HIGH BLOOD PRESSURE; FEMALE TONIC; NERVOUS TENSION*

# OTHER NUTRIENTS

*It has only been during the past decade that serious attention has been paid to dietary factors other than cholesterol in the regulation of serum cholesterol levels. We therefore have a long way to go before a clear understanding of all dietary factors is obtained. Obviously, you must provide a proper internal environment for the metabolism of all nutrients, especially the oils and fats.*

## VITAMINS

Vitamin B Complex
Vitamin C *1,000-3,000 mg*
Vitamin E *200-600 I.U.*
Bioflavonoids *100-300 mg*
Inositol *1,000 mg*
Choline *1,000 mg*
Niacinamide *100 mg*

## MINERALS

Calcium/Magnesium
Phosphorous
Potassium
Zinc

**MISCELLANEOUS**

GLA
Essential Fatty Acid
Cod Liver Oil
Walnut Oil
Lecithin
Brewer's Yeast

# REFERENCES

1. Ginter, E., Kubec, F.J., Vozar, J. & Bobek, R. "Natural hypocholesterolemic agent: pectin plus ascorbic acid." **International Journal of Vitamin and Nutrition Research,** 21(1), 51-54, 1982.
2. Lin, T.M., Kim, K.S., Karvinen, E. & Ivy, A.C. "Effect of dietary pectin, 'protopectin' and gum arabic on cholesterol excretion in rats." **American Journal of Physiology,** 188(1), 66-70, 1957.
3. Kay, R.M. & Truswell, A.S. "Effect of citrus pectin on blood lipids and fecal steroid excretion in man." **American Journal of Clinical Nutrition,** 30, 171-175, 1977.
4. Leveille, G.A. & Sauberlich, H.E. "Mechanism of the cholesterol-depressing effect of pectin in the cholesterol-fed rat." **Journal of Nutrition,** 88, 209-217, 1966.
5. Kay, R.M. "Effects of dietary fiber on serum lipid levels and fecal bile acid excretion." **Canadian Medical Association Journal,** 123, 1213-1217, 1980.
6. Story, J.A., Kritchevsky, D., & Eastwood, M.A. **Dietary fibers. Chemistry and Nutrition.** Academic Press, N.Y., 1979, p. 49.
7. Reddy, B.S., Watanabe, K. & Sheinfil, A. "Effect of dietary wheat bran, alfalfa, pectin and carrageenan on plasma cholesterol and fecal bile acid and neutral sterol excretion in rats." **Journal of Nutrition,** 110, 1247-1254, 1980.
8. Kay, R.M. & Truswell, A.S. "The effect of wheat fiber on plasma lipids and fecal steroid excretion in man." **British Journal of Nutrition,** 37, 227-235, 1977.
9. Jenkins, D.J.A., Leeds, A.R., Newton, C. & Cummings, J.H. "Effect of pectin, guar gum and wheat fiber on serum cholesterol." **Lancet,** 1, 1116-1117, 1975.
10. Tsai, A.C., Elias, J., Kelley, J.J., Lin, R.S.C. & Robson, J.R.K. "Influence of certain dietary fibers on serum and tissue cholesterol levels in rats." **Journal of Nutrition,** 106, 118-123, 1976.

11. Apostolov, I. Goranov, I., Balabanski, L., Krasteva, A. & Popova, D. "Studies on serum lipids in patients with hyperlipoproteine-mia on pectin preparations diet-treatment." **Vutreshni Bolesti,** 21(1), 51-54, 1982.
12. Idem: "Dietary fibre: effects on plasma and biliary lipids in men." in **Medical Aspects of Dietary Fibre,** Spiller, G.A., Kay, R.M., eds., Plenum Press, N.Y., 1980, p. 153.
13. Heaton, K. in **Refined carbohydrate Foods and Disease.** Bur-kett, D.P. & Trowell, H.C., eds. Academic Press, London, 1975., p. 173.
14. Sharma, R.V., Sharma, S.C. & Prasad, Y. "Effect of pectin on carbohydrate and fat metabolism." **Indian Journal of Medical Research,** 76, 771-775, 1982.
15. Jenkins, D.J.A, Leeds, A.R., Goff, D.V., et al. "Unabsorbable carbohydrates and diabetes increased postprandial hypergly-caemia." **Lancet,** ii, 172, 1976.
16. Sharma, R.V. "Effect of dietary fiber on postprandial hyperg-lyceamia, lipid metabolism (serum cholesterol and serum trig-lycerides)." **M.D. Thesis (Physiology).** Argra University, Agra, India, 1978.
17. Burkitt, D.P., Walker, A.R.P, & Painter, N.S. "Dietary fiber and diseases." **Journal of the American Medical Association,** 229, 1068-1074, 1974.
18. Jenkins, D.J.A., Leeds, A.R., Gassull, M.A., Cochet, G., Alberti, K.G.M.M. "Decrease in postprandial insulin and glucose con-centrations by guar and pectin." **Annals of Internal Medicine,** 86, 20-23, 1977.
19. Miranda, P.M., & Horwitz, D.L. "High-fiber diets in the treatment of diabetes mellitus." **Annals of Internal Medicine,** 88, 482-486, 1978.
20. Sambaiah, K & Satyanarayana, N. "Hypocholesterolemic effect of red pepper & capsaicin." **Indian Journal of Experimental Biology,** 18, 898-899, 1980.
21. Sambaiah, K. Satyanarayana, N. & Rao, M.V.L. **Nutrition Re-ports,** 18(5), 521-529, 1978.
22. Srinivasan, M.R., Sambaiah, K., Satyanarayana, M.W. & Rao, M.V.L. "Influence of red pepper and capsaicin on growth, blood constituents and nitrogen balance in rats." **Nutrition Reports International,** 21(3), 455-467, 1980.
23. Mowrey, D.B. Unpublished data accumulated from June, 1978 to August, 1978 at the Nebo Institute for Herbal Sciences, Span-ish Fork, Utah.

24. Valette, G., Sauvaire, Y., Baccou, J.-C., & Ribes, G. "Hypocholesterolaemic effect of fenugreek seeds in dogs." **Atherosclerosis,** 50, 105-111, 1984.
25. Ribes, G., Sauvaire, Y., Baccou, J.C., Valette, G. Chenon, D., et al. "Effects of fenugreek seeds on endocrine pancreatic secretions in dogs." **Annals of Nutrition and Metabolism,** 28, 37-43, 1984.
26. Shani, J., Goldschmied, A., Joseph, B., Ahronson, Z. & Sulman, F.G. "Hypoglycaemic effect of Trigonella foenum graecum and Lupinus termis seeds and their major alkaloids in alloxan-diabetic and normal rats." **Arch. Intern. Pharmacodyn. Ther.,** 210, 27-37, 1974.
27. Bever, B.O. & Zahnd, G.R. "Plants with oral hypoglycaemic action." **Quarterly Journal of Crude Drug Research,** 17, 139, 1979.
28. Singhal, P.C., Gupta, R.K. & Joshi, L.D. "Hypocholesterolemic effect of trigonella foenum graecum." **Current Science,** 51, 136, 1982.
29. Kritchevski, D. "Soya, saponins, and plasma-cholesterol." **Lancet,** 1, 610, 1979.
30. Sauvaire, Y., Baccou, J.C., & Besandcon, P. "Nutritional value of the proteins of a leguminous seed—fenugreek (trigonella foenum graecum L.)" **Nutrition Reports,** 14, 527, 1976.
31. Guglielmi, G, Spagnoletto, P., & Messina, B. "Risultati clinici e comportamento di alcuni parametri biologici in ocrso di trattamento con mucillagine idrofila." **Clinica e Terapeutica,** (San Paulo) 87, 27, 1978.
32. Enzi, G. Inelmen, E.M. & Crepaldi, G. "Effect of a hydrophilic mucilage in the treatment of obese patients." **Pharmatherapeutica,** 2(7), 421-428, 1980.
33. Fahrenbach, M.J., Riccardi, B.A. & Grant, W.C. "Hypocholesterolemic activity of mucilaginous Pol. in white leghorn cockerels." **Proceedings of the Society of Experimental and Biological Medicine,** 123, 321, 1966.
34. Forman, D.T., Garvin, G.E., Forestner, J.E. & Taylor, C.B. "Increased excretion of fecal bile acids by an oral hydrophilic colloid." **Proceedings of the Society of Experimental and Biological Medicine,** 127,1060, 1968.
35. Maksiutina, N.P., Nikitina, N.I., Lipkan, G.N., Gorin, A.G. & Voitenko, I.N. "Chemical composition and hypocholesterolemic action of some drugs from plantago major leaves." **Famatsevtychnyi Zhurnal,** 4, 56-61, 1978.

36. Salerno, **Minerva Otorinolaringologica,** 5, 12, 1955.
37. Genazzani, E. & Sorrentino, L. "Vascular action of acteina: active constituent of actaea racemose L." **Nature,** 194(4828), 544-545, 1962.
38. Benoit, P.S., Fong, H.H.S, Svoboda, G.H. & Farnsworth, N.R. "Bilogical and phytochemical evaluation of plants. XIV. Antiinflammatory evaluation of 163 species." **Lloydia,** 39(2-3), 160-171, 1976.
39. Farnsworth, N.R. & Segelman, A.B. "Hypoglycemic plants." **Till and Tile,** 57(3), 52-56, 1971.
40. Costello, C.H., Lynn, E.V. "Estrogenic substances from plants." **Journal of the American Pharmaceutical Association,** 39, 177-180, 1950.
41. Gizicky, H. "Arzneiplfanzen in ihren beziehungen zum weiblichen gentalsystem, versuche an weissen ratten und maeusen mit cimicifuga racemosa."**Zeitschrift fuer die Gesamte Experimentelle Medizin,** 113, 633-635, 1944.

# CIRCULATION

## HERBS

**Form:** Capsule.

**CONTENTS:** **CAYENNE** *(Capsicum annum)*, **Kelp** *(Saminaria, Macrocystis, Ascophyllum)*, **Gentian root** *(Gentiana lutea)*, **Ginger root** *(Zingiber officinale)*, **Blue Vervain** *(Verbena hastata)*.

**PURPOSE: Blood. To stimulate circulation.**

**Other Applications:** Frostbite, hypothermia, varicose veins, colds, flu, fevers, sore throat, indigestion, heartburn.

**USE:** 1. Poor Circulation: 2-4 capsules per day.
2. Infectious Ailments: 4-6 capsules per day. Use in conjunction with blends for FEVERS & INFECTIONS, and INFLUENZA:
3. Hypothermia: 2 capsules per hour until body temperature stabilizes.
4. Indigestion: 2 capsules every 2-3 hours.
5. To supplement blend for HEART: 2-3 capsules per day.
6. To supplement blend for HIGH BLOOD PRESSURE: 2-3 capsules per day.

**Contraindications:** None. Do not exceed recommended use. For a discussion of Cayenne, see Appendix A.

It is vital to all of the body's cells that they receive an adequate supply of oxygen and nutrients. How important the need for oxygen is can be seen by the fact that if the brain is deprived of oxygen for just 5 minutes, irreparable damage to that organ can occur. Carbon dioxide must be removed. If it isn't, other problems ensue. Many factors can reduce the blood's ability to deliver the goods and take away the wastes. Examples include injuries and diseases of the brain, heart, lungs, adrenal glands and kidneys, damage to the tissues themselves, intensive exercise, change of altitude, and cold. Under such conditions, the circulation can use a boost from external sources. Use this blend when you have a cold, or when you're cold, or if you have generally poor circulation. Use it to supplement various other blends as noted above. Under normal circumstances, please adhere to the suggested dosage. Only in case of hypothermia, bad colds, and/or severe fevers should greater quantities be consumed.

**CAYENNE** pepper will get your blood moving posthaste, especially in the gustatory regions. Other foods ingested along with Cayenne will be assimilated faster and more easily. The research data to support this fact is voluminous (e.g. **1-4**). One suggested explanation for this effect is that the herb releases endogenous gastric secretagogues which increase both tissue perfusion by blood and secretory activity (**1**). A little goes a long way, so don't overdo it. Remember, Nature made the stuff hot and pungent for a reason. If you can't swallow too much outside of a capsule, don't swallow too much inside of a capsule either. *See Also BLOOD PURIFICATION; HIGH BLOOD PRESSURE; FATIGUE*

**GINGER ROOT** will stimulate circulation in the G.I. tract and other parts of the body, and will help the body digest and the blood assimilate the Cayenne. My own research on Ginger root, as well as that of other researchers, notably German, documents the ability of this herb to stimulate gastric motility, relieve indigestion and promote digestion (**5-6**). Ginger, therefore, will hasten the delivery of Cayenne and other nutrients into the blood stream. Another study found that the herb has a powerful positive stimulating effect on muscular contractions of the atria (**7**); this effect should increase overall circulation. The active principles have been identified as gingerols (**8**). It has also been shown experimentally that Ginger root stimulates the vasomotor and respiratory centers of the central nervous system. as well as the heart (**9**). Ginger root also helps reduce serum cholesterol levels, an effect that would promote long term circulatory improvement (**10**). Finally, in a very recent test-tube study, another mechanism by which Ginger root may improve circulation was discovered. In that study, a water extract of Ginger root significantly reduced platelet aggregation (the tendency of blood cells to stick together or clot) (**11**). Agents found to possess this property are generally beneficial to the circulation. The authors of the above study are currently investigating this property in humans. Eventually, other properties of Ginger root may be discovered that will help explain its positive effects on the circulatory system. *See Also BLOOD SUGAR; FATIGUE; STOMACH/INTESTINAL; DIGESTION; LAXATIVE; NAUSEA; NERVOUS TENSION*

**GENTIAN ROOT** is invaluable to the body's circulation and overall health by bolstering its ability to digest and assimilate food. In the studies cited above (**4-5**), Gentian root was as important as Ginger root in terms of stimulating the digestive process and eliminating or overcoming the causes of digestive problems. In good health or bad, it increases absorption, assimilation and resorption. The effect of Gentian on the vascular system is to help insure that the abdominal organs receive a rich supply of blood. It has also been found that Gentian root increases the sensitivity of many glands and organs to the effect of adrenalin—the endogenous hormone that is secreted when the body needs quick energy (**12**). *See Also STOMACH/ INTESTINAL; DIABETES; NERVES & GLANDS*

**KELP** possesses cardiotonic principles of its own. In one study, it was found that Kelp increases contractile force in the atria (much like Ginger root as noted above) (**13**). In another study, two cardiac principles were isolated from Laminaria that stimulated the hearts of frogs (**14**). These sorts of findings vindicate the wisdom of including Kelp in a blend designed to increase healthy circulation. In addition, Kelp adds that measure of nutritive support that the body needs to maintain proper health. It helps offset the effects of stress, protects against sickness, aids digestion and respiration, and generally promotes well-being. *See Also FEVERS & INFECTIONS; WEIGHT LOSS; FATIGUE; THYROID; DIABETES; ENVIRONMENTAL POLLUTION; MENTAL ALERTNESS/SENILITY; PAIN; INFERTILITY; HEART; BLOOD PURIFICATION/DETOXIFICATION*

**BLUE VERVAIN** is valued by many herbalists as an agent that will help to rectify poor circulation problems (**15**). But among its many uses, this is perhaps its most obscure, a practice cherished by those who use it, but ignored by others. I am aware of no published research, experimental or clinical, that bears directly on this particular use of Blue Vervain. However, extrapolating from its proven *parasympathetic* properties (**16**), it should have a normalizing or stabilizing effect. Also, its anti-inflammatory principles (**17**) would make it a valuable ingredient in a blend designed to improve the circulation of blood going to infected, feverish areas. *See Also NERVES & GLANDS; FEVERS & INFECTIONS*

## OTHER NUTRIENTS

*The circulation can get bogged down when wastes and toxins accumulate, as well as under other conditions. Proper nutrition and nutritional supplementation can significantly aid in maintaining clear, healthy, unobstructed circulation. The following recommendations may vary widely from individual to individual.*

### VITAMINS

*(Daily requirements unless otherwise noted)*

Vitamin A *25,000 I.U. daily*
Vitamin B-1 *25 mg*
Vitamin B-2 *25 mg*
Vitamin B-6 *25 mg*
Vitamin B-12 *25 mcg*
Vitamin C *1,000 mg*
Vitamin D *200-400 I.U.*
Vitamin E *200-500 I.U.*
Pantothenic Acid *100 mg*
PABA *15 mg*

### MINERALS

Calcium/Magnesium
Potassium
Iodine
Zinc

## REFERENCES

1. Limlomwongse, L., Chaitauchawong, C. & Tongyai, S. "Effect of capsaicin on gastric acid secretion and mucosal blood flow in the rat." **Journal of Nutrition,** 109, 773-777, 1979.

2. Kolatat, T. & Chungcharcon, D. "The effect of capsaicin on smooth muscle and blood flow of the stomach and the intestine." **Siriraj Hospital Gazette,** 24, 1405-1418, 1972.
3. Ketusinh, O., Dharanintra, B. & Juengjareon, K. "Influence of capsaicin solution on gastric acidities." **American Journal of Proceedings,** 17, 511-515, 1966.
4. Molnar, E., Baraz, L.A. & Khayutin, V.M. "Irritating and depressing effect of capsaicin on receptors and afferent fibers of the small intestine." **Tr. Insst. Norm. Patol. Fiziol. Akad. Med. Nauk SSSR,** 10, 22-24, 1967.
5. Glatzel, H. "Treatment of dyspeptic disorders with spice extracts: practical use of a new therapeutic principle." **Hippokrates,** 40(23), 916-919, 1969.
6. Mowrey, D. Unpublished manuscript that essentially replicates and extends the work of Glatzel.
7. Masada, Y., Inoue, T., Hashimoto, K., Fujioka, M. & Uchino, C. "Studies on the constituents of ginger (Zingiber officinale) by GC-MS." **Yakugaku Zasshi,** 94(6), 735-738, 1974.
8. Shoji, N., Iwasa, A., Takemoto, T., Ishida, Y. & Ohizumi, Y. "Cardiotonic principles of ginger (Zingiber officinale, Roscoe), **Journal of Pharmaceutical Sciences,** 71(10), 1174-1175, 1982.
9. Ally, M.M. "The pharmacological action of zingiber officinale." **Proceedings of the Pan Indian Ocean Scientific Congress, 4th, Karachi, Pakistan,** Section G, 11-12, 1960.
10. Gujral, S., Bhumka, H. & Swaroop, M. "Effect of ginger (Zingiber officinale roscoe) oleoresin on serum and hepatic cholesterol levels in cholesterol fed rats." **Nutrition Reports International,** 17(2), 183-189, 1978.
11. Srivastava, K.C. "Effects of aqueous extracts of onion, garlic and ginger on platelet aggregation and metabolism of arachidonic acid in the blood vascular system." **Prostaglandins Leukotrienes and Medicine,** 13, 227-235, 1984.
12. Deininger, R. "Amarum—bittere arznei." **Krankenpflege,** 29(3), 99-100, 1975.
13. Searl, P.B., Norton, T.R., & Lum B.K.B. "Study of a cardiotonic fraction from an extract of the seaweed Undaria pinnatifida." **Proceedings of the Western Pharmacology Society,** 24, 63-65, 1981.
14. Kosuge, T., Nukaya, H., Yamamotoa, T. & Tsuji, K. "Isolation and identification of cardiac principles from laminaria." **Yakugaku Zasshi,** 103(6), 683-685, 1983.

15. Hutchens, A.R. **Indian Herbalogy of North America,** Merco, Ontario, Canada, 1973.
16. Thomson, W.R. **Herbs that Heal,** Charles Scribner's Sons, New York, 1976, pp.156-157.
17. Sakai, S. "Pharmacological actions of verbena officinalis extracts." **Gigu Ika Daigaku Kiyo,** 11(1), 6-17, 1963.

# DETOXIFY/NURTURE

**HERBS**

**Form:** Capsule, Tea

**CONTENTS:** **RED CLOVER** *(Trifolium pratense)*, **CHAPARRAL** *(Larrea divaricata)*, **Licorice root** *(Glycyrrhiza glabra)*, **Oregon Grape root** *(Mahonia aquifolium)*, **Stillingia** *(Stillingia sylvatica)*, **Burdock root** *(Arctium lappa)*, **Cascara Sagrada bark** *(Rhamnus purshiana)*, **Sarsaparilla root** *(smilax officinalis)*, **Prickly Ash bark** *(Zanthoxylum americanum)*, **Buckthorn bark** *(Rhamnus frangula)*, & **Kelp** *(Laminaria, Macrocystis, Ascophyllum)*.

**PURPOSE: A nutritive supplement for degenerative disorders.**

**Examples of Applications:** Arthritis, cancer, post-surgery trauma, neural degeneration, heart disease, senility, Addison's disease.

**USE:** 1. 3 capsules, 3 to 4 times per day, with plenty of liquid.
2. To supplement the BLOOD PURIFICATION Blend: 1-2 capsules, 3 times per day.
3. To supplement the FEVERS & INFECTIONS Blend: 2 capsules, twice per day.

**Contraindications:** None. Chaparral, though sometimes called creosote bush, contains no creosote. For discussion of licorice root, see Appendix A.

The purpose of this blend is to provide nutritive and therapeutic support to the body during the course of, and during recuperation from, any debilitating condition, be it arthritis or appendicitis, major surgery or frostbite, pneumonia or polio. These herbs provide a comprehensive cleansing and detoxification program including nutrition, stimulation, rejuvenation, and remedy. Red Clover alone, if used throughout a period of convalescence, will achieve most of those purposes. Red Clover, combined with Kelp, Stillingia and Burdock root is one of the most powerful blood cleansers known. This action is even believed by some to cure cancer, though proof of that theory has never been satisfactorily shown. Other important groupings of these herbs can be made. For example, on the basis of specific activity, we group Buckthorn and Cascara Sagrada according to their influence on the G.I. tract; Licorice root, Burdock root and Sarsaparilla root on the basis of their mild and gentle strengthening, toning and stimulating properties; Chaparral, Oregon Grape root and Prickly Ash according to the beneficial effect they have on glands and mucous membranes. The alkaloids, glycosides, amino acids, carbohydrates, volatile oils, antibiotics, acids and enzymes contained in these herbs present a consummately impressive array of vital physiological and metabolic activity.

**RED CLOVER** has been used in America for over 100 years to treat and prevent cancer. There is little scientific data available to support this use, but it is firmly entrenched in American medicinal folklore. In Europe, where the plant originated, it is used extensively as a diuretic to treat gout, and as an expectorant (**1**). Once introduced to America, it found widespread use as a sedative for whooping cough (**2-4**). In the course of routine laboratory screenings Red Clover has shown some estrogenic activity; this effect is probably due to the presence of the plant-estrogen coumerol found in Red Clover tops (**5**). Many naturopathic physicians use the herb as an alterative, including it in regular cleansing programs. It is from this use that it has gained a reputation as a cancer remedy. Because of its high content of several important nutrients, including vitamins and minerals, Red Clover has become a dependable nutritive supplement in all forms of degenerative disease (**6**). Antibiotic tests on Red Clover have shown it to possess activity against several bacteria, the most significant of which is the pathogen that causes tuberculosis (**7**).

**CHAPARRAL** and its properties are covered extensively in the chapters on ARTHRITIS, BONE-FLESH-CARTILAGE, and SKIN DISORDERS. Here, I will only discuss the research on the herb's possible role in curing cancer. Evidence shows that some people with certain types of cancer in certain stages of development may benefit from Chaparral, but it is not clear who may benefit, which cancers are most susceptible or at which stage of cancer development the herb is most effective. One study in rats found that NDGA (nordihydroguaiaretic acid), the purported active principle in Chaparral, produced almost complete inhibition of aerobic and anaerobic glycolysis and respiration in some kinds of cancer cells while normal cells were not affected (**8**). Since most cancer cells are anaerobic while normal cells are aerobic, NDGA may kill cancer cells by shutting down the anaerobic respiratory pathway. Since NDGA is used as an antioxidant in oils and vitamins because of its ability to shut down anaerobic pathways that lead to fermentation (**9**), its potential use in cancer therapy seems all the more likely. There is a good deal of recent research involving the role that cellular enzymatic pathway disruption plays in the etiology or cause of cancer. The faulty metabolism of arachidonic acid and, to a lesser extent, other unsaturated fatty acids (e.g., linoleic and oleic) may produce carcinogenic by-products. How that occurs is not clear at this time. But it has been repeatedly shown that NDGA (technically classified as a lipoxygenase inhibitor) prevents the formation of cancerous cells (**10-15**). This line of research is brand new, making generalizations difficult, but it promises to validate the use of Chaparral, and elucidate the mechanism by which it may kill and/or prevent cancerous growth.

An important case study was reported in the late 1960's by a medical team from the University of Utah about a man who had cured his own case of skin cancer (of the face) by drinking large quantities of Chaparral tea (**10**). The following year the same team published a follow-up study which began with the following statement, "On January 12, 1969...a Surgical Resident at the University of Utah presented a prize winning paper on an interesting regression of melanoma in a patient taking 'Chaparral Tea.' This unfortunately was covered by the news media and released internationally through the United Press" (**11**). The key word in that statement is "unfortunately," because it exposed the physicians' bias about the plant. And indeed, the paper which followed was a hastily constructed and transparent attempt by the authors to extricate themselves from a politically and professionally embarrassing situation: they were being cast as the heroes of the health food movement. The study reveals the fates of 36 *"incurable"* patients who were given two to three glasses of Chaparral tea daily, and 23 who received 250 to 3,000 mg of pure NDGA per day. Some patients improved; most stayed the same or got worse. The physicians concluded that nobody should treat themselves with Chaparral tea.

But the study does not indicate which patients received which treatment, nor which received high or low doses, nor which improved or which didn't, nor even how long each patient was treated. In other words, very little attempt was made to experimentally discover anything. We are not even informed if this study was double-blind or not; I know what my guess would be. The study was successful in accomplishing its major purpose of suppressing further experimental research with humans using Chaparral. Publishing the results of the first study was not "unfortunate;" publishing the second study was, for we still do not know for sure under what conditions the use of Chaparral will impede the progress of carcinoma. Many anecdotal accounts, and some research, vouch for its effectiveness, but we don't yet know when it will work, for whom it will work, how much is required, or how long treatment must be given. *See Also SKIN DISORDERS; BONE-FLESH -CARTILAGE; ARTHRITIS*

**LICORICE ROOT** is a plant of major medicinal importance. Discussed elsewhere in this book are its many properties: anti-inflmmatory, antitussive, antiulcer, mineralcorticoid, sedative, bronchiodilatory, diuretic, laxative, antibacterial, antiviral, antimicrobial, antiarthritic, antirheumatic, antiallergic, antitoxic, anticonvulsive, and estrogenic. All of those properties combine to make Licorice root one of the great detoxifiers in nature. In fact, in China, Licorice root is known as "The Great Detoxifier." A group of Russian researchers have found that Licorice root inhibits the growth of certain tumors (sarcoma-45 and Ehrlich ascites cells) (**18**). This is hardly surprising, and I expect we will see more reports of this nature in the future. Another recent study, in an attempt to elucidate the mechanism by which Licorice root remedies hepatitis (in conjunction with the amino acids cysteine and glycine), found that the herb actually stimulates the production of interferon, that critical chemical in the immune system that could be the key to preventing and treating many immune-response deficiency diseases in the future (**19**). The search for non-toxic and effective interferon inducers has been in progress for several years. Licorice root is now prominent on that list. *See Also FEMALE TONIC; SKIN DISORDERS; INFERTILITY; ARTHRITIS; RESPIRATORY AILMENTS; BLOOD PURIFICATION/DETOXIFICATION; CIRCULATION; FATIGUE; WEIGHT LOSS; ENVIRONMENTAL POLLUTION; FEVERS & INFECTIONS; THYROID; WHOLE BODY TONIC; MENTAL ALERTNESS/SENILITY*

**OREGON GRAPE ROOT** has a direct action on the skin. Therein it behaves unlike any other herb known. The early American physicians quickly learned of this property and used the plant to restore the skin to a smooth, clear condition following any kind of skin disease or other illness that may have dried out the skin or produced sores. Oregon Grape is also a good source of berberine which, along with hydrastine, are the active principles in Goldenseal. In fact, the findings relating to Goldenseal, discussed in the Chapters on FEVERS & INFECTIONS, VAGINAL YEAST INFECTION, AND NERVES & GLANDS, should apply to Oregon Grape as well. Formal studies on the Oregon Grape found a strong bacteriacidal effect **(20)**. In one study berberine chloride and two other constituents, oxycanthine chloride and columbamine chloride, proved effective against several forms of bacteria **(21)**. Berberine was more effective than chloramphenicol against some bacteria. Historically, like many other medicinal herbs, Oregon Grape gradually fell into disuse in medicine, being replaced by various topical cortisone preparations and the like. The use of blood purifiers to treat skin disorders from within is a practice appreciated only by a minority of people in today's world. But, as the debilitating side effects of drug usage become better understood (e.g., that prostate cancer is caused by cortisone), perhaps we will witness a gradual return to the use of natural methods. Until then, let's hope that we can prevent some of our little known but effective herbs, like Oregon Grape, from slipping into forgotten history.

**STILLINGIA ROOT** is a North American plant that, following its introduction to medicine in 1828, became the alterative of choice among the eclectic physicians of that century. It was hailed by many, but not all, of these doctors as the best treatment for syphilis known. Gradually, its other properties were explored and substantiated; the final result was its acceptance as a treatment for tuberculosis and cancer, as well as all other conditions for which an alterative could be recommended **(2-3,22)**. Indians of the Southern United States used this herb for venereal disease before the whites became aware of it. Stillingia root was official in the USP from 1831 to 1926, and in the National Formulary from 1926-1947, much longer and later in both volumes than many of the more well-known medicinal plants. *See Also BLOOD PURIFICATION/DETOXIFICATION; SKIN DISORDERS.*

**BURDOCK ROOT** is another classic blood purifier, or alterative. It is also diuretic and diaphoretic. So, in three different ways it helps cleanse the body of toxins and wastes, especially those that accumulate during illness. These three mechanisms are further enhanced by the herb's proven restorative effects on the liver and gallbladder (**23**). Antibiotic and antifungal principles have been discovered in Burdock root (**24-25**), and at least one study found anti-tumor principles in the herb (**26**). Add to these a strong hypoglycemic action (**27**) and you have an herb with a great deal of potential value in the prevention and remedy of, and recuperation from, disease. *See Also BONE-FLESH-CARTILAGE; BLOOD PURIFICATION/DETOXIFICATION; SKIN DISORDERS*

**CASCARA SAGRADA** is the primary laxative in this blend. The laxative in any detoxification blend is meant to aid in the removal of consolidated, bacteria-laden waste matter that accumulates in the large intestine during periods of illness. Cascara eases the passage of such material without producing griping, cramping, diarrhea or constipative rebound. Cascara is especially well suited for the elderly (**28**). Cascara is also an important source of aloe-emodin which, as referenced under BUCKTHORN below, has antileukemia properties. Additional therapeutic properties, not commonly known, have been attributed to several of the constituents of Cascara. Cascara is rich in tri- and dihydrooxyanthraquinones (emodin, frangulin, iso-emodin, aloe-emodin, and chrysophanol), rhein, and aloins. Rhein derivatives are used in Africa to expel worms (**27**). Anthraquinones have potent antibacterial properties against pathogenic intestinal gram positive and gram negative bacteria (**28-30**). It has been proposed that emodin, rhein and related compounds demonstrate antibiotic activity by inhibiting the biosynthesis of nucleic acids and the respiration processes of bacteria (**31**). Liver diseases are prevented or cured by these same chemicals (**32**). Hydroxyanthraquinones have also been used against leukemia and as an immunosuppressant during skin graft operations (**33**). Finally, Cascara constituents can serve as chelating agents to prevent the formation of calcium-containing urinary stones (**34**). *See Also LAXATIVE; LIVER DISORDERS*

**SARSAPARILLA** is used in the United States and China for about the same purposes: rheumatism, arthritis, skin disease, venereal disease, fevers, digestive disorders and as a general tonic. Other countries, including Mexico and Honduras, use the plant in a similar way. But there is not a great deal of experimental evidence to support all of these uses, just the interesting fact that countries from around the world use the plant in the same way. One Chinese clinical study found a 90% degree of effectiveness against primary syphilis as determined by a negative blood assay (**6**). And a couple of studies have verified the presence of antibiotic principles (**7, 37**).

We can expect that further research will demonstrate the validity of other folklore claims for this universal tonic and remedy. In this blend, its primary purpose is to tone up the body and provide nutritive and therapeutic support for the convalescent patient. *See Also BLOOD PURIFICATION/DETOXIFICATION; INFERTILITY; ARTHRITIS; WHOLE BODY*

**PRICKLY ASH BARK** is a native American medicinal food that has earned itself an incredible reputation at certain times during the last 200 years. For example, in 1849-1850, during an outbreak of Asiatic Cholera in the Midwest, a preparation of Prickly Ash was used as a remedy with what was uniformly considered great success. On another occasion it was used as a main ingredient in a very popular compound, known as "Trifolium Compound," that was used in syphilis to speed up tissue repair. On yet another occasion, Prickly Ash was chosen for inclusion in Hoxey's famous cancer cure. However, in spite of these famous successes, Prickly Ash has never been one of the "Big Ten," i.e., those herbs everybody knows about and are widespread in use, such as Cayenne, Ginseng, Alfalfa, Licorice root or Goldenseal. Nevertheless, there have been individual physicians who, once having learned of this plant's powers, have made it a major item in their materia medica. Speaking of typhoid pneumonia and typhus fever, one 19th century physician wrote, "I am compelled to say that I consider the tincture of Prickly Ash berries superior to any other form of medication." (**22, p. 127**). Prickly Ash has been used extensively to remedy conditions like rheumatism, neural and gastrointestinal flaccidity, gonorrhea, debilitating fevers, cholera, dysentery, neuritis, lumbago and ulcers. Though it is known that the herb contains coumarins, alkaloids, lignans and other substances, no one knows how it works its miracles. It is supposed that the plant is a direct nervous system stimulant, operating most likely on the pituitary-hypothalamic pathway, and that most of its medicinal properties are achieved indirectly through stimulation of glandular systems. Common observations on its use emphasize the warm glow, the nervous tingling, and the electric feeling produced upon ingestion. Prickly Ash was used also by the North American Indians in a medicine called Hantola, to remedy colic, gonorrhea and rheumatism (**22**). From the modern laboratory has come little research (we might wish the herb grew in Europe and Asia—then there would probably be considerable available documentation). However, Merck does report that asarinin, one of the lignans in Prickly Ash, has anti-tubercular properties (**38**). The herb was official in the USP for a considerable time: 1820-1926, and in the NF from 1916-1947.

**BUCKTHORN BARK** is included in this blend on the basis of its reputation as a part of the famous Hoxey cancer cure. There is, in fact, some small support for this claim in the form of a study in which certain Buckthorn preparations showed significant inhibition of P-388 lymphocytic leukemia in mice (**39**). The active principle was identified as aloe emodin. The major constituents of Buckthorn are anthraquinone glycosides, which are mildly laxative in nature. Buckthorn is the mildest anthraquinone-containing herb, with Cascara being next mildest (**1, 40**). The anthraquinones reflexively stimulate peristalsis and mucous secretion in the intestine, and thereby contribute a certain measure toward ridding the body of accumulations of toxic waste (as explained above under CASCARA). Buckthorn is a very popular remedy in Europe, where basic research has determined that the active principles of this herb are not released in the stomach, but first in the small intestine; from that point, their next major locus of activity is in the large intestine, and to a lesser extent on the rectum (**41**). France and Rumania have also performed experiments which elucidated the nature of Buckthorn glycosides (**42-45**).

**KELP** belongs in any blend dedicated to restoring the sick and maintaining the healthy. It supplies an incredible number of nutrients and possesses numerous medicinal properties of its own. Note especially its anti-cancer, anti-rheumatic, anti-inflammatory, hypotensive and fibrous qualities, all discussed more fully in other chapters.


## OTHER NUTRIENTS

*Proper detoxification and nurturing of the glands and systems of the body demand an extremely healthy intake of daily nutrients. Individual needs may depart significantly from the following general recommendations.*

### VITAMINS

*(Daily requirements unless otherwise noted)*

Vitamin A *50,000 I.U.*
Vitamin B Complex
Vitamin B1 *25-100 mg*
Vitamin B2 *25-100 mg*
Vitamin B6 *25-100 mg*

Vitamin B12 *150 mcg*
Vitamin C *3,000-5,000 mg*
Vitamin D *800 I.U.*
Vitamin E *400-600 I.U.*
Niacinamide *100 mg*
PABA *30 mg*
Pantothenic acid *200 mg*

**MINERALS**

Calcium/Magnesium
Phosphorous
Zinc
Iodine

**MISCELLANEOUS**

HCl

# REFERENCES

1. List, P.H. & Hoerhammer, L. **Hagers Handbuch der Pharmazeutischen Praxis.** Volumes 2-5, Springer-Verlag, Berlin.
2. Ellingwood, F. **American Materia Medica, Therapeutics and Pharmacognosy.** Eclectic Medical Publications, Portland, Oregon, 1983.
3. Felter, H. W. **The Eclectic Materia Medica, Pharmacology and Therapeutics.** Eclectic Medical Publications, Portland, Oregon, 1983 (first published 1922).
4. Hartwell, J.L. "Plants used against cancer: a survey." **Lloydia,** 33, 97, 1970.
5. Schultz, G. "Content of estrogenic isoflavones in red clover (trifolium pratense) cultivated in sand with different mineral supplies." **Deutsche Tieraerztliche Wochenschrift,** 74(5), 118-120, 1967;
6. Leung, A.Y. **Encyclopedia of Common Natural Ingredients.** New York, 1980.
7. Fitzpatrick, F.K. "Plant substances active against mycobacterium tuberculosis." **Antibiotics and Chemotherapy,** 4(5), 528-536, 1954.
8. Sporn, A. & Schobesch, O."Toxicity of nordihydroquaiaretic acid." **Igiena (Bucharest),** 15(12), 725-726, 1966.
9. Olivetto, E.P. "Nordihydroguaiaretic acid: a naturally occurring antioxidant." **Chemistry and Industry,** Sep., 677-679, 1972.

10. Schwarz, M., Peres, G., Kunz, W. et al "On the role of superoxide anion radicals in skin tumor promotion." **Carcinogenesis,** 5(12), 1663-1670, 1984.
11. Carine, K., & Hudig, D. "Assessment of a role for phospholipase A2 and arachidonic acid metabolism in human lymphocyte natural cytotoxicity." **Cellular Immunology,** 87(1), 270-283, 1984.
12. Nemoto, N, Takayama, S. "Arachidonic acid-dependent activation of benzo(a)pyrene to bind to proteins with cytosolic and microsomal fractions from rat liver and lung." **Carcinogenesis,** 5(7), 961-964, 1984.
13. Valone, F.H., Obrist, R., Tarlin, N. & Bast, R.C. "Enhanced arachidonic acid lipoxygenation by K562 cells stimulated with 12-0-tetradecanoylphorbol-13-acetate." **Cancer Research,** 43(1), 197-201, 1983.
14. Thomson, D.M.P. "Various authentic chemoattractants mediating leukocyte adherence inhibition." **Journal of the National Cancer Institute,** 73(3), 595-606, 1984.
15. Nakamura, Y., Colburn, N.H., & Gindhart, T.D. "Role of reactive oxygen in tumor promotion implication of superoxide anion in promotion of neoplastic transformation in JB-6 cells by 12-0-tetradecanoylphorbol-13-acetate." **Carcinogenesis,** 6(2) 229-236, 1985.
16. Smart, C.R., Hogle, H.H., Robins, R.K., Broom, A.D. & Bartholomew, D. "An interesting observation on nordihydroguaiaretic acid (NSC-4291; NDGA) and a patient with malignant melanoma—a preliminary report." **Cancer Chemotherapy Reports,** Part 1, 53(2), 147-151, 1969.
17. Smart, C.R., Hogle, H.H., Vogel, H., Broom, A.D. & Bartholomew, D. "Clinical experience with nordihydroguaiaretic acid—Chaparrel (sic) tea in the treatment of cancer." **Rocky Mountain Medical Journal,** November, 1970, 39-43.
18. Shvarev, I.F. Konovalova, N.K. & Putilova, G.I. "Effect of triterpenoid compounds from glycyrrhiza glabra on experimental tumors." **Voprosy Izucheniya Ispol'zovaniy. Solodki v SSSR, Akademi Nauk SSSR,** 167-170, 1966.
19. Abe, N., Eina, T. & Ishida, N. "Interferon induction by glycyrrhizin and glycyrrhetinic acid in mice." **Micorobiology and Immunology,** 26(6), 535-539, 1982.
20. Kowalewski, Z., Kedzia, W. & Mirska, I. "Effect of berberine sulfate on staphylococci." **Archives of Immunology and Experimental Therapeutics,** 20(3), 353-360, 1972.

21. Andronescu, E., Petcu, P. Goina, T. & Radu, A. "Antibiotic activity of the extract and the alkaloid isolate from berberis vulgaris." **Clujul Medical (Romania),** 46(3), 627-631, 1973.
22. Millspaugh, C. F. **American Medicinal Plants.** Dover Publications, Inc. New York, 1974 (first published 1892).
23. Chabrol, E. & Charonnat, R. "Therapeutic agents in bile secretion." **Ann. Med.,** 37, 131-142, 1935.
24. Vincent, E. & Segonzac, G. "Higher plants having antibiotic properties."**Toulouse Medicale,** 49, 669, 1948.
25. Schulte, K.E., Ruecker, G. & Boehme, R. "Polyacetylenes in burdock roots." **Arzneimittel-Forschung,** 17(7), 829-833, 1967.
26. Foldeak S. & Dombradi, G.A. "Tumor-growth inhibiting substances of plant origin. I. Isolation of active principle of Arctium lappa." **Acta Physiology & Chemistry (Szeged).,** 10, 91-93, 1964.
27. Lapinina L.O. & Sisoeva, T.F. "Investigation of some plants to determine their sugar-lowering action." **Farmatsevticcheski Zhurnal,** (Kiev), 19(4), 52-58 , 1964.
28. Marchesi, M., Marcato, M. & Silvestrini, C. "A laxative mixture in the therapy of constipation in aged patients." **Giornale di Clinica Medica,** (Bologna) 63, 850-863, 1982.
29. Anton, R. & Duquenois, P. "Cassia marilandica in therapy with medicinal plants." **Quarterly Journal of Crude Drug Research,** 9(4), 1469-1472, 1969.
30. Lindemann, G. **Acta Phytotherapeutica,** 14, 75-76, 1967.
31. Patel, R.P. & Patel, K.C. "Antibacterial activity of cassia tora and cassia obovata." **Indian Journal of Pharmacology,** 19, 70-73, 1957.
32. Cudlin, J., Blumauerova, M. Steinerova, N., Mateju, J. & Zalabak, V. "Biological activity of hydroxyanthraquinones and their glucosides toward microorganisms." **Folia Microbiologica (Prague),** 21(1), 54-57, 1976.
33. Chen, C.H., Cheng, W.F., Su, H.L., et. al. "Studies on chinese rhubarb. I. Preliminary study on the antibacterial activity of anthraquinone derivatives of chinese rhubarb (rheum palmatum)." **Acta Pharmaceutica Sinica (Yao Hsueh Hsueh Pao),** 9, 757-762, 1962.
34. Kerharo, J. & Bouquet, A. **Plantes Medicinales et Toxiques de la Crote d'Ivoire, Haute-Vota,** (Vigot, Paris), 1950.
35. Hilgert, I., Cudlin, J., Steinerova, N. & Vanek, Z. "Antitumor and immunosuppressive activity of hydroxyanthraquinones and their glucosides." **Folia Biologica (Prague),** 23(2), 99-109, 1977.

36. Berg, W., Hesse, A., Hensel, K., et.al. "Einfluss von anthrachinonderivaten auf die tierexperimentelle hernsteinbildung." **Urologe,** Part A, 15(4), 188-191, 1976.
37. D'Amico, M.L. "Ricerche sulla presenza di sostanze ad azione antibiotica nelle piante superiori." **Fitoterapia,** 21(1), 77-79, 1950.
38. **The Merck Index. An Encyclopedia of Chemicals and Drugs.** 9th ed., 1976, Merck. Rahway, NJ.
39. Kupchan, S.M. & Karim, A. "Tumor inhibitors 114: Aloe emodin: antileukemic principle isolated from Rhamnus frangula L." **Lloydia,** 39, 223-224, 1976.
40. Youngken, H.W. **Textbook of Pharmacognosy,** 5th ed. Blakiston, Philadelphia, PA, 1943.
41. Behrens, P. "Healing remedies in word and illustration." **Krankenpflege,** 29(3), 101-104, 1975.
42. Dauguet, J.C. & Paris, R.R. "Flavanoid glycosides of Rhamnus frangula." **Plantes Medicinales et Phytotherapie,** 8(11), 32-43, 1974.
43. Rosca, M. & Cucu, V. "Naphthalin glycosides from the bark of Rhamnus frangula." **Planta Medica,** 28, 178-181, 1975.
44. Rosca, M. & Cucu, V. "About a monoglucoside of emodine from the bark of Rhamnus frangula." **Planta Medica,** 28, 343-345, 1975.
45. Savonious, K. "Isolation and identification of emodin glucoside B from Frangula alnus." **Farmaseuttinen Aikakauslehti, (Finnish),** 82(9-10), 136-139, 1973.

# DIABETES

## HERBS

**Form:** Capsule, Tea

**CONTENTS: UVA-URSI** *(Arctostaphylos uva-ursi),* **DANDELION root** *(Taraxacum officinale),* **Parsley** *(Petroselinum sativum),* **Gentian root** *(Gentiana lutea),* **Huckleberry leaves** *(Vaccinum myrtillus),* **Raspberry leaves** *(Rubus idaeus),* **Buchu leaves** *(Barosma crenata),* **Saw Palmetto berries** *(Serenoa repenssabal),* **Kelp** *(Laminara, Macrocystes, Ascophyllum),* & **Bladderwrack** *(Fucus vesiculosus).*

**PURPOSE:** To promote the body's ability to reduce high blood sugar (hyperglycemia), To help store and sustain liver, spleen, kidney, gallbladder and pancreas funcion.

**Other Applications:** Diuretic.

**USE:** 1. For Hyperglycemia: 3 capsules, 3 times per day.
2. For Glandular Health: 2-4 capsules per day.
3. Use 2-4 capsules per day of the NERVE & GLAND TONIC Blend for added benefit to glands.
4. This blend also works well in conjunction with recommended dosages of the WHOLE BODY TONIC blend.
5. If used with the DIURETIC Blend, use 2-4 capsules per day of each.

**Contraindications:**
1. Do not use if nephritis exists.
2. Should not be used by hypoglycemics.
3. Persons who use diuretics often, who are generally run-down, or have a known potassium deficiency, should use caution when using any diuretic product, and should definitely take potassium supplements.
4. Avoid sodium rich diets.
5. Frequent consultation with your physician is recommended to adjust insulin-intake requirements, as this blend may significantly reduce necessary insulin supplementation.

   Diabetes is a defect in carbohydrate metabolism that results from insufficient pancreatic insulin production. The hormone insulin is required to transport glucose into cells where the sugar is converted to energy. Without insulin, glucose continues to circulate and accumulate in the blood until it is eventually excreted in the urine. Dangerous symptoms occur when the body attempts to dilute very high blood glucose levels. The water is pulled from cells and with it comes potassium. A severe potassium deficiency may produce coma and even death. The diabetic often requires a daily insulin injection so that he can consume moderate amounts of carbohydrate. If the diabetic does not ingest enough carbohydrate to use up most of the injected insulin, a glucose insufficiency results which causes the body to draw energy from stored fat deposits. Poisonous substances are produced during that process that can lead to a state of shock. It is thus a delicate tightrope the diabetic must walk. Any dietary treatment that can reduce or eliminate the need for insulin injections will increase the diabetic's ability to avoid serious symptoms and will decrease his susceptibility to heart disease and other common complications of insulin therapy.
   The diabetic, while under the care of a qualified physician, may find this blend to be about the best adjunctive aid Mother Nature can supply, but it is not meant to supplant qualified medical care. As a supplement to insulin therapy, it will provide sound functional support to the physiological systems involved, and in some cases may lessen the need for insulin. It may depress the blood sugar level in any given individual (and should therefore not be used by hypoglycemics) and may ameliorate pre-diabetic or sub-diabetic conditions. Beyond that effect, however, the blend invigorates several of the body's most important organs, glands and glandular organs, especially the liver, pancreas, kidneys and gallbladder. Used regularly, together with blends WHOLE BODY and NERVE &

GLAND TONICS, the effect of these herbs can be extraordinary, leading ultimately to the dependable service of healthy glands and organs even into old age. The hypoglycemic effect is due primarily to the Dandelion and Uva Ursi, and secondarily to Gentian, Parsley and Raspberry leaves.

**UVA URSI** contains a group of compounds called phenolic glycosides that were known as early as the 13th century to have diuretic and urinary antiseptic action (**1**). This activity helps relieve pain from bladder stones and gravel, relieves cystitis, nephritis and kidney stones (**2**). Early in American history, Uva-ursi was felt to be of great benefit in numerous ailments, as an astringent and anti-scorbutic, and was used as food by Indians and the English (**3**). These observations and findings led to the inclusion of the herb in American and English pharmacopoeias. Shortly thereafter, other American researchers found that Uva-ursi was effective against nephritis and kidney stones, and possessed all around tonic properties (**4-5**). Today, the herb is used as a tonic and specific in cases involving weakened liver, kidneys and other glands. *See Also DIURETIC; MENSTRUATION*

**DANDELION ROOT** exhibits hypoglycemic effects in experimental animals (**6**). Some authors believe, though with a paucity of evidence, that the inulin content of Dandelion contains insulin-like principles that may actually substitute, on a limited basis, for insulin (**7-8**). It is at least an interesting hypothesis that deserves to be tested. The more probable explanation is that because inulin is a concentrated source of dietary fiber whose carbohydrate substructure is fructose, it buffers blood glucose levels, preventing sudden and severe fluctuations. In addition, it probably benefits the diabetic by improving kidney function, especially that organ's ability to cleanse the blood and resorb nutrients. Dandelion's beneficial effects on liver complaints have been documented by both Asian practitioners (**9**) and American physicians (**5**). It stimulates bile production and helps the body get rid of excess water produced by the diseased liver. Dandelion extracts are said to also benefit the spleen and improve the health of the pancreas. *See Also LIVER DISORDERS; NERVES & GLANDS; BLOOD PURIFICATION/DETOXIFICATION; SKIN*

**PARSLEY** is commonly used to treat jaundice and gallstones. Though many properties of Parsley have been experimentally established (e.g.: laxative, hypotensive, antimicrobial, uterine tonic (**10**)), its effects on the liver have not been experimentally investigated.

However, the claims of clinical physicians, over the past 100 years or so, that the herb is very effective in remedying liver diseases (**11**), suggest that it is time research efforts be expanded to include this aspect of Parsley's medicinal nature. *See Also PROSTATE; DIURETIC; BONE-FLESH-CARTILAGE*

**GENTIAN ROOT** has been used by both Western and Eastern societies as a potent bitter. Its focus of activity is on those glands and organs involved in digestion, such as the gallbladder and pancreas, with secondary affects on other organs such as the liver and kidneys. It has been found experimentally to promote the secretion of bile (**12**) and to possess anti-inflammatory properties (**13**). The diabetic or pre-diabetic will experience increased pancreatic health. Gentian root may delay the onset of "brittle" diabetes, or prevent its occurrence completely. Heartburn, gastritis, various forms of upset stomach, and even cancer have yielded to the effects of Gentian root (**14**). Gentian, today, is regarded as one of the premier herbs to use when anyof the above ailments exist. *See Also NERVES & GLANDS; CIRCULATION; STOMACH/INTESTINAL; THYROID*

**HUCKLEBERRY LEAF** is used by many naturopathic physicians to treat sugar diabetes, and ailments of the kidneys and gallbladder (**15-16**). This is not surprising since the Huckleberry is a close cousin, if not brother, to Uva-ursi, its leaves containing very similar compounds as that plant. The active principle is neomyrtilicine. The herb is one of the best for mild diabetes; and may be especially beneficial for use in "senile" diabetes.

**RASPBERRY LEAF** is primarily used for diarrhea and for problems associated with female biology, but is used frequently in folk medicine to relieve urethral and kidney irritation (**17**). There is some experimental support for using Raspberry leaf to treat diabetes: the leaf has a proven hypoglycemic action. (**18**). *See Also EYES; MEN-STRUATION; FEMALE TONIC*

**BUCHU LEAF** is aromatic and carminative. It helps to relieve irritation of the bladder, urethra and kidneys (**11**). *See Also PROSTATE; DIURETIC; VAGINAL YEAST INFECTION*

**SAW PALMETTO BERRY,** although specific for certain disorders of the prostate and reproductive organs, is generally effectively used for nutritional support of all bodily systems. It helps build new tissue and restore function. Its inclusion in this blend is precisely for the reason that diabetes and other diseases of the glands and organs require the kind of nutritive and chemical support that these berries provide. *See Also THYROID; INFERTILITY; RESPIRATORY AILMENTS; FEMALE TONIC; PROSTATE; NERVES & GLANDS; DIGESTION*

**KELP,** due to its high iodine content, is a necessary inclusion in any product that purports to help the glands (esp. thyroid and liver) of the body. Kelp contains a sugar named mannitol that imparts some degree of sweetness but does not raise blood sugar levels. It is thought that Kelp may someday become a source for a sweetening agent that diabetics can use. Presently, however, nobody is raving about the "sweet" taste of Kelp. *See Also FEVERS & INFECTIONS; WEIGHT LOSS; FATIGUE; BLOOD PURIFICATION/DETOXIFICATION; HEART; INFERTILITY; PAIN; MENTAL ALERTNESS/SENILITY; ENVIRONMENTAL POLLUTION; THYROID; CIRCULATION*

**BLADDERWRACK,** another product of the sea,, has been effective against nephritis, bladder inflammation, cardiac degeneration, obesity, thyroid problems, and menstrual problems (**19-20**).

## OTHER NUTRIENTS

*Diabetes has been known to respond well to proper nutrition. Among other things, the diabetic should be certain to maintain as strong a nutrition program as possible. The following recommendations are provided as guidelines only. Individual requirements may vary significantly.*

**VITAMINS**

*(Daily requirements unless otherwise noted)*

Vitamin A *25,000 I.U.*
Vitamin B1 *25-50 mg*
Vitamin B2 *25-50 mg*
Vitamin B6 *25-100 mg*
Vitamin B12 *50-100 mg*
Vitamin C *1,000-3,000 mg*
Vitamin D *400 I.U.*
Vitamin E *200-600 I.U.*
Niacinamide 100 mg
Pantothenic Acid 50 mg
Biotin

**MINERALS**

Potassium
Zinc
Chromium
Manganese
Calcium/Magnesium

**MISCELLANEOUS**

Water
Essential Fatty Acids
Complex Carbohydrate
Lecithin
Yeast
Protein

# REFERENCES

1. Trease, G.E. & Evans, W.C. **Pharmacognosy.** 1978. 11th Edition, Bailliere Tindall. London.
2. Lust, J. **The Herb Book.** 1974. Benedict Lust. Sini Valley, Calif.
3. Josselyn, J. "New England's Rarities Discovered, in Birds, Beasts, Fishes, Serpents, and Plants of that Country", **Archaeologica Americana, Transactions and Collections of the American Antiquarian Society.** Boston, 1860, Vol IV,105-238.
4. Barton, B.S. **Collections for an Essay towards a Materia Medica of the United States.** 3rd Ed., with additions. Philadelphia, printed for Edward Earle and Co., 1810.
5. Clapp, A. "Report on Medical Botany...A synopsis, of systematic catalogue of the indigenous and naturalized, flowering and filicoid...medicinal plants of the United States..." **Transactions of the American Medical Association,** Vol V, 1852, Philadelphia.
6. Farnsworth, N.R. & Segelman, A.B. "Hypoglycemic plants" **Till and Tile.** 1971, 57, 52-55.
7. **Nutrition Almanac.** Nutrition Search, Inc. John D. Kirschmann, ed. McGraw Hill Book Co., New York, 1979, 178.
8. **Bestways,** May 1980, p. 75.
9. Li Shih-chen, **Chinese Medicinal Herbs.** Translated by F. Porter Smith and G.A. Stuart. Georgetown Press, San Francisco, 1973.

10. Leung, A.Y. **Encyclopedia of Common Natural Ingredients.** New York, 1980, 257-259.
11. Culbreth, D.M.R. **A Manual of Materia Medica and Pharmacology,** Philadelphia, 1927.
12. Sadritdinov, F. "Comparative study of the antiinflammatory properties of alkaloids from gentiana plants." **Farmakologia Alkaloidov Serdechnykh Glikozidov,** 146-148, 1971.
13. Chi, H-C., Liu, K-T. & Sung, C-Y. "The pharmacology of gentianine. II. The antiphlogistic effect of gentianine and its comparison with some clinically effective drugs." **Sheng Li Hsueh Pao,** 23, 151-157, 1959.
14. Hartwell, J.L. "Plants used against cancer. A survey." **Lloydia,** 32, 153, 1969.
15. Shoemaker, J.V. **A Practical Treatise on Materia Medica and Therapeutics.** Philadelphia, 1908, p. 910.
16. Turova, M.A. **Lekarstvennye Sredstava Iz Rastenyi** (Medical-Herbal Preparations). Publisher: Medicinskaya Literatura, Moscow, 1962.
17. Leek, S. **Herbs, Medicine & Mysticism.** Chicago. Henry Regnery Co. 1975.
18. **Plant Medica.** 11, 159, 1963.
19. Felter, H.W. **The Eclectic Materia Medica, Pharmacology and Therapeutics.** Eclectic Medical Pubs, Portland, Oregon, 1983 (first published, 1922).
20. Ellingwood, F. **American Materia Medica, Therapeutics and Pharmacognosy.** Eclectic Medical Pubs, Portland, Oregon, 1983.

# DIGESTION

## HERBS

**Form:** Capsule, Tea, Poultice

**CONTENTS: PAPAYA leaves** *(Carica papaya)* **PEPPER-MINT leaves** *(Mentha piperita,* **Ginger root** *(Zigiber officinale),* **Catnip** *(Nepeta cataria),* **Fennel seed** *(Foeniculum vulgare),* & **Saw Palmetto berries** *(Serenoa repens-sabal).*

**PURPOSE: A digestive aid; To relieve intestinal gas (flatulence), enteritis, colic, heartburn, etc.**

**Other Applications:** Ulcers; Worms.

**USE:** 1. For indigestion, use 2 capsules with each meal.
2. To supplement the STOMACH/INTESTINAL Blend: 2 capsules of each blend, with meals.
3. To supplement the PARASITES & WORMS Blend: 1-2 capsules per day.
4. For deficient digestive enzymes, or bile production, also use the LIVER PROBLEMS blend.

**Contraindications:** None.

Cars need fuel, and so does the human body. Combustion is the process a car uses to turn fuel (gasoline) into forms of energy that make it go. Digestion is the process by which fuel (food) is converted to forms of energy the body can use to make it go. But the similarities between car and man end when we begin discussing the biological nature of humans. Digestion, for example, is an amazingly complex process that involves and depends upon the proper functioning of a series of valves, gates, enzyme secreting plants, properly buffered processing facilities, microscopic filtration, absorption, resorption, motoric churning, pumping and crunching. This herbal blend focuses mainly on the chemical processes involved, though some tonic strengthening of the motoric functions is also involved. Many digestive complaints can be traced to the simple problem of not enough enzyme production, or to an unhealthy chemical milieu that either destroys the enzymes before they can work, or neutralizes them so they can't work. Indigestion (dyspepsia) is both a physiological state and a feeling. The state is one of faulty digestion. The feeling is one of discomfort, being "stuffed", pain, cramps, heartburn, gas and nausea. Indigestion may often be a symptom of a greater problem, in which case the advice of a physician should be obtained. Simple indigestion, however, can usually be remedied quite easily. A change of diet, eating less, smoking less, and avoiding coffee and alcohol are good ways to reduce indigestion. Supplemental niacin and HCl should be considered. This blend of herbs will help reduce digestive and intestinal complaints in two distinct ways. First it enhances digestion itself. Second, it remedies the various side-effects of poor digestion: flatulent gas, colic, heartburn, etc. Keep this blend handy and use it frequently. Don't forget to also use the LIVER PROBLEMS blend.

**PAPAYA LEAF** contains the powerful proteolytic enzymes papain and chymopapain, sulfhydryl proteases that hydrolyze (digest) proteins, small peptides, amides and esters. Their activity extends also to carbohydrate and fat. The optimum pH range is 3 to 12 at 10 - 70 degrees centigrade. These agents can be found currently in dozens of commercial digestive aids since they are more effective than naturally occurring proteases like pepsin and trypsin. Since many stomach ailments are the direct result of indigestion, Papaya may help prevent and remedy these by increasing digestive processes. Papaya enzymes are for all other stomach problems also, including those that come about through inadequate fat digestion, liver and bile duct ailments and pancreas disease. Papain is commercially extracted from the papaya fruit, but is contained in the leaf also. The digestive properties of papain are so well established that they need no documentation (a few are included here anyway as **1-3**). Papaya has acquired the reputation of 'biological scalpel' because it selectively digests dead tissue without affecting the surrounding live tissue. In an interesting extension of that principle, medical teams are now injecting chymopapain directly into herniated lumbar disks where it immediately begins to dissolve proteins in the problem area, reduce protrusions and relieve pressure that produces pain. In this case Papaya is truly replacing the scalpel as a surgical requirement. Doctors who have worked in South Africa and witnessed first hand and native use of Papaya to treat many sorts of skin disease, wounds and ulcers, often bring the technique back to England, Canada and Australia where they use it themselves to speed the healing process of similar conditions. One popular case involved a postoperative infection that wouldn't yield to antibiotics. Strips of Papaya laid over the wound healed it within 48 hours (**4**). *See Also STOMACH/INTESTINAL; MENSTRUATION*

**PEPPERMINT LEAF,** Fennel, Ginger root, and Catnip contain volatile oils and other constituents that absorb intestinal gas, calm upset stomach, inhibit diarrhea as well as constipation, aid digestion, eliminate heartburn, and prevent and remedy childhood colic. These properties are integral to the folk medicine of North and South America, all of Europe and Asia, Africa, Australia, the Pacific Islands—is there anybody left? In tea or capsule, with cream or milk, in small and large quantities these herbs have served their intended purpose for centuries. Peppermint is probably the best known remedy for stomach problems. Its use can be traced back almost as far as the beginnings of recorded history. It is used for both chronic and acute indigestion, gastritis and enteritis, acting in two distinct ways to remedy these problems. First, its essential oils enhance digestive activity by stimulating contractile activity in the gallbladder and by encouraging the secretion of bile (**5**). Secondly, Peppermint leaf oils normalize gastrointestinal activity, removing flaccidity and reducing cramps (**6**). Other research has found antiulcer, anti-inflammatory and choleretic principles in this herb (**7-8**). Of no small importance is the ability of Peppermint to inhibit and kill many kinds of micro-organisms that, among other things, might create severe digestive problems (**9-15**). A few of these bugs need special mention: Influenza A viruses, the cause of much Asian flu; *Herpes simplex,* the source of cold sores; Mumps virus; *Streptococcus pyogenes,* the cause of sore throat, scarlet fever, rheumatic fever, ottitis media, cystitis, cellulitis, etc; *Staphlococcus aureus,* from which we acquire pneumonia, sinusitis, impetigo and endocarditis, etc; *Psuedomonas acruginosa,* which produces a great variety of suppurative and other infections; and *Candida albicans,* the cause of vaginal yeast infection. Altogether, more than 30 pathogenic micro-organisms have yielded to the influence of Peppermint. *See Also MENTAL ALERTNESS/SENILITY; FATIGUE*

**GINGER ROOT** is another incredibly active and effective gastrointestinal aid, whose primary activity is described elsewhere in this book (see STOMACH/INTESTINAL, CIRCULATION, NAUSEA). Of great importance here are these findings: (**1**) Ginger root contains a digestive enzyme, zingibain, whose effectiveness even exceeds that of papain (**16**); (**2**) the herb stimulates the flow of saliva and increases dramatically the concentration of the digestive enzyme (amylase) in the saliva (**17**); (**3**) it activates peristalsis and increases intestinal muscle tone (**17**); and (**4**) it is a featured herb in European proprietary digestive aids (**18**). The ability of Ginger root to clear up gas, flatulence, indigestion, stomachache and other stomach problems has been repeatedly confirmed in my own experimental investigations (**19**). *See Also FATIGUE; NERVOUS TENSION; LOW BLOOD SUGAR; NAUSEA; CIRCULATION; LAXATIVE; STOMACH/INTESTINAL*

**CATNIP,** often called Catmint, indeed is a member of the mint family, and acts in much the same manner as Peppermint. It is a soothing carminative to the gastrointestinal tract, a mild tonic, and a favorite tea for young children. North American Indians used the tea for childhood colic (**20**), while Europeans used it for similar complaints as well as colds and bronchial infections. Like Peppermint, it has been shown to have antibiotic properties, though the amount of research is not nearly as extensive (**21**). Used before meals, it stimulates appetite; after meals it stimulates digestion. Catnip is sometimes called "Nature's Alka Seltzer," though that term aptly describes the whole Mint family.

**FENNEL SEEDS** contain aromatic or essential oils that are very similar in structure and activity to those of Catnip and Peppermint (**22-23**). Whereas Catnip oils are better suited for use in infants, Fennel oils appear to be just as effective in adults. Fennel is especially effective against flatulence in adults. Like other essential oil-bearing carminative plants, Fennel is used for the same purposes wherever it grows (e.g., North America, Europe, Asia, Japan, Russia, China, Africa, Australia, New Zealand). Perhaps we should heed the admonition of an old Welsh doctor, that "He who sees fennel and gathers it not, is not a man, but a devil!" (**24**). Fennel was official in the U.S. Pharmacopoeia for many years and is still official in over a dozen major foreign pharmacopoeias worldwide. *See Also WEIGHT LOSS*

**SAW PALMETTO BERRY** comes to us from a more limited historical pattern of use. Its inclusion in this blend is based on the recommendations and celebrations of people who have used it, and doctors who have prescribed it, to stimulate the appetite, improve digestion and increase assimilation. Their enthusiasm has been justified by at least one corroborating study in which young albino rats, to whose daily feed crushed Saw Palmetto berries were added, experienced a significantly more rapid weight gain than control litter mates (**25**). That result could have been due to the nutritional properties of the berries themselves or to their effect on appetite, digestion and assimilation. *See Also INFERTILITY; FEMALE TONIC; RESPIRATORY AILMENTS; DIABETES; PROSTATE; NERVES & GLANDS; THYROID*

## OTHER NUTRIENTS

*Digestion is a complex mechanism that requires good health from many different parts of the body, including the liver, spleen, gall-bladder, stomach, intestines, and blood. It is important, therefore, to make sure these structures receive adequate health-giving nutrition. Individual needs may depart substantially from the following recommendations.*

### VITAMINS

*(Daily requirements unless otherwise noted)*

Vitamin B Complex
Vitamin B1 *25-50 mg*
Vitamin B2 *25-50 mg*
Vitamin B6 *25-50 mg*
Folic Acid *400 mcg*
Niacinamide *100 mg*
Pantothenic Acid *50 mg*

### MINERALS

Calcium/Magnesium

### MISCELLANEOUS

Betain HCl
Pepsin
Pancreatin
Ox Bile
Yogurt/Acidophilus

# REFERENCES

1. Yamamoto, A. in **Enzymes in Food Processing,** 2nd Ed., G. Geed, ed., Academic Press, New York, 1975, p.123.
2. Arnon, R. **Methods in Enzymology,** VI 19, G.E. Perlmann and L. Lorand, eds., Academic Press, New York, 1970, p. 226.
3. Kunimatsu, D.K. & Yasunobu, K.T., in **Methods in Enzymology,** Vol 19, G.E. Perlmann and L. Lorand, eds., Academic Press, New York, 1970, p. 244.
4. Rudge, C. "African Folk Medicine", and interview, **Parade Magazine,** Salt Lake Tribune, June 5, 1977.
5. List, P.H. & Hoerhammer, L. Hagers Handbuch der **Pharmazeutischen Praxis.** Volumes 2-5, Springer-Verlag, Berlin.
6. Demling, L., et. al., **Fortschritte der Medizin,** 37, 1305, 1969.
7. Pasechnik, I.K. "Study of the choleretic properties specific to flavonoids from Mentha piperita leaves." **Farmakologiia i Toksikologiia,** 29(6), 735-737, 1966
8. Maksimenko, G.N. "Antipyretic effect of azulene from peppermint oil." **Farmakologia i Toksikologia,** 27(5), 571-573, 1964.
9. Sanyal, A, & Varma, K.C. "In vitro antibacterial and antifungal activity of mentha arvensis var. piperascens oil obtained from different sources." **Indian Journal of Microbiology,** 9(1), 23-24, 1969.
10. Herrman, E.C. & Kucera, L. "Antiviral substances in plants of the mint family (labiatae). III. Peppermint (mentha piperita) and other mint plants." **Proceedings of the Society of Experimental Biology and Medicine,** 124, 874-875, 1967.
11. Abdullin, K.K. "Bactericidal effect of essential oils." **Uchenye Zapiski Kazanskogo Veterinarnogo Instituta,** 84, 75-79, 1962.
12. Pizsolitto, A.C., Mancini, B., Fracalanzza, L. et al. "Determination of antibacterial activity of essential oils officialized by the Brazilian Pharmacopeia 2nd. Ed." **Revista da Faculdade de Famacia e Odontologia de Araragwara,** 9(1), 55-61, 1975.
13. Marauzella, J.C. & Sicurella, N.A. "Antibacterial activity of essential oil vapors." **Journal of the American Pharmaceutical Association,** 49(11), 692-694, 1960.
14. Maruzella, J.C. & Lichtenstein, M.B. "The in vitro antibacterial activity of oils." **Journal of American Pharmaceutical Association,** 45(6), 378-381, 1956.
15. Tanner, P.W. & Davis, E. "Some observations on the sanitary condition of confections." **American Journal of Public Health,** 12, 605-607, 1922.

16. Thompson, E.H., Wolk, I.D. & Allen, C.E. "Ginger rhizome: a new source of proteolytic enzyme." **Journal of Food Science,** 38(4), 652-655, 1973.
17. Glatzel, H. **Deutsche Apotheker Zeitung,** 110, 5, 1970.
18. Glatzel, H. "Treatment of dyspeptic disorders with spice extracts." **Hippokrates,** 40(23), 916-919, 1969.
19. Mowrey, D.B. Work performed between 1975-1979 on animals and in humans, some of which has been published (see references in STOMACH/INTESTINAL chapter.
20. Vogel
21. D'Amico, L. "Ricerche sulla presenza di sostanze ad azione anatibiotica nelle piante superiori." **Fitoterapia,** 21(1), 77-79, 1950.
22. Shipochliev, T. **Veterinarno-Meditsinski Nauki,** 5(6), 63-69, 1968.
23. Ramadan, F.M., El-Zanfaly, R.T., Aian, A.M. & El-Wakeil, F.A. "Antibacterial effects of some essential oils. I. Use of agar diffusion method." **Chemie Mikrobiologie Technologie der Lebensmittel,** 2, 51-55, 1972.
24. Curtain, L.S.M. **Healing Herbs of the Upper Rio Grande,** Santa Fe, New Mexico.
25. Mowrey, D.B. Unpublished study, performed during routine toxicological screenings, 1978, Spanish Fork, Utah.

# DIURETIC

## HERBS

**Form:** Capsule.

**CONTENTS: CORNSILK** *(Stigmata maydis)*, **Parsley** *(Petroselinum sativum)*, **Uva-Ursi leaves** *(Arctostaphylos uva-ursi)*, **Cleavers** *(Galium aparine)*, **Buchu leaves** *(Barosma crenata)*, **Juniper berries** *(Juniperus communis)*, **Kelp** *(Laminaria, Macrocystis Ascophyllum)*, **Cayenne** *(Capsicum annuum)*, & **Queen-of-the-Meadow Root** *(Eupatorium purpureum)*.

**PURPOSE:** **Diuretic; For edema and all edematous conditions; Also a treatment for urinary deficiency and infection.**

**Other Applications:** Arthritis, For Cleanses and Detoxification Programs, Gout.

**USE:** 1. Acute irritation and edematous conditions: 5-8 capsules per day while condition persists.
2. Urinary tract infections: 3 capsules, 3 times per day.
3. Arthritis supplement: 3-4 capsules per day maximum while using the ARTHRITIS Blend.
4. Cleanses & Detoxification: 5-8 capsules per day; 3-4 capsules per day of the SKIN DISORDERS and BLOOD PURIFICATION/DETOXIFICATION Blends.
5. Obesity: Do not exceed 2 capsules per day. Use recommended amount of the WEIGHT LOSS Blend.

**Contraindications:**
1. Do not use if nephritis exists.
2. Persons who use diuretics often, who are often rundown, or have a known potassium insufficiency should exercise caution and consider the use of supplemental potassium when using diuretics.
3. Avoid using this blend on a continuous basis.
4. Avoid high sodium foods when using this blend.
5. See appendix A for discussion of Cayenne.

A diuretic is any substance that increases the rate of formation and secretion of urine by the kidneys. Many common substances have some diuretic action, including water, glucose, caffeine, and alcohol. Decreased excretion of water and electrolytes by the kidneys leads to edema (increase in extracellular body fluid). Congestive heart failure is one of the most dangerous causes of edema. Other causes include poor lymphatic drainage, inflammation, and protein-deficient blood Edema is treated with diuretics. There are, fortunately, literally hundreds of natural diuretics. This blend includes some of the most effective, yet mild acting, diuretic herbs available. Herbal diuretics seem to work in different ways. Some are believed to act directly on the kidneys. Others operate by inhibiting salt reabsorption in body tissues. This blend is also a potent urinary aid, affecting all forms of urinary infection, inflammation, and disease. This product can easily be recommended ahead of many prescription medications, because treatments involving the body's systems as a totality rather than as discrete isolated entities usually yield much better results. When using diuretics you should be under a physician's care. **Note:** Ingestion of large quantities of this blend could turn the urine dark—a harmless condition.

**CORNSILK** has been shown in recent research to be highly diuretic yet mild and non-toxic (**1-2**). Of course, Chinese and early eclectic physicians knew that already (**3-4**). In China, the herb is also used to treat diabetes and hypertension (**5**). Dropsical conditions are especially susceptible to the moderate diuretic principles in Cornsilk. *See Also PROSTATE*

**PARSLEY,** judging by its related pharmacological properties, including laxative, hypotensive and expectorant (**6-7**), probably obtains its diuretic activity by directly inhibiting salt reabsorption by body tissues. Parsley is also used to treat jaundice, asthma, menstrual problems and digestive problems (**8**). *See Also BONE-FLESH-CARTILAGE; DIABETES; PROSTATE*

**UVA URSI LEAF** is recognized by medical authorities as diuretic, astringent and antiseptic (**9**). Arbutin, the primary active principle, has been shown to be an effective urinary disinfectant if the urine is alkaline (**10**). Uva ursi leaves and extracts have been included in many commercial diuretic preparations, and the leaves are used in folk medicine around the world to treat nephritis, kidney stones and chronic cystitis (**11**). Uva ursi is thought to act directly on the kidneys to achieve its diuretic effect. *See Also DIABETES; MENSTRUATION*

**CLEAVERS** probably acts directly on the kidneys much like Uva-ursi. Its action is weaker and more mild, although its specific action on acute inflammation or irritation of the urinary tract is stronger than most treatments. The use of cleavers was known to the early eclectic physicians (**12**), who often combined it with Buchu and Uva ursi for maximum benefit, including the elimination of gallstones and kidneystones. Hypotensive principles have been isolated from Cleavers (**13**). Hypotensive activity could be important if you use this blend in a treatment program for heart disease. Cleavers also possess some antibiotic acitivity (f05214).

**BUCHU LEAF** acts directly on the kidneys and the urinary apparatus in general, increasing the fluids and solids of the urine (**15**). Though not as powerful as some of the other diuretics, it definitely enhances the tonic, restorative nature of any diuretic blend that contains it. Buchu was used by the Hottentots of South Africa long before the white man came along. It is still widely used in South Africa, usually as a vinegar or tincture. It is used mainly for diseases of the kidney and urinary tract, but has been applied for scores of other ailments in that country. Its diuretic action is due to a volatile oil that promotes diuresis and imparts its recognized odor to the urine. *See Also PROSTATE; VAGINAL YEAST INFECTION*

**JUNIPER BERRY** also acts directly on the kidneys, stimulating the flow of urine by raising the rate of glomerulus filtration (the process by which blood is purified and wastes filtered out) (**16**). Glomerulus filtration refers to the main detoxification procedure used by the kidneys. This effect is due principally to its high volatile oil content (especially terpenol). Juniper berries and extracts are found in certain over-the-counter drugstore diuretic and laxative preparations

**(11)**. The herb is particularly soothing to the kidneys and is therefore a valuable component of this blend. After acute nephritic illness, Juniper will return the renal epithelium to normal secretory action and normalize blood pressure **(7)**. Overdoses may irritate the kidneys, but this blend is formulated to obtain the maximum benefit from Juniper berries without the risk of overdose. *See Also VAGINAL YEAST INFECTION*

**QUEEN-OF-THE-MEADOW ROOT,** an indigenous plant of North America, has found widespread use on this continent from the earliest years until present. Investigators of Indian medicine found that several tribes used this herb in the same manner as the whites **(17)**. It is used primarily as a diuretic (for which reason it is often called gravel root), stimulant and astringent tonic, directly influencing chronic renal and cystic problems, especially where uric acid levels are high **(18)**. It produces reliable urine flow in cases where the desire is there, but the product is being suppressed. *See Also ARTHRITIS*

**KELP & CAYENNE** import nutritional and chemical support for this blend. They possess little diuretic action, but are included in recognition of the fact that diuretics deplete the body of several nutrients and electrolytes that these herbs can replace.

## OTHER NUTRIENTS

*The use of a diuretic may deplete the body of all kinds of water soluble vitamins. Only vitamins A,D,E,K and essential fatty acids are safe. Minerals, especially potassium, may also be lost and should be replaced by supplementation. The following general recommendations are provided as guidelines only.*

### VITAMINS

Vitamin B Complex
Vitamin B1 *25-100 mg*
Vitamin B2 *25-100 mg*
Vitamin B6 *25-100 mg*
Vitamin C *2,000-5,000 mg*
Vitamin E *200-400 I.U.*

## MINERALS

Potassium
Copper
Magnesium

# REFERENCES

1. Li Shih-Chen. **Chinese Medicinal Herbs.** Georgetown Press, San Francisco. Translated by F. P. Smith and G.A. Stuart, 1973.
2. Ellingwood, F. **American Materia Medica, Therapeutics and Pharmacognosy.** Eclectic Medical Pubs., Portland, Oregon, 1983.
3. Kiangsu, ibid. 556.
4. Opdyke, D.L.J. "Parsley seed oil." **Food and Cosmetics Toxicology** 13(Suppl.), 897-898, 1975.
5. Kaczmarek, F., Ostrowska, B. & Szpunar, K. "Spasmolytic and diuretic activity of the more important components of petroselinum sativum." **Biuletyn Instytutu Roslin Leczniczych (Poznan),** 8, 111-117, 1962.
6. Rosengarten, F., Jr. **The Book of Spices.** Livingston, Wynnewood, Pa.
7. Kiangsu Institute of Modern Medicine. **Encyclopedia of Chinese Drugs.** 2 vols. Shanghai Scientific and Technical Publications. Shanghai Peoples Republic of China, 555.
8. Hahn, S.J. "Pharmacological action of maydis stigma." **K'at'olik Taehak Uihakpu Nonmunjip,** 25, 127-141, 1973.
9. **Martindale: The Extra Pharmacopoeia.** The Pharmaceutical Press. London. 1977.
10. List, P. H. & Hoerhammer, L. **Hagers Handbuch der Pharmazeutishcen Praxis.** Vols. 2-5, Springer-Verlag. Berlin. 1969-1976.
11. Leung, A.Y. **Encyclopedia of Common Natural Ingredients.** New York. 1980.
12. Felter, H.W. **The Eclectic Materia Medica, Pharmacology and Therapeutics.** Eclectic Medical Pubs, Portland, Oregon, 1983 (first published, 1922).
13. Knott, R.P. & McCutcheon, R.S. "Phytochemical investigation of a rubiaceae, galium triflorum." **Journal of Pharmaceutical Sciences,** 50(11), 963-965, 1961.

14. Fitzpatrick, F.K. "Plant substances active against mycobacterium tuberculosis." **Antibiotics and Chemotherapy,** 4(5), 528-536, 1954.
15. Claus, E.P. **Pharmacognosy.** 4th ed. Lea & Febiger. Philadelphia, Pa. 1974.
16. Racz-Kotilla, E. & Racz, G. **Farmacia,** 19, 165, 1971.
17. Mooney, J. "The Sacred Formulas of the Cherokees," **Seventh Annual Report of the Bureau of American Ethnology,** 1885-86, 301-397.
18. King, J. **The American Dispensatory.** Cincinnati, 1866.

# ENVIRONMENTAL POLLUTION

## HERBS

**Form:** Capsule.

**CONTENTS: ALGIN** (from seaweed and algae), **Wheat bran, Apple pectin, Alfalfa** *(Medicago sativa),* & **Kelp** *(Laminaria, Macrocytes, Ascophyllum).*

**PURPOSE:** **To increase the body's ability to resist the effects of Environmental pollution and Heavy metal toxicity.**

**Other Applications:** To lower serum cholesterol levels; radiation, microwave exposure; to obtain sufficient fiber (colitis, obesity, appendicitis, constipation, gallstones, etc.); vitamin A absorption, colds, flu, cancer prevention, atherosclerosis.

**USE:** 1. Prevention and General Purpose: 2-4 capsules per day.
2. Treatment: 2 capsules every 8 hours as needed.
3. Vitamin C supplementation will enhance this blend's effectiveness.

**Contraindications:** None. Be sure to supplement with Vitamin E (200 I.U. daily) when using any product that contains raw Alfalfa. In addition, some individuals may demonstrate a normal allergic reaction to alfalfa. Diabetics may experience lowered insulin requirements as a result of using this blend (see CHOLESTEROL REGULATION), and should inform their physicians of this dietary change.

Illustrating the plant kingdom's ability to serve the evolving needs of humankind, this blend helps the body protect itself against the debilitating effects of a peculiarly modern problem: environmental (air, land and water) pollution. Though historical perspectives for herbal manipulation of this problem are irrelevant, we can rely on modern research findings that indicate it is possible to battle the effects of pollution with sound herbal methods. This blend also works well with the CHOLESTEROL REGULATION blend to reduce excessively high serum cholesterol levels.

**ALGIN & KELP** offer incredibly good protection from many kinds of modern day pollutants, carcinogens and toxins. Canadian researchers have found, for example, that Algin, though non-digestible, can prevent living tissue from absorbing radioactive materials, including strontium-90, barium, mercury, zinc, tin, cadmium, manganese and zinc (**1**). These results have been replicated in other labs (**2**). Strontium-90 is so dangerous because it has a great affinity for calcium and will accumulate in food substances high in that mineral (e.g., milk and green leafy vegetables). Contaminated calcium will carry this pollutant directly to the bones where it damages bone marrow. Kelp blocks this mechanism by preventing the Strontium-90 from being absorbed in the body. The principle of the method lies in the formation of insoluble salts when Kelp particles (sodium alginates) strip the metal ions from the calcium molecule. The salts are unabsorbable and are harmlessly excreted in the urine and feces. Kelp encourages the action of dietary fiber, by supplying nutrients, and by normalizing bowel functions. Brown Kelp is the only source of Algin. The Algin used in the strontium-90 tests was obtained from Pacific Brown Kelp. Many species of Kelp have been found to possess antioxidant, anticarcinogenic, and antitoxic properties. For example, although the specific mode of action is not yet known, Kelp has been conclusively proven to prevent breast cancer in women (especially Japanese women for whom Kelp is viewed as a food, not as a medicinal food) (**3-7**). Ways that Kelp could prevent cancer and reduce the risks of poisoning from many sources of environmental pollution can be listed as follows: 1. By providing a source of nondigestible fiber (**8**) it increases fecal bulk: for example, alginate powder has been used successfully, without irritation or side-effects, to treat constipation in humans (**9**); 2. By reducing cholesterol levels through the inhibition of bile acid absorption (**10**), it may prevent cancer caused by faulty metabolism of bile acids, sterols and steroid hormones (**11**); 3. By altering the nature of fecal flora, it may render harmless the colonic bacteria that could be carcinogenic (**12**); 4. By a direct cytotoxic effect, it may mediate enhancement of the immune response system (**13-14**).

**BRAN** and **PECTIN,** as obtained from dietary sources, have been experimentally shown to protect blood and tissue against various environmental toxins by ensuring the regular cleansing of the bowel, and by complexing with certain air and water-borne pollutants. Bran and Pectin are types of fiber. Dietary fibers are usually defined as those vegetable substances which are not digested by the enzymes of the human alimentary tract (**15**). They are derived from plant cell walls and from the nonstructural polysaccharides in natural foods. Low fiber intake has been conclusively related to obesity, diabetes mellitus, coronary heart disease, diseases of the colon—including cancer, and to various other ailments of industrialized, civilized, pasteurized and otherwise Westernized man (**16-17**). Fiber-rich diets lead to decreases in body weight, blood sugar levels, serum cholesterol and total triglycerides (**18-19**), with corresponding improvements in health. Low concentrations of serum lipids and low incidence of coronary heart disease are found in Seventh Day Adventists, Trappist monks, strict vegetarians, lacto-vegetarians and persons using the Zen macrobiotic diet (**20-23**).

Not all dietary fibers produce the same metabolic effects. It is helpful, therefore to sub-divide fibers into groups according to their mode of action. 1. *Cellulosics* and *Hemicellulosics* include those non-digestible portions of many plants, including Bran, cereals, grains, beans, peppers, carrots and cabbage, that absorb water, and increase in bulk (the key word). They have a normalizing effect on the bowel, prevent constipation by accelerating the passage of material through the large intestine, and protect the body from several diseases, including cancer, colitis, and spastic colon. 2. *Gums* include the extremely water loving material found in oats, guar, Irish Moss and locust beans, to name a few. Gums are also inert, simply absorbing water, swelling, and serving much the same purpose as the cellulosics. 3. *Pectins* are the water soluble substances that bond adjacent cell walls in the tissues of many plants, including apples, citrus fruits, potatoes, strawberries and green beans. They yield a gel which is the basis of fruit jellies. Pectins and gums bind with bile acids, and decrease cholesterol levels and fat absorption. 4. *Lignins* are plant polymers that combine with cellulose to form plant cell walls and the cementing material between them. Lignin has been found to reduce time of passage of stomach contents, bind with bile acids and lower cholesterol levels.

Pectin has the greatest effect on cholesterol levels (see

CHOLESTEROL REGULATION for complete discussion). A few studies indicate that Bran from wheat, corn and sugar beets lower serum cholesterol levels, but most data fail to show a significant effect in that direction (**24-25**). The presence or absence of other dietary factors may finally determine to what extent Bran is effective. Oat bran, which is partly mucilaginous, does lower cholesterol levels substantially (**26**). Cellulose does not lower cholesterol levels except in large quantities (**27**), and lignins have variable effects (**28**). In summary, it appears that mucilaginous fiber (pectin, oat bran) rather than particulate fiber (cellulosics, most brans, lignins) is responsible for decreased serum cholesterol levels.

Several mechanisms have been postulated to explain the effects of fiber. It may alter gastric emptying and intestinal transit rates, thereby decreasing the availability of carbohydrates to be absorbed. Or, since dietary fibers swell (each part of a polysaccharide may hold 100 parts of water), they may simply be filling, limiting the amount of food that can be eaten. In this manner the fiber actually displaces foods that contribute saturated fat and cholesterol to the diet. By modulating glucose absorption, dietary fiber could prevent or reduce obesity. The most likely explanation is that the mucilaginous fibers form gels in the small intestine that interfere with the absorption of both cholesterol and bile acids. This idea is supported directly by the finding that Pectin reduces lymphatic cholesterol absorption best when the diet contains cholesterol (**29**). Pectin also increases the excretion of neutral bile acids (**30**). The ionic charge of Pectin is such that it has a great affinity for biliary salts (**31**). These Pectin-salt complexes are excreted as waste. As a result, there are fewer biliary salts present to form micelles, and therefore absorbed cholesterol decreases. This, in turn, may stimulate the production of biliary acids from endogenous (non-dietary) cholesterol. The final result is greatly lowered cholesterol levels.

Bran, though it doesn't lower cholesterol levels as surely as Pectin does, has nevertheless been shown to help prevent the precipitation of cholesterol from the bile that produces gallstones. Bile is a finely balanced solution of cholesterol, bile salts and phospholipids. The oversecretion of cholesterol or the undersecretion of bile salts leads to supersaturation of cholesterol that then precipitates as gallstones. Bran increases the size of the bile salt pools (**32-33**) when necessary and otherwise normalizes the balance between the major components of the bile. Thirty grams of Bran per day was shown to significantly improve the bile composition in several patients with cholesterol gallstones (**34-35**). Pectin and lignin are also effective in preventing gallstones (**36**), and Pectin can even produce regressions in gallstones. For more information on the above principles see CHOLESTEROL REGULATION.

According to Soviet investigators, heavy metals, such as lead and mercury, are excreted harmlessly from the body much more efficiently when Pectin is included in the diet (**37**). Apple pectin, Rice Bran, Wheat Bran, Alfalfa fiber and Burdock root fiber, along with other sources of dietary fiber, have been shown to protect the body, and especially the gut, against the toxic effects of several common food additives, including amaranth (FD & C No. 2), Tween 60 (polyoxyethylene sorbitan monostearate), sodium cyclamate, tartrazine (FD & C Yellow No. 5), and Sunset Yellow (FD & C Yellow No. 6) (**38-42**). Possible modes of action include a binding of the additives with the fiber, thereby preventing absorption, or perhaps the fiber prevents adverse effects through an action on the digestive process or gut bacteria.

**ALFALFA** is one of the most studied plants. We know it contains many important substances, including several saponins, many sterols, flavanoids, coumarins, alkaloids, acids, vitamins, amino acids, sugars, proteins (25% by weight), minerals, trace element and other nutrients. Overall, it is one of the most nutritious foods known. Recent research has found that Alfalfa saponins inhibit increases in blood cholesterol levels by 25% when high cholesterol diets are fed to monkeys (**43**), rats (**44-45**), and rabbits (**46-47**). Other components of Alfalfa probably enhance the action of the saponins by binding the bile acids that are necessary for cholesterol absorption. French scientists have shown that Alfalfa can reduce tissue damage caused by another modern hazard, radiotherapy (**48**). Also of interest are the effects of Vitamin K, found in high concentrations in Alfalfa. In man, a bleeding disorder occurs when the delivery of bile to the bowel is hindered, as for example in obstructive jaundice or biliary fistula. Other bleeding disorders result from the use of artificial formulas to feed newborn children, protracted antibiotic therapy, pancreatic insufficiency, chronic diarrhea and steatorrhea, and from the use of anticoagulants, aspirin and anticonvulsant drugs. Most of these conditions are the result of misuse of modern medical technology. Dietary Vitamin K has the effect of remedying all of the above conditions (**49-52**). Alfalfa has also been shown to possess antibacterial action against gram negative bacteria (such as Salmonella typhi) (**53**), and it contains at least one protein with known antitumor activity (**54**). It is important to realize that Alfalfa is also fiber. As such it has been shown, along with Bran and Pectin to bind and neutralize various types of agents carcinogenic to the colon (**55**).

Finally, some work suggests that Alfalfa induces activity in a complex cellular system that inactivates dietary chemical carcinogens in the liver and small intestine before they have a chance to do the body any harm (**56**). *See Also ARTHRITIS; WHOLE BODY TONIC*

# OTHER NUTRIENTS

*While dietary fiber is certainly one of the most important sources of the substances needed to reduce your chances of disease through ingesting environmental toxins, keeping a healthy immune system is also very important. That is done by maintaining a daily adequate intake of some crucial vitamins and minerals as well as some other nutrients. Individual requirements may depart substantially from these recommendations.*

### VITAMINS

*(Daily requirements unless otherwise noted)*

Vitamin A *10,000 I.U.*
Vitamin B Complex
Vitamin B1 *25 mg*
Vitamin B2 *25 mg*
Vitamin B6 25 mg
Vitamin B12 *3 mcg*
Vitamin C *500-1,000 mg*
Vitamin D *400 I.U.*
Vitamin E *400 I.U.*
Choline *1,000 mg*
Inositol *1,000 mg*
PABA *30 mg*
Folic Acid *400 mcg*
Pantothenic Acid *50 mg*

### MINERALS

Calcium/Magnesium
Phosphorous

### MISCELLANEOUS

GLA
Essential Fatty Acid
Brewer's yeast
Yogurt/acidophilus

# REFERENCES

1. Tanaka, Y., Hurlburt, A.J., Argeloff, L, Skoryna, S.C. & Stara, J.F. "Application of algal polysaccharides as in vivo binders of metal pollutant." in **Proceedings of the Seventh International Seaweed Symposium,** Wiley & Sons, New York, 1972, 602-607.
2. Humphreys, E.R. & Howells, G.R."Degradation of sodium alginate by gamma-irradiation and by oxidative-reductive depolymerization." **Carbohydrate Research,** 16(1), 65-69, 1971.
3. Hirayama, T. "Epidemiology of breast cancer with special reference to the role of diet." **Preventive Medicine,** 7, 173-195, 1978.
4. Wynder, E.L. "Dietary habits and cancer epidemiology." **Cancer,** supplement, 43(5), 1955-1961, 1979.
5. Kagawa, T. "Impact of westernization on the Japanese. Changes in physique, cancer longevity and centerians." **Preventive Medicine,** 7, 205-217, 1978.
6. Fujimoto, I., Hanai, A & Oshima, A. "Descriptive epidemiology of cancer in Japan: current cancer incidence and survival data." **National Cancer Institute Monographs,** 53, 5-15, 1979.
7. Nomura, A., Henderson, B.E. & Lee, J. "Breast cancer and diet among the Japanese in Hawaii." **American Journal of Clinical Nutrition,** 31, 2020-2025, 1978.
8. Mendelof, A.I. "Current Concepts: dietary fiber in human health." **New England Journal of Medicine,** 297, 811-814, 1977.
9. Mulinos, M.G. & Glass, G.B.J. "The treatment of constipation with a new hydrosorbent material derived from kelp." **Gastroenterology,** 24, 383-393, 1953.
10. Iritani, N. & Nogi, J. "Effect of spinach and wakame on cholesterol turnover in the rat." **Atherosclerosis,** 15, 87-92, 1972.
11. Bokkenhause, V.D., Winter, J. & Kelly, W.G. "Metabolism of biliary steroids by human fecal flora." **American Journal of Clinical Nutrition,** 31, S221-S226, 1978.
12. Salyers, A.A., Palmer, J.K. & Wilkins, T.D. "Degradation of polysaccharides by intestinal bacterial enzymes." **American Journal of Clinical Nutrition,** 31, S128-S130, 1978.
13. Yamamoto, I. Nagumo, T, Yagi, K. Tominaga, H. & Aoki, M. "Antitumor effect of seaweeds. 1. Antitumor effect of extracts from Sargassum and Laminaria." **Japanese Journal of Experimental Medicine,** 44(6), 543-546, 1974.
14. Jolles, B., Remington, M & Andrews, P.S. "Effects of sulphated degraded laminarin on experimental tumor growth." **British Journal of Cancer,** 17, 109-115, 1963.

15. Trowell, H. "The development of the concept of dietary fiber in human nutrition." **American Journal of Clinical Nutrition,** 31(10), S3-S11, 1978.
16. Southgate, D.A.T. "Dietary fiber: analysis and food sources." **American Journal of Clinical Nutrition,** 31, S107, 1978.
17. Levin, B, Horwitz, D. "Dietary fiber." **Medical Clinics of North America,** 63(5), 1043-1055, 1979.
18. Albrink, M.J. "Dietary fiber, plasma insulin and obesity." **American Journal of Clinical Nutrition,** 31(10), S277S278, 1978.
19. Reiser, S. "Effect of dietary fiber on parameters of glucose tolerance in humans." In Inglett, G.E.; Falkehag, S.I.: **Dietary fibers. Chemistry and nutrition.** Academic Press, New York, 1979, p. 173.
20. Phillips. R.L., Lemon, F.R., Beeson, W.L., et al. "Coronary heart disease mortality among Seventh-Day Adventists with differing dietary habits: a preliminary report." **American Journal of Clinical Nutrition,** 31 (supple), S191, 1978.
21. Barrow, J.G., Quinlan, C.B., Edmando, R.E., et al. "Prevalence of atherosclerotic complications in Trappist and Benedictine Monks (abstract)." **Circulation,** 24, 881-882, 1961.
22. Hardinger, M.G., Chambers, A.C., Crooks, H., et al. "Nutritional studies of vegetarians. III. Dietary levels of fiber." **American Journal of Clinical Nutrition,** 6(5), 523525, 1958.
23. Sacks, F.M., Castelli, W.P., Donner, A., et al. "Plasma lipids and lipoproteins in vegetarians and controls." **New England Journal of Medicine,** 292(22), 1148-1151, 1975.
24. van Berge-Henegouwen, G.P., Huybregts, .W., van de Werf, S., Demacker, P. & Schade, R.W. "Effect of a standardized wheat bran preparation on serum lipids in young healthy males." **American Journal of Clinical Nutrition,** 32, 794-798, 1979.
25. Heaton, K.W., Pomare, E.W. "Effects of bran of blood lipids and calcium." **Lancet,** 1, 49-50, 1974.
26. Anderson, J.W., Lin Chen, W. J.L. "Plant fiber. Carbohydrate and lipid metabolism." **American Journal of Clinical Nutrition,** 32(2), 346-363, 1979.
27. Idem: "Dietary fibre: effects on plasma and biliary lipids in men." in **Medical Aspects of Dietary Fiber,** Spiller, G.A., Kay, R.M., eds. Plenum Press, New York, 1980, p. 153.
28. Lindner, P. Moeller, B. "Lignin: a cholesterol-lowering agent?" **Lancet,** 2, 1259, 1973.
29. ibid.
30. Kay, R.M. & Truswell, A.S. "Effect of citrus pectin on blood lipids and fecal steroid excretion in man." **American Journal of Clinical Nutrition,** 30(2), 171-175, 1977.

31. Story, J.A., Kritchevsky, D. & Eastwood, M.A. **Dietary fibers. Chemistry and Nutrition,** Academic Press, 1979. p. 49.

32. Pomare, E.W., Heaton, K.W., Low-Beer, T.S. & Espiner, H.J. "The effect of wheat bran upon bile salt metabolism and upon the lipid composition of bile in gallstone patients." **American Journal of Digestive Diseases,** 21(7), 521-526, 1976.

33. Watts, J.M., Jablonski, P., & Toouli, J. "The effect of added bran to the diet on the saturation of bile in people without gallstones." **American Journal of Surgery,** 135(March), 321324, 1978.

34. McDougall, R.M., Ykymyshyn, D., Walker, K., et al. "Effect of wheat bran on serum lipoproteins and bilieary lipids." **Canadian Journal of Surgery,** 21(5), 433435, 1978.

35. Pomare, E.W., Heaton, K.W. "Alteration of bile salt metabolism by dietary fibre (bran)." **British Medical Journal,** 4, 262-264, 1973.

36. Heaton, K. in **Refined Carbohydrate Foods and Disease.** Burkett, D.P. & Trowell, H.C., eds. Academic Press, London, 1975, p. 173.

37. O.D. Livshits, "Prophylactic role of pectin-containing foods during lead poisonings." **Voprosy Pitaniya,** 28(4), 76-77, 1969. And O.G. Arkhipova & Zorina, L.A. **Professional'nye Zabolevaniya V Khimicheskoi Promyshlennosti,** 210-213, 1965.

38. Ershoff, B.H. & Thurston, E.W. "Effects of diet on amaranth (FD & C Red NO. 2) toxicity in the rat." **Journal of Nutrition,** 104, 937, 1974.

39. Ershoff, B.H. & Marshall, W.E. "Protective effects of dietary fiber in rats fed toxic doses of sodium cyclamate and polyoxyethylene sorbitan monostearate (Tween 60)." **Journal of Food Science,** 40, 357, 1975.

40. Ershoff, B.H. "Synergistic toxicity of food additives in rats fed a diet low in dietary fibre." **Journal of Food Science,** 41, 949, 1976.

41. Ershoff, B.H. "Effects of diet on growth and survival of rats fed toxic levels of tartrazine (FD &C Yellow No. 5) and Sunset Yellow FCF (FD & C Yellows No. 6.)." **Journal of Nutrition,** 107, 822, 1977.

42. Kimura, T., Furuta, H., Matsumoto, Y. & Yoshida, A. "Ameliorating effect of dietary fiber on toxicities of chemicals added to a diet in the rat." **Journal of Nutrition,** 110, 513, 1980.

43. Malinow, M.R., Mclaughlin, P. & Papworth, L. "Hypocholesterolemic effect of alfalfa in cholesterol-fed monkeys." **IVth International Symposium on Atherosclerosis,** Tokyo, Japan, 1976.

44. Malinow, M.R., McLaughlin, P., Papworth, L., Stafford, C., et al. "Effect of alfalfa saponins on intestinal cholesterol absorption in

rats." **American Journal of Clinical Nutrition,** 30, 2061-2067, 1977.

45. Malinow, M.R., McLaughlin, P., Stafford, C, et al. "Comparative effects of alfalfa saponins and alfalfa fiber on cholesterol absorption in rats." **American Journal of Clinical Nutrition,** 32, 1810-1812, 1979.
46. Cookson, F.B. & Federoff, S. "Quantitative relationships between administered cholesterol and alfalfa required to prevent hyper-cholesterolaemia in rabbits." **British Journal of Experimental Pathology,** 49, 348-355, 1968.
47. Cookson, F.B., Altshcul, R. & Fedoroff, S. "The effects of alfalfa on serum cholesterol and in modifying or preventing cholesterol induced atherosclerosis in rabbits." **Journal of Atherosclerosis Research,** 7, 69-81, 1967.
48. De Froment, P. "Unsaponifiable substance from alfalfa for pharmaceuticals and cosmetic use." **French Patent 2,187,328,** 1974.
49. Almquist, H.J. "The early history of vitamin K." **American Journal of Clinical Nutrition,** 28, 656-659, 1975.
50. Greaves, J.D., Schmidt, C.L.A. "Nature of the factor concerned in loss of blood coagulability of bile fistula rats." **Proceedings of the Society of Experimental Biology and Medicine,** 37, 43-45, 1937.
51. Warner, E.D., Brinkhous, K.M., & Smith, H.P. "Bleeding tendency of obstructive jaundice: prothrombin deficiency and dietary factors." **Proceedings of the Society for Experimental Biology and Medicine,** 37, 628-630, 1938.
52. Vest, M. "Vitamin K in medical practice." **Vitamines and Hormones NY,** 24, 649-663, 1966.
53. Gestetner, B., Assa, Y., Henis, Y., Birk, Y. & Bondi, A. "Lucerne saponins. IV. Relation between their chemical constitution and hemolytic and antifungal activities." **Journal of Science, Food and Agriculture,** 22(4), 168-172, 1971.
54. Tyihak, E. & Szende, B. "Basic plant proteins with antitumor activity." **Hungarian Patent 798,** 1970.
55. Smith-Barbaro, P., Hanson, D. & Reddy, B.S. "Carcinogen binding to various types of dietary fiber." **Journal of the National Cancer Institute,** 67(2), 495-497, 1981.
56. Wattenberg, L. "Effects of dietary constituents on the metabolism of chemical carcinogens." **Cancer Research,** 35, 3326-3331, 1975.

# EYES

## HERBS

**Form:** Capsule, Tea

**CONTENTS: EYEBRIGHT herb** *(Euphrasia officinalis)*, **Goldenseal root** *(Hydrastis canadensis)*, **Bayberry root bark** *(Myrica cerifera)*, **Red Raspberry leaves** *(Rubus idaeus)*, & **Cayenne** *(Capsicum annum)*.

**PURPOSE: A tonic for poor or unhealthy vision: (NOT INTENDED FOR EXTERNAL APPLICATION).**

**Other Applications:** To help prevent cataracts; for relief of inflamed eyes, stinging and weeping eyes, over-sensitivity to light.

**USE:** 1. Normal use: 2-4 capsules per day.
2. Acute problems: 2-3 capsules, three times per day.
3. Use the INFLUENZA or FEVERS & INFECTIONS blends to supplement this blend whenever infection is present.

**Contraindications:** None. NOT INTENDED FOR EXTERNAL APPLICATION.

The principle purpose of this blend is to be tonic for the eyes; the major effect is supplied by Eyebright and Goldenseal. The other herbs in the blend are antibiotics, astringents and stimulants. They provide the "housekeeping" chores for the blend: toning, warding off bacteria, delivering nutrients, and eliminating wastes. Although from time to time one hears reports that blends such as this have cured blindness, cataracts and other severe vision problems, documentation of the diagnostic measures and exact mode of treatment in·such cases has been lacking.

**EYEBRIGHT,** as its name indicates, is one of the primary herbal sources of eye care. But even though Eyebright has been depended upon for at least 2000 years in the treatment of eye problems, modern science has avoided the study of this plant like the plague. Periodically, its effectiveness has been questioned, even by herbalists, but nay-sayers have made little impact. They are quickly buried and forgotten and the traditional use continues unabated. Some naturalists, spooked by the obvious correlation between the Doctrine of Signatures and the appearahce and use of Eyebright, have been quick to call attention to this puported superstitious connection. Are they right? Is this herb a fraud? Not according to the majority of those who have investigated its properties for themselves. Positive clinical cases abound, and glowing personal reports are received by doctors continually. Most cases involve sore and/or inflamed eyes in which there is considerable stinging and irritation associated with watery-to-thick discharges, or conjunctivitis (pink eye). The herb may help to relieve other symptoms that often accompany inflammed eyes, such as runny nose, earache and sneezing. Science, it appears, has been remiss in refusing to investigate this herb. Eyebright may be procured and used by itself as an eyewash or compress to potentiate the effects of this blend (do not use powdered herb for this purpose; use whole herb). Its mode of action is not known, but used internally, it probably affects the liver among other organs in such a way as to cleanse the blood supply to the eyes.

**GOLDENSEAL ROOT,** because of its potent antibiotic and antiseptic nature, will greatly help reduce infection and inflammation of the eyes (**1-2**). These properties of Goldenseal are discussed fully in the INFLUENZA chapter. Pertinent to this blend, it can be noted that herbalists have used Goldenseal in America for over a hundred years for inflammation of eyes (**3**) and to soothe and tone catarrhal and follicular conjunctivitis (**4**). The American Indians were the first to use it for sore eyes. White doctors did not pick up the use of this herb until about 1800 (**5-6**). Early pioneers, along with many Indian tribes, used it as a general tonic, but thought of it as being a specific treatment for the eyes. *See Also INFLUENZA; STOMACH/*

*INTESTINAL; VAGINAL YEAST INFECTION; NERVES & GLANDS; FEVERS & INFEC-
TIONS; HEMORRHOIDS*

**BAYBERRY ROOT BARK** is provided in this blend as a stimulating tonic for the good of the whole system. It works well in conjunction with Cayenne to increase the body's ability to ward off infections of all kinds. The tonic and astringent properties of this herb are discussed in the INFLUENZA chapter.

**RED RASPBERRY LEAF,** in the small quantities found in this blend, imparts a certain amount of astringency to the blend, and is included for that reason. Astringency helps lessen the severity of mucous discharge from, in this case, the eyes and nose. *See Also DIABETES; MENSTRUATION; FEMALE TONIC*

**CAYENNE** insures the rapid delivery of nutrients to infected areas as well as the efficient removal of waste material. Such service can be extremely important in cases of eye infection and other eye-related problems. The mode of action of Cayenne is to stimulate the cardio-vascular system as a whole, but is felt predominantly in the capillaries, i.e., precisely where needed for proper infusion of the diseased area with a constant fresh supply of blood-borne nutrients. *See Also CIRCULATION; BLOOD PURIFICATION/DETOXIFICATION; FATIGUE; HIGH BLOOD PRESSURE*

## OTHER NUTRIENTS

*The roles played by Vitamin A, Provitamin A and B-Carotene on eyesight cannot be overemphasized. But other nutrients are important. This table may serve as a reference guide for the most important nutrients you can obtain from supplemental sources.*

### VITAMINS

*(Daily requirements unless otherwise noted)*

*Vitamin A 25,000-50,000 I.U.*
Vitamin B Complex
Vitamin B1 *25-50 mg*
Vitamin B2 *25-50 mg*
Vitamin B6 *25-50 mg*
Vitamin C *3,000-5,000 mg*

Vitamin D *400-1,000 I.U.*
Pantothenic Acid *100 mg*
Niacinamide *50 mg*

## MINERALS

Calcium/Magnesium
Phosphorous

## MISCELLANEOUS

B-Carotene

## REFERENCES

1. Gibbs, O.S. "On the curious pharmacology of hydrastis." **Federation of American Societies for Experimental Biology. Federation Proceedings,** 6(1), 332, 1947.
2. Nandkarni, A.K. **Indian Materia Medica.** Popular Book Depot, Bombay-7. Dhootopapeshwar Prakashan Ltd, Panvel 1954, Vol 1. 3rd ed., 189-190.
3. Ellingwood, F. **American Materia Medica, Therapeutics and Pharmacognosy.** Eclectic Medical Publications, Portland, Oregon, 1983.
4. Felter, H. W. **The Eclectic Materia Medica, Pharmacology and Therapeutics.** Eclectic Medical Publications, Portland, Oregon, 1983 (first published 1922).
5. Culbreth, D.M.R. **A Manual of Materia Medica and Pharmacology.** Philadelphia, 1927, p. 99.
6. Millspaugh, C. F. **American Medicinal Plants.** Dover Publications, Inc. New York, 1974 (first published 1892).

# FATIGUE

## HERBS

**Form:** Capsule.

**CONTENTS: CAYENNE** *(Capsicum annum),* **Siberian GIN-SENG** *(Eleutherococcus senticosus),* **Gotu Kola** *(Hydrocotyle asiatica),* **Kelp** *(Laminaria, Macrocystis, Ascophyllum),* **Peppermint leaves** *(Mentha piperita),* **Ginger root** *(Zingiber officinale).*

**PURPOSE: To help they body overcome fatigue, physical weakness, lack of sthrength, etc. To increase stamina.**

**Other Applications:** Depression, emotional exhaustion.

**USE:** 1. Routine Maintenance: 2-4 capsules per day.
2. Severe stress: 4-6 capsules per day.
3. As adjunct to NERVOUS TENSION blend: 1-2 capsules/day.
4. As adjunct to MENTAL ALERTNESS/SENILITY blend: 2 caps/day.
5. As adjunct to LOW BLOOD SUGAR blend: 1-2 capsules/day.

**Contraindications:** None. For a discussion of Cayenne, see Appendix A.

Everybody feels worn out at one time or another. Some more than others. Constant fatigue is a sign of physiological stress, which may be caused by a wide variety of conditions, including poor nutrition, anemia, obesity, emotional stress, infectious disease, and lack of sleep. Overcoming chronic fatigue requires that you either get well, if sick, or change lifestyle, if the fatigued condition is stress-induced. This means you must eat better, use dietary supplements, get more exercise, and learn to relax. This herbal blend is designed to be a part of such a program. It promotes both short-term and long-term anti-fatigue properties and enhancement of physical strength and stamina. The Cayenne and Peppermint provide a quick stimulant effect, and when the blend is used daily, the Ginseng, Gotu Kola, Kelp and Ginger root gradually increase stamina.

**CAYENNE**'s stimulant effects have been shown through animal studies to be rapid but transient. Animals, stressed under various conditions, perform better if Cayenne is added to their diet on the day before the tests, but not if added three days before the test (**1**). Animal tests have also demonstrated long-term resistance to stress when Ginseng and Gotu Kola form a semi-permanent part of the diet (**1-2**). In addition, Cayenne has been proven to have a strong effect on circulation and respiratory reflexes (**3**). Other evidence for a stimulant, anti-fatigue effect in Cayenne has been provided by a French team (**4**). *See Also CIRCULATION; HIGH BLOOD PRESSURE*

**SIBERIAN GINSENG** resembles other Ginseng species in overall activity, though there are some minor differences, none of which justifies the tremendous price difference between this species and the exotic, practically deified varieties. Ginseng is properly the number one tonic herb in the world. Other herbs are used more, but none is so highly regarded. In a blend such as this it contributes remarkable properties, and its effects are enhanced further by the other herbs. However, taken as a quick antidote to fatigue, Ginseng is not that effective. Used on a daily basis, it gradually builds up the body's ability to resist fatigue. You may find yourself just as tired at the end of the day, but you will have done so much more for it. That is the marvel of Ginseng. Studies on the anti-fatigue (or anti-stress) properties are substantial (e.g.,**5-8**). Resisting the onset of fatigue requires an intact, healthy, fully functioning adrenocortical system, for it is this system that regulates the chemistry of stress. Ginseng directly stimulates this system (**9**), helping to prevent the cumulative effect of hundreds of different kinds of daily stress from overwhelming the body's ability to fight back. In the aged, Ginseng saponins (the active principles) have an additional important effect. They influence cellular enzyme activity in such a way to impart to vital organs an increased ability to tolerate anaerobic conditions. The result is that ageing heart and brain tissues, in a reversal of normal patterns, are better able to withstand sustained work (**10**). Americans, Chinese, Russians and other Europeans and Asians all agree: Ginseng is the wonder food of the plant kingdom. *See Also INFERTILITY; WHOLE BODY; MENTAL ALERTNESS/SENILITY; LOW BLOOD SUGAR*

**GOTU KOLA** is another tonic of Asian origin. It does not have the reputation of Ginseng, however. In fact, very little experimental work has been done. Several years ago I studied Gotu Kola, Ginseng and Capsicum in a blend and separately. I noticed that Gotu Kola behaved similar to Ginseng with regard to effects on fatigue, i.e., in a long term test on a gerbil in an activity cage, I noticed gradually increasing levels of activity that could not be accounted for by maturation alone. What little other research has been done agrees with that finding (**11,2**). Contrary to the misconceptions of some writers, including university professors in California and Utah, Gotu Kola is not related to the Kola nut, nor does it owe its anti-fatigue properties to caffeine, a stimulant not found in Gotu Kola. *See Also WHOLE BODY; MENTAL ALERTNESS/SENILITY*

**KELP** influences the body first through nutritive excellence, supplying a long list of essential vitamins and mineral salts (**12**). Secondly, Kelp contains cardiac principles which stimulate the heart ever so gently (**13-14**). Hypotensive principles have also been isolated from Kelp (**15**). Finally, iodine, the primary constituent of Kelp activates and regulates metabolism (**12**).

**PEPPERMINT LEAF** provides a refreshing aromatic principle to the blend, and its inclusion adheres to good blend-making guidelines. An aromatic in every blend would make herbal preparations much more acceptable to the body, more digestible, and would increase assimilation and utilization by the body's major systems. In addition, the volatile oils of Peppermint are said to be directly stimulating to the entire body. A mechanism to explain this effect is not known, but the subjective feeling of energy and vitality imparted by the herb is well-known. *See Also DIGESTION; MENTAL ALERTNESS/SENILITY*

**GINGER ROOT** produces a generalized stimulant effect which diffuses slowly from the G.I. tract, and gently energizes the blood, producing a feeling of warmness throughout the body. Ginger root also has some specific effects that contribute to the blend's effectiveness in a more direct manner. For example, in one study in the

Soviet Union, it was discovered that patients with various chronic lung and heart insufficiencies experienced considerable cardiotonic benefits from ingesting a species of wild ginger similar to Zingiber officinale (**16**). Cardiotonic principles in Ginger root have been discovered by Japanese researchers also (**17**). The cholinergic activity of Ginger root discussed in the chapter on NERVOUS TENSION is also important in this blend, since it helps the body recover from the effects of stress and fatigue more rapidly than otherwise (**18**). According to another study, Ginger root stimulates the vasomotor and respiratory centers (**19**). In my own experience and that of acquaintances, I have observed that Ginger root effectively relieves headaches of a wide assortment, but for years I was not aware that the herb is or ever was popularly used for this problem. Then I learned that East African peoples use it regularly for headaches (and also for rheumatism). It has also come to my attention that a shop in Groeningen, Germany, sells a Ginger preparation for treating, among other things, toothache and headache (**11**). So, one never knows.... *See Also NERVOUS TENSION; LOW BLOOD SUGAR; CIRCULATION; LAXATIVE; STOMACH/INTESTINAL; NAUSEA; DIGESTION*

## OTHER NUTRIENTS

*One of the most important aids to overcoming fatigue is to keep the body well supplied with the nutrients it needs for tissue repair, oxygen transport and waste disposal. These recommendations are meant as guidelines only. Individual differences in nutrient requirements can be substantial.*

### VITAMINS

*(Daily requirements unless otherwise noted)*

Vitamin B-1 *25-100 mg*
Vitamin B-2 *25-100 mg*
Vitamin B-6 *25-100 mg*
Vitamin C *500-1000 mg*
Vitamin D *400 I.U.*
Vitamin E *500-600 I.U.*
Niacinamide *100 mg*
Folic acid *400 mcg*
Pantothenic Acid *100 mg*

## MINERALS

Calcium/Magnesium
Phosphorus
Zinc

# REFERENCES

1. Mowrey, D.B. "Capsicum, ginseng and gotu kola in combination." **The Herbalist,** premier issue, 22-28, 1975.
2. Mowrey, D.B. "The effects of capsicum, gotu kola and ginseng on activity: further evidence." **The Herbalist,** 1(1), 51-54, 1976.
3. Molnar, E., Baraz, L.A. & Khayutin, V.M. "Irritating and depressing effect of capsaicin on receptors and afferent fibers of the small intestine." **Tr. Inst. Norm. Patol. Fiziol. Akad. Med. Nauk SSSR,** 10, 22-24, 1967.
4. Roquebert, J., Canellas, J., Demichel, P. & Dufour, Ph. "Study on vasculotropic properties of Capsicum annuum." **Annales Pharmaceutiques Francaises,** 36(7-8), 361-368, 1978.
5. Baubrin, Y.F. "Eleutherococcus's effect on telegraph operators work results and audial sensitivity." **Eleutherococcus and other Adaptogenic Plants of the Far East,** 7th ser., 179-184, 1966.
6. Brandeis, S.A. & Pilovitskaya, V. N. "The effectiveness of using eleutherococcus root extract during protracted work and inhaling gas mixtures rich with oxygen." **Eleutherococcus and other Adaptogenic Plants of the Far East,** 7th ser., 179-184, 1966.
7. Berdyshev, V.V. "Effect of Eleutherococcus on body functions and the work capacity of sailors on a cruise." **Voenno Meditsinskii Zhurnal,** 2, 48-51, 1981.
8. Batin, V.V, Popov, I., Lifar, V.K. "Experience in using sugar and an Eleutherococcus extract with the workers of the hot shops and the night shifts of the Raichikhinsk glass plant." **Gigiena Truda i Professional'nye Zabolevaniya,** 5, 36-38, 1981.
9. Kirilov, O.I. "The effect of fluid extract of eleutherococcus root on the pituitary-adrenocortical system." **Slb. Otd. Acad. Nauk S.S.S.R.,** 23, 3-5, 1964.
10. Shia, G.T.W., Ali, S. & Bittles, A.H. "The effects of Ginseng saponins on the growth and metabolism of human diploid fibroblasts." **Gerontology,** 28, 121-124, 1982.
11. List, P.H. & Hoerhammer, L. **Hagers Handbuch der Pharmazeutischen Praxis.** Volumes 2-5, Springer-Verlag, Berlin.

12. Binding, G.J. & Moyle, A. **About Kelp.** Thorsons Publishers Limited. Wellingborough, Northamptonshire, England, 1974.
13. Kosuge, T., Nukaya, H., Yamamoto, T. & Tsuji, K. "Isolation and identification of cardiac principles from laminaria." **Yakugaku Zasshi,** 103(6), 683-685, 1983.
14. Searl, P.B., Norton, T.R. & Lum, B.K.B. "Study of a cardiotonic fraction from an extract of the seaweed undaria pinnatifida." **Proceedings of the Western Pharmacology Society,** 24, 63-65, 1981.
15. Funayama, S. & Hikino, H. "Hypotensive principle of Laminaria and allied seaweeds." **Planta Medica,** 41, 29-33, 1981.
16. Khmetova, B.K. "The electrocardiographic changes in patients with chronic pulmonary and pulmonary-cardiac insufficiency treated with European wild ginger." **Sbornik Nauchnykh Trudov Bashkirskii Meditsinskii Institut,** 17, 113-118, 1968.
17. Shoji, N., Iwasa, A., Takemoto, T., Ishida, Y. & Ohizumi, Y. "Cardiotonic principles of ginger (Zingiber officinale, R)." **Journal of Pharmaceutical Science,** 71(10), 1174-1175, 1968.
18. Suzuki, Y., Taguchi, K., Hagiwara, Y., & Kajiyama, K. "Pharmacological studies on Zingiber mioga Roscoe (2)." **Folia Pharmacologia Japonica,** 75(7), 731-746, 1979.
19. Ally, M.M. "The pharmacological action of zingiber officinale." **Proceedings of the Pan Indian Ocean Scientific Congress, 4th, Karachi, Pakistan,** Section G, 11-12, 1960.

# FEMALE
# TONIC

## HERBS

**Form:** Capsule, Tea, Douche

**CONTENTS: BLACK COHOSH root** *(Cimicifuga racemosa),* **LICORICE root** *(Glycyrrhiza glabra),* **Raspberry leaves** *(Rubus idaeus),* **Passion Flower** *(Passiflora incarnata),* **Chamomile** *(Matricaria chamomilla),* **Fenugreek** *(Trigonella Foenum-graecum),* **Black Haw bark** *(Viburnum prunifolium),* **Saw Palmetto berries** *(Serenoa repens-sabal),* **Squaw vine** *(Mitchella repens),* **Wild Yam root** *(Dioscorea villosa),* & **Kelp** *(Laminaria, Macrocystis, Ascophyllum).*

**PURPOSE:** Female Tonic. For use during pregnancy, delivery, menses, menopause; also for pain, cramp, atony, etc., related to birth, pregnancy, menstruation and menopause.

**Other Applications:** Morning sickness; hot flashes; infertility; mild sedative; rheumatism; insominia.

**USE:** 1. As a Tonic: 2-3 capsules per day along with 2 capsules per day of the NERVE & GLAND TONIC.
2. Menses: 4-6 capsules per day.
3. Pregnancy: 3-5 capsules per day. Supplement with the NERVE & GLAND TONIC and WHOLE BODY TONIC, 2-3 capsules each, per day.
4. Other applications: 4 capsules as needed, up to 12 per day.

5. To supplement the VAGINAL YEAST INFECTION Blend: 3-4 capsules per day.
6. To supplement the MENSTRUATION Blend: 5-6 capsules per day.
7. To supplement the INFERTILITY Blend: 3-7 capsules per day.
8. For morning sickness: use NAUSEA blend as directed; supplement with 3-5 capsules per day of this blend.

**Contraindications:**
1. Persons with low blood sugar should be sure to use supplemental capsules of the LOW BLOOD SUGAR Blend.
2. For a further discussion of Licorice Root, see Appendix A.

The focus of this blend is on sustaining and reinforcing the woman during difficult physical times, such as pregnancy, birth, menopause, menstruation, etc. It reduces pain, cramping, uterine atony, and related problems, and helps maintain good hormonal health and balance. Most of the herbs in this blend are designed to complement and extend the activity of Black Cohosh. The blend will serve best when used moderately on a regular basis. An Important Note: Although estrogenic and other neurohormonal agents are present in some of the herbs, the estrogenic action of blends like this has been grossly overestimated by some individuals. While some estrogenic activity may be present, exaggerated assertions along those lines are unwarranted. Clinical observations of medicinal effects support a variety of interpretations, of which the estrogenic theory is but one.

**BLACK COHOSH** was introduced to American medicine by the Indians, who called it squaw root in reference to one of its common uses: to treat uterine disorders. Among clinical findings are the following: it promotes and/or restores healthy menstrual activity; it soothes irritation and congestion of the uterus, cervix and vagina; it relieves the pain and distress of pregnancy; it contributes to quick, easy and uncomplicated deliveries; and it promotes uterine involution and recovery (**1-3**). In support of the above clinical evidence, laboratory research has found hypotensive principles, vasodilatory, anti-inflammatory, and uterine contractile activity in Black Cohosh (**4-7**). Though the exact mode of action remains a mystery, Black Cohosh appears to act both directly on the tissues of the reproductive apparatus and indirectly through the nervous system. *See Also NERVOUS TENSION; HIGH BLOOD PRESSURE*

**LICORICE ROOT**'s estrogenic activity has been clearly established by experimental investigation (**8-11**), but the exact nature of that effect remains elusive (**12**). Some researchers have tentatively identified beta-sitosterol and stigmasterol as the active principles (**13**), but other steroid chemicals have been identified that may also be responsible for part of the action: estriol (**9**); glizestrone, phytosterol and 22,23-dihydrostigmasterol (**14**). In a typical animal study, castrated mice and infantile rats are administered various Licorice root extracts, after which the effects of the extracts are measured as, for example, by increased uterine weight. In a study involving women who could not ovulate, normal ovulation was successfully induced, by utilizing an extract of Licorice Root (**15**). As a uterine tonic, Licorice root has been used by cultures as divergent as Asia, Europe and North America, and is recognized today as a premier herb for such applications in wholistic medicine. Users of this blend will also benefit from Licorice Root's anti-inflammatory, anti-viral, and detoxification properties, all discussed fully in other chapters. *See Also ARTHRITIS; RESPIRATORY AILMENTS; SKIN; BLOOD PURIFICATION/DETOXIFI-CATION; CIRCULATION; FATIGUE; WEIGHT LOSS; ENVIRONMENTAL POLLUTION; FEVERS & INFECTIONS; THYROID; DETOXIFY/NURTURE; WHOLE BODY; MENTAL ALERTNESS/SENILITY*

**RASPBERRY LEAF** is one of those herbs that just seem to be peculiarly well-suited for women. Its effect can best be described as normalization. Tonus is sometimes viewed as a state of tension. But ideally it is a state of relaxed health, of tissue prepared to deal with stress. Raspberry leaf tempers the effects of hormonal runaway, such as might occur during menstruation, pregnancy and delivery. One study showed that Raspberry leaf prevented the typical hypergrowth effects of chronic gonadotrophin on ovaries and uterus (**16**), while another study demonstrated that Raspberry leaf will, in fact, relax uterine muscles (**17**). In the latter study tea concentrates were tested on several species of animal, with very interesting results. If the smooth muscle of the uterus was "in tone," the water extract of Raspberry leaf relaxed it. If the muscle was relaxed, the herb caused contractions. The relaxing response is probably what makes the herb so valuable in aiding parturition, a use for which this herb has been famous for hundreds of years.

**PASSION FLOWER** is used primarily as a sedative (see NERVOUS TENSION), but, in a related fashion, can be used to calm nerves that get on edge during the periods of hormonal adjustment common to most women (**18**). A related use for Passion Flower is to relieve pain. This analgesic (pain-killing) effect has been demonstrated in laboratory and clinical tests (**19-20**). Together, the analgesic and sedative effects of Passion Flower eliminate many of the discomforts and nervous manifestations associated with menses, parturition and menopause. *See Also NERVOUS TENSION; INSOMNIA*

**CHAMOMILE** possesses a definite and proven uterine tonic property. In one carefully controlled study, Russian researchers were able to isolate and document the tonus effects of several herbal extracts on uterine tissue (from animals). Of those yielding positive results, Chamomile had the greatest activity (**21**). Also well-documented are the mild sedative and anti-inflammatory properties of Chamomile (**22-24**). In one study, for example, mice were given amounts of Chamomile infusions comparable to normal human consumption. The sedative effect was seen in the rapid depression of several behavioral indices of activity (**25**). One can expect a nice positive interaction between the effects of Passion Flower and Chamomile. A few years ago, a symposium was held in Germany during which several papers addressed the tremendous amount of clinical, therapeutic and experimental work that had been done on Chamomile. Of the many therapeutic properties substantiated during this symposium, only a few are listed here: antiinflammatory (due to chamazulene), antispasmotic, carminative, antibacterial, antimycotic, nontoxic, dermatological (**26**). These properties all contribute toward making Chamomile one of the few medicinal plants that still retain a prominent role in traditional medicine. *See Also NERVES & GLANDS*

**FENUGREEK SEED** imparts tonus to the uterus through a general stimulant action (**27**). The seeds also lower blood sugar levels, and dramatically lower cholesterol levels (**28**), probably as a result of their high saponin and fiber content (see CHOLESTEROL REGULATION). While yams are the main source of substances (diosgenin) from which sex hormones are made (see below), Fenugreek seeds, which contain considerable quantities of diosgenin and tigogenin, are currently being cultivated for this purpose (**29-30**). The plant is native to the soils of the Mediterranean countries, where it is often used to stimulate lactation. As a specific for female problems, Fenugreek thus commands a high position. Interestingly, it has also at times been used for male fertility problems. The only modern study into this area, however, suggests that Fenugreek seeds may in fact be spermicidal (**31**). *See Also CHOLESTEROL REGULATION; STOMACH/INTESTINAL*

**BLACK HAW BARK** is an effective treatment for dysmenorrhea, amenorrhea, and threatened abortion (**32**). From a variety of tests on guinea pigs, rats and human uterus, a definite antispasmodic property has been established (**33**). The herb stabilizes tonus and reduces the severity of contractions (**34**). The active principles appear to be the coumarins scopoletin and asculetin, but other constituents have been shown to also be active on the uterine muscle (**35**). Additionally, extracts of whole bark have a sedative effect on the central nervous system (**32**). We would expect this herb to be particularly effective against all forms of menstruation disorders, the anemia of pregnancy, disrupted estrus cycles, and disorders of sexual performance. More research is needed to determine this herb's effectiveness in combatting threatened abortion. However, it was used for this purpose extensively in the 19th century in Canada (**31**) and the United States (**32**), and is still used for that purpose in some parts of Europe, where leading naturopathic physicians enthusiastically endorse it, even using it successfully to counteract the effects of abortificient drugs (**32**).

**SAW PALMETTO BERRY** has had an important place in homeopathic herbal medicine in the United States for about 200 years. It functions as a nutritive tonic, increasing the size and secreting ability of the mammary glands, decreasing ovarian and uterine irritability, relieving dysmenorrhea resulting from lack of tonus, and ameliorating ovarian dysfunction. It is used to treat virtually all diseases of the reproductive system. *See Also INFERTILITY; RESPIRATORY AILMENTS; DIABETES; PROSTATE; NERVES & GLANDS; THYROID; DIGESTION*

**SQUAW VINE** is another of our native American plants that, with the exception of Japan, is practically unknown to the rest of the world. Therefore it has not been investigated in those countries that devote much effort to the investigation of medicinal plants. The herb figured so prominently in the native American medicine and in homeopathic medicine, however, that it has won a place among the most trusted of herbal remedies. *See Also VAGINAL YEAST INFECTION*

**WILD YAM ROOT**'s history could, sadly, have matched that of Squaw Vine, with which it was often combined to help prevent miscarriage, had someone not discovered its steroid constituents. As it was, in 1936 Japanese researchers discovered glycoside saponins of several Mexican Yam species from which steroid saponins, primarily diosgenin, could be derived. These derivatives could then be converted to progesterone, an intermediate in cortisone production. Steroid drugs derived from diosgenin include corticosteroids, oral contraceptives, androgens and estrogens (Yams do not contain, as sometimes believed, full-blown estrogens or other hormones—these substances are produced after four processing steps). Such findings might help explain why, during the previous two centuries of American medicine, Wild Yam roots had successfully been employed in treating dysmenorrhea, ovarian neuralgia and cramps, after pains, and other problems of menses and child-birth. *See Also LIVER DISORDERS*

**KELP** is included in this blend, not only for its considerable nutritive and tonic value, but because it performs one other function of great value for women. It prevents breast cancer (**38**). Mild protection for most people can be expected through use of this blend, but if you suspect you need extra protection or insurance, consider taking supplemental Kelp along with this blend. For more information on the anti-cancer properties of Kelp, see ENVIRONMENTAL POLLUTION. *See Also FEVERS & INFECTIONS; WEIGHT LOSS; FATIGUE; BLOOD PURIFICATION/DETOXIFICATION; HEART; INFERTILITY; PAIN; MENTAL ALERTNESS/ SENILITY; THYROID; CIRCULATION; DIABETES*

## OTHER NUTRIENTS

*The female genito-urinary, sexual and reproductive systems all benefit immensely from the intake of proper and essential nutrients. Individual needs may depart substantially from the following general recommendations.*

### VITAMINS

*(Daily requirements unless otherwise noted)*

*Vitamin A 25,000 I.U.*
Vitamin B1 *25-50 mg*
Vitamin B2 *25-50 mg*
Vitamin B6 *25-50 mg*
Vitamin B12 *up to 50 mcg*
Vitamin C *1,000 mg*
Vitamin D *4,000 I.U.*
Vitamin E *600-800 I.U.*

Folic Acid *400 mcg*
Bioflavanoids
PABA

**MINERALS**

Iron
Iodine
Calcium/Magnesium

**Miscellaneous**

Brewer's yeast
Kelp
Cod Liver Oll
Milk
Wheat germ

# REFERENCES

1. Porcher, F.P Report on the indigenous medical plants of South Carolina." **Transactions of the American Medical Association. Vol II,** 1849.
2. Millspaugh, C.F. **American Medicinal Plants.** Dover Publications, New York, 1974 (1st published in 1892).
3. Felter, H.W. **The Eclectic Materia Medica, Pharmacology and Therapeutics.** Eclectic Medical Pubs, Portland, OR, 1983 (1st published in 1922).
4. Young, J. **American Journal of Medical Science.** 9,310, 1831.
5. Farnsworth, N.R. & Seligman, A.B. "Hypoglycemic plants." **Tile and Till,** 57(3), 52-56, 1971.
6. Benoit, P.S., Fong, H.H.S., Svoboda, G.H. & Farnsworth, N.R. "Biological and phytochemical evaluation of plants. XIV. Antiinflammatory evaluation of 163 species of plant." **Lloydia,** 39(2-3), 160-161, 1976.
7. List, P.H. & Hoerhammer, L. **Hager's Hanbuch der Phaermazeutischen Praxis,** 6 Vols., 169-79, Springer Verlag, Berlin.
8. Sharaf, A., Gomaa, N., El-Camal, M.H.A. "Glycyrrhetic acid as an active estrogenic substance separated from glycyrrhiza glabra (liquorice)." **Egyptian Journal of Pharmaceutical Science,** 16 (2), 245-251, 1975.

9. Costello, C.H. & Lynn, E.V. "Estrogenic substances from plants: glycyrrhiza glabra." **Journal of the American Pharmaceutical Association,** 39, 177-180, 1950.
10. Pointet-Guillot, U. "Contribution a l'etude chimique et pharmacologique de la reglisse, These, Paris, 1958.
11. Murav'ev, I.A., & Kononikhina, N.F. "Estrogenic properties of Gycyrrhiza glabra." **Rastitel'nye Resursy,** 8(4), 490-497, 1972.
12. Dekanski, J.B., Gottfried, S. "Oestrogenic acitivity of enoxolone in rodents." **Journal of Pharmacy and Pharmacology,** 31, 62, 1979.
13. Van Hulle, C. "Ueber die oestrogen Wirkung der Suessholzwurzel." Pharmazie. 25, 260-261, 1970.
14. Lutomski, J. "Chemistry and the therapeutic use of licorice (glycyrrhiza glabra L.)." **Pharmazie in Unserer Zeit,** 12(2), 49-54, 1983.
15. Yaginuma, T, Izumi, R., Yasui, H., Arai, T. & Kawabata, M. "Effect of traditional herbal medicine on serum testosterone levels and its induction of regular ovulation in hyper-androgenic and oligomenorrhetic women." **Nippon Sanka Fujinka Gakkai Zasshi,** 34(7), 939-944, 1982.
16. Kurzepa, S. & Samojlik, E. "The effect of extracts from some Rosaceae plants upon the gonadotrophic and thyrotrophic activities in rat." **Endokrynologia Polska,** 15(2), 143-150, 1963.
17. Burn, J.H. & Withell, E.R. "A principle in rasberry leaves which relaxes uterine muscles." **Lancet,** 2(6149), 1-3, 1941.
18. Lutomski, J. "Die bedeutung der Pasionsblume in der heilkunde." **Pharmazie in unsere Zeit,** 10(2), 45-49, 1981.
19. Ambuhl, H. "Anatomische und chemische untersuchungen an Passiflora coerulea L., und Passiflor incarnata L." Dissertation Number 3830 ETH, Zurich, 1966.
20. Lutomski, J. "Alkaloidy Passiflora incarnata L." **Diss. Institut fur Heilpflanzenforschung,** Poznan. 1960.
21. Shipochliev, T. "Extracts from a group of medicinal plants enhancing uterine tonus." **Veterinary Sciences (Sofia),** 18(4), 94-98, 1981.
22. Breinlich, J. & Scharnagel, K. "Pharmacological properties of the ene-yne dicycloethers from matricaria chamomilla. antiinflammatory , antianaphylactic, spasmolytic, and bacteriostatic activity." **Arzneimittel-Forschungen,** 18(4), 429-431, 1968.
23. Jelicic-Hadzovic, J. & Stern, P. "Azulene and bradykinin." **Arzneimittel-Forschungen,** 22(9), 1210-1211, 1972.

24. Szelenyi, I., Isaac, O. & Thiemer, K. "Pharmacological experiments with components of chamomile. III. Experimental animal studies of the ulcer-protective effect of chamomile." **Planta Medica,** 35(2), 218-227, 1979.
25. Loggia, R.D., Traversa, U., Scarcia, & Tubaro, A. "Depressive effects of Chamomilla recutita (L.) Rausch, tubular flowers, on central nervous system in mice." **Pharmacological Research Communications,** 14(2), 153-162, 1982.
26. Demling, L. **Erfahrungstherapie—spaete Rechtfertigung,** Verlag G. Braun, Karlsruhe, West Germany, 1975.
27. Arbo & Al-Kafawi. **Plant Medica,** 17, 14, 1969.
28. Valette, G. Sauvaire, Y., Baccou, J-C, & Ribes, G. "Hypocholesterolaemic effect of fenugreek seeds in dogs." **Atherosclerosis,** 50, 105-111, 1984.
29. Thomson, W.A.R. **Herbs that Heal.** Charles Scribner's Sons, New York, 1976, pp. 160-161.
30. Sauvaire, Y. & Baccou, J.C. "L'obtention de la diosgenine (25R)-Spirost-5-ene-3Beta-ol—Problemes de l-hydrolyse acide des saponines." **Lloydia,** 41, 247, 1978.
31. Setty, B.S., Kamboj, V.P. Khanna, N.M. "Screening of Indian plants for biological activity. VII. Spermicidal activity of Indian plants." **Indian Journal of Experimental Biology,** 15, 231, 1977.
32. List, P.H. & Hoerhammer, L. **Hagers Handbuch der Pharmazeutischen Praxis.** Volumes 2-5, Springer-Verlag, Berlin.
33. Hoerhammer, L., Wagner,H. & Reinhardt, H. "New methods in pharmacognosy. XI. Chromatographic evaluation of commercial viburnum drugs." **Deutsche Apotheker Zeitung,** 105(40), 1371-1372, 1965.
34. Horhammer, L., Wagner, H. & Reinhardt, H. "Chemistry, pharmacology, and pharmaceutics of the components from viburnam prunifolium and v. opulus." **Botanical Magazine (Tokyo),** 79, 510-525, 1966.
35. Jarboe, C.H., Schmidt, C.M., Nicholson, J.A. & Zirvi, K.A. "Uterine relaxant properties of viburnum." **Nature,** 212(5064), 837, 1966.
36. "Canadian Medicinal Plants. A list." **Canadian Pharmaceutical Journal,** Shuttleworth, ed., Toronto, 1868.
37. Gunn, J.D. **New Domestic Physician,** Moore, Wistach, Keys, Cincinnati, 1857.
38. Teas, J. "The dietary intake of Laminaria, a brown seaweed, and breast cancer prevention." **Nutrition and Cancer** 4(3), 217-223, 1983.

# FEVERS & INFECTIONS

## HERBS

**Form:** Capsule, Tea, Compress, Poultice

**CONTENTS: ECHINACEA root** *(Echinacea augustifolia)*, **MYRRH gum** *(Commiphora myrrha)*, **Goldenseal root** *(Hydrastis canadensis)*, **Licorice root** *(Glycyrrhiza glabra)*, **Blue Vervain** *(Verbena hastata)*, **Cinchona** *(Peruvian bark)*, **Butternut root bark** *(Juglans cinerea)*, **Garlic** *(Allium sativum)* & **Kelp** *(Laminaria, Macrocystis, Ascophyllum)*.

**PURPOSE: To alleviate fevers (general ailments due to common colds and influenza); Infections.**

**Other Applications:** Parasites, amoebic infections.

**USE:** 1. Fevers: 3 capsules, 4 times per day with plenty of liquid. Consider using these blends: BLOOD PURIFICATION/DETOXIFICATION (3 capsules/day), FATIGUE (2-3 capsules/day), and INFLUENZA (2-3 capsules/day).
2. Infections: *Internal*—anywhere from 2 - 12 capsules per day as desired.
   *External*—2-3 capsules may be applied as a poultice or wash to open wounds and sores. Consider adding Chaparral to this poultice.
3. If nausea or diarrhea is present, use the NAUSEA blend according to directions.
4. For cleanses, use 2-3 capsules per day in conjunction with the DETOXIFY/NURTURE blend, as directed.

**Contraindications:**    None.


The symptoms of a body battling against bacterial and viral invaders would be a welcome sign of a healthy defense system, were those symptoms not so painful and irritating. It may be some consolation to know that fever is a sign that the body is "feverishly" manufacturing white blood cells to counterattack the invaders, and it may be comforting to view a sore throat (due to swelling lymph nodes) as a battleground upon which the carcasses of the enemy are strewn. Neither of those imaginative exercises makes the pain more bearable. So we rely on medications such as this blend and the RESPIRATORY AILMENTS blend, and the INFLUENZA blend to treat infections and fevers, and/or to subdue the worst symptoms. This blend kills germs that cause fevers and infections. It increases the body's resistance, increases the body's capacity to withstand a successful invasion, and boosts the body's ability to recuperate. Fevers of all kinds, including the rare typhoid, malaria, and meningitis, have been successfully treated and/or prevented by these herbs. It is hoped that the reader is using good herbal products to not only treat colds and infections but to prevent them as well. During cold weather or other periods of stress, the body requires a well-rounded health regimen, including herbs, to maintain health (**1**).

**ECHINACEA,** one of the primary medicinal agents of the past century, was used to treat common fevers and minor infections, as well as typhoid, meningitis, malaria, diptheria, etc., and is still an expedient treatment of infectious diseases today. It destroys the germs of infection directly, and bolsters the body's defenses by magnifying the white blood cell count. It equalizes body temperature, lowering elevated temperatures, raising subnormal temperatures. It is antiseptic and anesthetic. These properties were all experimentally verified on humans in 19th century studies conducted in major hospitals (**2**). In recent years, research has discovered the mechanisms by which Echinacea may work to prevent infection. One of the primary defense mechanisms of the body is known as the hyaluronidase system (we'll call it the H-system). Hyaluronic acid (HA) is the stuff that occurs in the tissues between cells to "cement" them together. It forms a very effective barrier against infection. There is an enzyme that attacks HA in a way not fully understood. When it does, the HA quickly loses viscosity, like jello turning to water. This is the weak link in the system. If the enzyme is allowed to destroy the integrity of the HA barrier, pathogenic bacteria such as staph and strep penetrate the tissues and make you sick. A similar mechanism is thought to be involved in rheumatism and tumor formation and at the beginnings of malignancy. Echinacea has been shown to prevent the enzyme from dissolving HA (**3-4**). It's that simple. The herb acts to effectively close down one of the major routes of bug-invasion. It inhibits the spread of infection that may have already occurred. A possible mode of action is that Echinacea and HA combine together to form a complex that is resistant to enzyme invasion and that facilitates fibrous connective tissue regeneration (**5-6**). Cortisone-like activity has also been discovered in Echinacea (**7**) that could help account for some of its anti-inflammatory activity. In addition, Echinacea accelerates the production of granulomatous tissue (necessary for healing) and has a stimulating effect on the lymph system (**8**), increasing its ability to carry waste tissue away from areas of infection. Echinacin, the active constituent of Echinacea, exhibits interferon-like activity. It protects cells against virus related diseases, such as herpes, influenza, canker sores, etc. (**8a**). German research on Echinacea has supported all the claims made in this paragraph plus demonstrated another immunostimulating property of the plant: namely, its ability to stimule T-cell activity. This cell is an important mediator in the body's immune system (**8b**). *See Also SKIN DISORDERS; BLOOD PURIFICATION/DETOXIFICATION*

**MYRRH GUM** contains many of the familiar volatile oils, including limonene, eugenol and pinene. These oils make the herb ideally suited for promoting free breathing during congestive colds, and for clearing out mucous-clogged passages throughout the body (**9**). It increases circulation by stimulating capillary activity, restores tone and normal secretion, increases digestion, promotes the absorption and assimilation of nutrients, increases the number of white blood cells, and through all of these means is helpful in treating feverish symptoms like cold skin, weak pulse, and so on (**2,8,10**). *See Also STOMACH/INTESTINAL*

**GOLDENSEAL ROOT** is a proven antibiotic and antiseptic. To avoid repeating the same information, however, a full discussion of these properties is presented in the INFLUENZA chapter.

**LICORICE ROOT**'s effects in regard to fevers and infections are also easy to substantiate. Historically, the herb has been used by many cultures for these purposes, having achieved the status of a major tonic in China (**11**). Licorice root has the ability to prevent and remedy infections, inflammations and fevers. One of the earliest studies along these lines, from China (**12**), found that Licorice root possessed antibacterial activity against several common gram negative intestinal pathogens. Later, in 1979-80, a team of Italian researchers reported a series of experiments in which they discovered several different antiviral mechanisms attributable to licorice root, such as the extracellular destruction of virus particles, the prevention of intracellular 'uncoating', or activation, of infecting viruses, and the impairment of the assembling ability of virus structural components (**13-14**). Recently, a team of scientists in China noted the similarity of action against infectious hepatitis between a Licorice root compound (**20**) and interferon. Their experiments along those lines revealed that Licorice root constituents actually activate the interferon mechanism (**21**). We can expect further study on this mechanism. A United States team of investigators carried out a thorough, very carefully executed study in which they verified Licorice root's antimicrobial properties, especially against staph and mycobacterium smegmatis (**22**). And another impeccable trial, this time from Japan, demonstrated Licorice root to be effective against both an original *staphylococcus aureus* strain that had already been made resistant to penicillin and streptomycin, and against succeeding drug resistant cultures or generations of that strain (which were continuing to develop ever greater resistance to the standard drugs) (**23**). Several Russian and English papers have appeared that underscore the anti-inflammatory property of Licorice root (**15-19**), an effect that is directly related to the herb's corticosteroid-like action. It is an important characteristic for it helps the body deal with the inflammation that often accompanies various infections. *See Also INFERTILITY; WHOLE BODY; ARTHRITIS; THYROID; WEIGHT LOSS; RESPIRATORY AILMENTS; SKIN DISORDERS; FEMALE TONIC; BLOOD PURIFICATION/DETOXIFICATION; CIRCULATION; FATIGUE; DETOXIFY/NURTURE; MENTAL ALERTNESS/SENILITY*

**BLUE VERVAIN** has not received much scientific attention though it has been used for hundreds of years by people in many countries. Hippocrates recommended it for the ague and plague. It has always remained in the background, yielding center stage to the more powerful stimulants, bitters, diuretics and astringents. But in every good herbalist's cabinet one can find Blue Vervain. It is added to many blends to impart its own special stimulant properties. During convalescence, one should be sure to include this herb in the diet. One medical study, carried out in Japan, found that Blue Vervain possessed noticeable anti-inflammatory and analgesic properties (**24**). Those properties are extremely useful to curb infectious swelling and pain. Listed in the National Formulary for ten years in the early 1900's, it was recommended as a diaphoretic (to make a feverish person sweat) and as an expectorant to relieve cold symptoms. During the drug shortages of the Revolutionary War, Blue

Vervain was often used by Army physicians as an emetic and expectorant (**25**). *See Also NERVES & GLANDS*

**CINCHONA,** the primary source for quinine until the drug was synthetically produced, possesses the same antiviral, antimalarial, antipyretic properties as the drug. This equivalency may surprise those who believe that patented, commercialized drugs are superior to natural medicines, but it has been proven. In one classic experiment, rats were injected with an infectious malarial agent and then fed or injected with quinine or fed Cinchona extract. An effective dose of Cinchona extract elicited the same antimalarial activity as an effective dose of quinine (**26**). Cinchona works probably by reducing tissue respiration through a direct influence on the enzymatic processes of the cell. This inhibition leads to a lowering of the nucleoprotein metabolism and the death of microorganisms. Most lower organisms, such as infusoria, are quickly killed by Cinchona; others, like bacteria, cocci, and bacilli, demonstrate variable sensitivity, some being very sensitive, and others very resistive to the herb. Though large doses of Cinchona have a depressant effect on the heart, small amounts are completely harmless. Before the advent of quinine-the drug, Americans used Cinchona not only for malaria and other fevers, but also as a tonic (**27**), and to stimulate the appetite and digestion (**28**). Quinine is a common ingredient in non-prescription remedies for headaches, leg cramps, and colds, and is also found in many gargles (**29**). Further proof of the non-toxic nature of Cinchona is its use in ice cream, baked goods, condiments, soft drinks and candy (**30**). As a historical note, before the discovery of quinine, exports of Cinchona bark from South America to Europe and the United States numbered in the millions of pounds each year.

**BUTTERNUT ROOT BARK** has the distinction of being one of the primary febrifuges used by the pioneers. It fell into disuse with the advent of quinine (and the absence of malaria). It is used in this blend, however, primarily for its mild laxative property. Its inclusion conforms to the principle of balance in herbal blending which states that in blends dealing with combat of infections, fevers and colds, some part of the treatment should be laxative to help the body rid itself of bacteria-laden wastes. *See Also LAXATIVE; PARASITES*

**GARLIC,** appropriately the current best-seller on the anti-fever hit parade, has been celebrated for thousands of years. It was heralded in the Bible, in the literature of ancient Hebrew, Babylonian, Greek and Roman civilizations, and was a favorite fare of the ancient Egyptians, Vikings and Phoenicians. Garlic was described by Virgil in the **Second Idyll,** as a treatment for snake bite, and Hippocrates used it to treat pneumonia and suppurating wounds. All around the world, Garlic has been used to treat such ailments as dysentery, cholera, gastritis, and typhoid fever. Several years ago, Garlic was reported to be more effective than penicillin for the treatment of throat infections (**31**). A 16th century herbalist makes this sanguine claim: "The virtue of this herb is thus. It will unbind all wicked winds within a man's body." Today, we know that Garlic prevents colds and fevers by increasing resistance to infection and stress. In addition, it is extremely nutritious, containing high levels of protein, vitamins A and C, thiamine, and trace minerals including copper, zinc, iron, tin, calcium, potassium, aluminum, sulfur, germanium and selenium. Garlic is a noteworthy antibiotic against bacilli and germs that cause any number of ailments. One mg of its major constituent, allicin, is estimated to equal 15 standard units of penicillin (**32**).Garlic's use during the great plague of Europe was therefore a wise course of action. Toward the end of the 19th century, American and European doctors noted a remarkably high cure rate in tuberculosis patients treated with Garlic. The herb was used successfully in World War I in the treatment of typhus and dysentery, and to prevent septic poisoning and gangrene in battle wounds. Dr. Albert Schweitzer used Garlic effectively against typhus, cholera and typhoid. During this time, in Russia, Garlic earned the appelation of "Russian penicillin." The antibacterial activity of Garlic has been proven against numerous organisms including many forms of *Staph* and *Strep, Brucella, Bacillus, Vibrio, Klebsiella, Proteus, Escherichia, Salmonella, Hafnia, Aeromonas, Citrobacter* and *Providencia* (**33-37**). Antifunal activity has also been shown (**38-42**). Of major significance in the anti-fungal studies was the discovery that Garlic is very effective against *Candida Albicans,* the organism that causes most cases of vaginitis (vaginal yeast infection). Athlete's foot fungus and at least 20 other pathogenic fungi are susceptible to destruction by the antimicrobial property of Garlic. One of the most remarkable studies was recently carried out in China against the usually fatal cryptococcal meningitis. Eleven patients were given Garlic extract orally plus an injection, either intramuscularly or intravenously, over a period of several weeks. Side effects were minimal, and all cases of that terrible disease were successfully treated (**42**). Of equal importance, are the findings of two researchers who independently (one in Japan, the other in Romania) determined that Garlic is able to protect living organisms from influenza virus (**43-44**). That's good to know come next flu season. The above review is but a sample of the available research along these lines, but sufficiently demonstrates the remarkable effectiveness of Garlic in preventing, treating and curing infectious disease. *See Also HIGH BLOOD PRESSURE; PARASITES*

**KELP** counts among its many beneficial properties the ability to ward off infections and fevers. Like Garlic and other herbs in this blend, it works by killing various gram positive and gram negative bacteria, including many of those already enumerated (**45-47**). Most researchers believe that the antibiotic property is due to brominated phenalic compounds in the herb and not to the iodine. In one study, the diets of one of each of seven pairs of monozygotic (identical) twin cows was supplemented with Kelp for seven years. During that period the cows with Kelp-supplemented diets yielded more milk and had a much lower incidence of mastitis than did the controls. Since mastitis in cows is usually caused by unsanitary conditions, the antibiotic property of Kelp was probably responsible for the difference (**48**). In addition to these direct effects, Kelp is, of course, very helpful in terms of supplying nutritional support for the ailing and convalescent patient. *See Also WEIGHT LOSS; FATIGUE; THYROID; CIRCULATION; ENVIRONMENTAL POLLUTION; MENTAL ALERTNESS/SENILITY; PAIN; BLOOD PURIFICATION/DETOXIFICATION; HEART; DIABETES; PROSTATE*

## OTHER NUTRIENTS

*Since appetites often wane during periods of fever and infectious illness when the body's needs are greater than ever, it is very important to supplement the diet whenever possible with good high potency vitamins, minerals and other nutrients. Individual needs may depart substantially from the following general recommendations.*

### VITAMINS

*(Daily requirements unless otherwise noted)*

Vitamin A  *25,000-50,000 I.U.*
Vitamin B Complex
Vitamin B1  *25-100 mg*
Vitamin B2  *25-100 mg*
Vitamin B6  *25-100 mg*
Vitamin C  *3,000-5,000 mg*
　　　　　*500 mg/hour—1st day*
Vitamin D  *400-600 I.U.*

Pantothenic Acid *50 mg*
Niacinamide *50 mg*

**MINERALS**

Calcium/Magnesium
Phosphorus
Potassium
Sodium

**MISCELLANEOUS**

Cod Liver Oil
GLA
Essential Fatty Acid
HCl

# REFERENCES

1. Mowrey, D.B. "Stocking your herb shelves for winter." **Whole Foods,** October, 1984, pp. 37, 53-54.
2. Ellingwood, F. **American Materia Medica, Therapeutics and Pharmacognosy.** Eclectic Medical Publications, Portland, Oregon, 1983.
3. Bonadeo, I., Bottazzi, G. & Lavazza, M. "Echinacina B: polisaccaride attiva dell' Echinacea." **Rev. Ital. Essenze Profumi,** 53, 281-295, 1971.
4. Bonadeo, I. & Lavazza, M. "Echinacina B: suo azione sui fibroblasti." **Rev. Ital. Essenze Profumi,** 54, 195, 1972.
5. Buesing, K.H. "Hyaloronidase inhibition of some natural substances used in therapy." **Arzneimittel-Forschung,** 5(6), 320-322, 1955.
6. Tragni, E., Tubaro, A., Melis, S. & Galli, C.L. "Evidence from two classic irritation tests for an anti-inflammatory action of a natural extract, Echinacina B." **Food And Chemical Toxicology,** 23(2), 317-319, 1985.
7. Keller, H. "Recovery of active agents from aqueous extracts of the species of echinacea." **Ger. 950,674,** Oct 11, 1956.
8. List, P.H. & Hoerhammer, L. **Hagers Handbuch der Pharmazeutischen Praxis.** Volumes 2-5, Springer-Verlag, Berlin.
8. (a) Wacker, A. & Hilbig, A. "Virus inhibition by Echinancea purpurea." **Planta Medica,** 33, 89-102, 1978.
8. (b) Wagner, H. Proksch, A. "An immunostimulating active principle from Echinacea purpurea." **A. Angew. Phytother.,** 2(5), 166-178, 1981.
9. Leung, A.Y. **Encyclopedia of Common Natural Ingredients.** New York, 1980.

10. Tyler, V.E., Brady, L.R. & Robbers, J.E. **Pharmacognosy,** 7th Edition, Lea & Febiger, Philadelphia, 1976.
11. Teeguarden, R. **Chinese Tonic Herbs,** Japan Publications, Inc., Tokyo & New York, 1984.
12. Kou-sheng, L. & Chang, P.W.H. "In vitro antibacterial activity of some common chinese herbs on gram negative intestinal pathogens." **Chinese Medical Journal,** 68, 307-312, 1950.
13. Pompei, R., Pnie, A., Flore, O., Marcialis, M.A., & Loddo, B. "Antiviral activity of glycyrrhizic acid." **Experientia,** 36, 304, 1980.
14. Pompei, R., Flore, O., Marccialis, M.A., Pani, A., & Loddo, B. "Glycyrrhetinic acid inhibits virus growth and inactivates virus particles." **Nature,** 281, 689-690, 1979.
15. Finney, S.H. & Somers, G.F. "The anti-inflammatory activity of glycyrrhetinic acid and derivatives." **Journal of Pharmacology and Pharmacodynamics,** 10(10), 613-620, 1958.
16. Tangri, K.K., Seth, P.K., Parmar, S.S. & Bhargava, K.P. "Biochemical study of anti-inflammatory and anti-arthritic properties of glycyrrhetic acid." **Biochemical Pharmacology,** 14(8), 1277-1281, 1965.
17. Nikitina, S.S. "Data on the mechanism of anti-inflammatory action of glycyrrhizic acid." **Farmakologiia i Toksikologiia,** 29(1), 67-70, 1966.
18. Parmar, S.S., Tangri, K.K., Seth, P.K. & Bhargava, K.P. "Biochemical basis for anti-inflammatory effects of glycyrrhetic acid and its derivatives." **International Congress of Biochemistry,** 6(5), 410, 1967.
19. Nasyrov, K.M. & Lazareva, D.N. "Study of the anti-inflammatory activity of glycyrrhizin acid derivatives." **Farmakologiia i Toksikologiia,** 43(4), 399-404, 1980.
20. Fujisawa, K., Watanabe, Y. & Kimura, K. "Therapeutic approach to chronic active hepatitis with glycyrrhizin." **Asian Medical Journal,** 23, 745-756, 1980.
21. Abe, N. Ebina, T. & Ishida, N. "Interferon induction by glycyrrhizin and glycyrrhetinic acid in mice." **Microbiology and Immunology,** 26(6), 535-539, 1982.
22. Mitscher, L.A., Park, Y.H., Clark, D. & Beal, J.L. "Antimicrobial agents from higher plants. Antimicrobial isoflavanoids and related substances from glycyrrhiza glabra l var typica." **Journal of Natural Products,** 43(2), 259-269, 1980.
23. Mano, D. "Studies on the inhibitory action of plant (licorice root) components on the growth of bacteria. III. A study on the

inhibitory action of radix liquiritiae fractions on bacterial growth and the increased potential of resistance in bacteria." **Japanese Journal of Bacteriology,** 17(12), 938-941, 1962.

24. Sakai, S. "Pharmacological actions of verbena officinalis." **Gifu Ika Daigaku Kiyo,** 11(1), 6-17, 1963.

25. Vogel, V.J. *American Indian Medicine.* Ballantine Books, New York, 1970.

26. Aviado, D.M., Rosen, T., Dacanay, H. & Plotkin, S.H. "Antimalarial and antiarrhythmic activity of plant extracts." **Medicina Experimentalis—International Journal of Experimental Medicine,** 19(2), 79-94, 1969.

27. der Marderosian, A. & Yelvigi, M.S. "Medicine and drugs in colonial America." **American Journal of Pharmacy,** July-August, 113-124, 1976

28. Osol, A., Pratt, R. & Altschule, M.D. **The United States Dispensatory and Physicians' Pharmacology,** 26 ed., J.B. Lippincott Co., Phila.

29. Trease, G.E. & Evans, W.C. **Pharmacognosy,** 11th Ed., Bailliere Tindall, London, 1978.

30. Furia, T.E. & Bellanca, N. **Fenaroli's Handbook of Flavor Ingredients.** The Chemical Rubber Co., Cleveland, Ohio, 1971.

31. Fortunatov, M.N. "Experimental use of phytoncides for therapeutic and prophylactic purpose." **Voprosy Pediatrii i Okhrany Materinstva: Detstva,** 20(2), 55-58, 1952.

32. Cavallito, C.J. & Bailey, J.H. "Allicin, the antibacterial principle of allium sativum. I. Isolation, physical properties and antibacterial action." **Journal of the American Chemical Society,** 66, 1950-1951, 1945.

33. Huddleson, I.F., DuFrain, J., Barrons, K.C., Giefel, M. "Antibacterial substances in plants." **Journal of the American veterinary Medical Association,** 105, 394-397, 1944.

34. Cavallito, C.J. & Bailey, J.H. & Buck, J.S. "The antibacterial principle of allium sativum. III. Its precursor and essential oil of garlic." **Journal of the American Chemical Society,** 67, 1032-1033, 1945.

35. Jezowa, L. Rafinski, T., Wrocinski, T. "Investigations on the antibiotic activity of allium sativum I." **Herba Polonica,** 12, 3, 1966.

36. Sharma, V.D., Sethi, M.S., Kumar, A. & Rarota, J.R. "Antibacterial property of allium sativum Linn.: in vivo and in vitro studies." **Indian Journal of Experimental Biology,** 15(6), 466-468, 1977.

37. Johnson, M.G. & Vaughn, R.H. "Death of salmonella typhimurium and escherichia coli in the presence of freshly reconstituted dehydrated garlic and onion." **Applied Microbiology,** 17, 903-905, 1969.
38. Appleton, J.A., Tansey, M.R. "Inhibition of growth of zoopathogenic fungi by garlic extract." **Mycologia,** 67(4), 882-885, 1975.
39. Tansey, M.R. & Appleton, J.A. "Inhibition of fungal growth by garlic extract." **Mycologia,** 67(2), 409-413, 1975.
40. Barona, F.E. & Tansey, M.R. "Isolation, purification, identification, synthesis of activity of the anticandidal compounds of allium sativum, and a hypothesis for its mode of action." **Mycologia,** 69, 793-824, 1977.
41. Yamada, Y. & Azuma, K. "Evaluation of the in vitro antifungal activity of allicin." **Antimicrobial Agents and Chemotherapy,** 11, 743-749, 1977.
42. Hunan Medical College, China. "Garlic in cryptococcal meningitis. A preliminary report of 21 cases." **Chinese Medical Journal,** 93, 123-126, 1980.
43. Nagai, K. "Experimental studies on the preventive effect of garlic extract against infection with influenza virus." **Japanese Journal of the Association for Infectious Diseases,** 47, 111-115, 1973.
44. Esanu, V. & Prahoveanu, E. "The effect of garlic extract, applied as such or in association with NaF, on experimental influenza in mice." **Revue Roumaine de Medecine, (Serie) Virologie,** 34(1), 11-17, 1983.
45. Mautner, H.G., Gardner, G.M. & Pratt, R. "Antibiotic activity of seaweed extracts." **Journal of the American Pharmaceutical Association,** 42(5), 294-296, 1953.
46. Pratt, R., Mautner, H.G., Sha, Y. & Dufrencoy, J. "Report on antibiotic activity of seaweed extracts." **Journal of the American Pharmaceutical Association,** 40(11), 575-579, 1951.
47. Chenieux, J.C., Verbist, J.F., Biard, J.F., Clement, E., LeBoterff, J., Maupas, P. & Lecocq, M. "Seaweeds of French Atlantic coast with antimitotic compounds." **Planta Medica,** Supplement, 163-169, 1980.
48. Vacca, D.D. & Walsh, R.A. "The antibacterial activity of an extract obtained from Ascophyllum nodosum." **Journal of the American Pharmaceutical Association,** 43, 24-26, 1954.

# HAYFEVER AND ALLERGIES

## HERBS

**Form:** Capsule, Gargle

**CONTENTS:** **CLAY** **(Montmorillonite), Wild Cherry bark** *(Prunus serotina),* **Mullein leaves** *(Verbascum thapsus),* & **Horehound** *(Marrubium vulgare).*

**PURPOSE:** **To prevent the symptoms of allergies: use if you are susceptible to hayfever, asthma, food allergies, chemical allergies, etc.**

**Other Applications:** None.

**USE:** 1. Hayfever: 1 capsule several times per day, starting two weeks before hayfever season. Reduce use to 1 capsule two to three times per day during the season.
2. Food Allergies: 3-4 capsules at first sign (or sooner if possible), and 1 capsule every 1-2 hours during reaction period.
3. Misc. Allergies (dust, animal, etc.): 1-2 capsules every 1-2 hours during exposure to allergen.
4. As a preventative supplement to the RESPIRATORY AILMENT blend.
**NOTE:** Drink 1/2 cup liquid whenever ingesting these capsules.

**Contraindications:** None.

This blend can best be described as preventive. The idea is to stop allergic reactions to inhalant and ingestive allergens before they happen. Antibodies are produced by an initial antigen-antibody reaction that occurs when a substance to which a person is hypersensitive enters the system and comes in contact with plasma cells embedded in the mucosa of the nasopharynx, respiratory and gastrointestinal tract as well as other areas of the lymphatic system. These antibodies await the next intrusion of the offending substance. Unfortunately when that invasion occurs, the body reacts in an extremely overprotective manner, releasing large amounts of histaminic substances which produce the typical reactions of hayfever and allergy. Once the antigen-antibody reaction takes place, there is little that can be done to prevent an allergic reaction. This blend is designed to prevent that reaction from taking place. Remember it will be most effective if used *prior* to as well as *during* hayfever season.

**MONTMORILLONITE CLAY** is highly a*d*sorbent (not a*b*sorbent), and is capable of adsorbing many times its weight and volume in an aqueous medium. The distinction between a*b*sorb and a*d*sorb is important. Absorption is the process by which substances are sucked up into the internal structure of other substances, such as cells. The foreign substances must actually penetrate a cell membrane or some other such barrier, and must usually undergo some sort of chemical change before they are allowed (or forced) to enter. Adsorption, on the other hand requires only that substances be able to stick to the outside of the adsorbent medium. This usually means that the two substances have opposite electrical (ionic) charges, or that some other physical or chemical bond be readily formable. The difference may seem a slight one, but the critical factor is the amount of *time* it takes the two processes to occur. Absorption is relatively slow, and would therefore allow allergens to elicit an allergic reaction before they were neutralized. Adsorption is a very rapid process, almost instantaneous in certain cases. By quickly neutralizing allergens before these foreign invaders can attach themselves to blood cells, adsorptive surfaces prevent the allergic reaction. In addition, any histamine produced by allergens that "got away" could also be rapidly adsorbed. And that is the purpose of the clay. Montmorillonite (bentonite) clay has a predominantly negative charge that is capable of attracting many kinds of positively charged particles. However, the bonding structure of this substance is relatively weak. Sodium and calcium ions (charged particles) in the lattice (step-ladder) structure of the clay are easily displaced by other, smaller positive ions, such as potassium and magnesium. Therefore, it can attract even positively charged particles. As if that were not enough, water soluble allergens are also bound up by the clay due to its intense hydrophyllic (water-loving) nature. Therefore, to ingest bentonite in a pre-hydrated gel form would be a mistake if you are trying to prevent allergies, since the gel would not be able to adsorb many more allergen-bearing water molecules. The substantiation of these facts comes from several different sources (e.g., **1-5**). The quality of the clay is important (**6**), with poorer clays having high proportions of kaolinite, illite, calcium-based bentonite, and attapulgite, and the better clays being predominantly sodium monmorillonite. The difference is the degree of ion exchange capacity—the more, the better.

**WILD CHERRY BARK** is an excellent calming and soothing agent for irritated mucosal surfaces, but would be of little value during an actual allergic reaction. In this blend its primary action is to soothe any mildly irritated surfaces that result from allergens escaping the adsorptive action of the clay. *See Also RESPIRATORY AILMENTS*

**MULLEIN LEAF** provides an ounce of mucilaginous protection to mucous surfaces, thereby inhibiting the absorption of allergens through those membranes. During a particularly strong exposure to a potent allergen, this bit of protection may make the difference between all allergenic particles being adsorbed or a few making it through and creating distress. *See Also RESPIRATORY AILMENTS; HEMORRHOIDS*

**HOREHOUND** affects the respiration directly by dilating vessels (**7**) and acting as a serotonin antagonist (**8**). It should help alleviate any respiratory distress that occurs. Be sure to also use the blend for RESPIRATORY AILMENTS should distress continue or get worse.

## OTHER NUTRIENTS

*Many of us have found that we can build considerable resistance to hayfever and allergy by increasing our intake of any of several vitamins and other nutrients, such as vitamins A, C and Pantothenic acid, bee pollen, and essential fatty acids. Individual requirements may depart greatly from the following recommendations.*

## VITAMINS

*(Daily requirement unless otherwise noted)*

Vitamin A *25,000-50,000 I.U.*
Vitamin B Complex
Vitamin B1 *25-50 mg*
Vitamin B2 *25-50 mg*
Vitamin B6 *25-100 mg*
Vitamin B12 *10 mcg*
Vitamin C *1,000-1,500 mg*
Vitamin D *600 I.U.*
Vitamin E *400-800 I.U.*
Pantothenic acid *150-200 mg*
Choline *1,000 mg*
Inositol *1,000 mg*
Niacinamide *50 mg*

## MINERALS

Calcium/Magnesium
Phosphorous
Manganese
Potassium
Sodium

## MISCELLANEOUS

Bee Pollen
Liver
HCl

## REFERENCES

1. Erschoff, B.H. & Bajwa, G.S. "Physiological effects of dietary clay supplements." Final report on contract number NAS 9-3905, 1965, available from NASA Manned Spacecraft Center, Houston, TX.
2. Smith, R.R. "Recent Advances in nutrition: clay in trout diets." Presented at the USTAFA Convention, no date.
3. Britton, R.A., Dolling, D.P. & Klopfenstein, T.J. "Effect of complexing sodium bentonite with soybean meal or urea in vitro ruminal ammonia release and nitrogen retention in ruminants." **Journal of Animal Science,** 46, 1738, 1978.

4. Quisenberry, J.H. & Bradly, J.W. "Sodium bentonite feeding experiments." **Feedstuffs,** 36, 23, 1964.
5. Rindsig, R.B., Schultz, L.H. & Shook, G.E. "Effect of addition of bentonite to high grain rations which depress milk fat percentage." **Journal of Dairy Science,** 52, 1770, 1969.
6. Lacy, W.J. "Decontamination of radioactively contaminated water by slurrying with clay." **Industrial and Engineering Chemistry,** 45(5), 1061-1065, 1954.
7. Karryev, M.O., Bairyev, C.B., & Ataeva, A.S. "Some therapeutic properties and phytochemistry of common horehound." **Izvestiya Akademiya Nauk Turkmenskoi SSR, Seriya Biologicheskikh Nauk,** 3, 86-88, 1976.
8. Cahen, R. "Pharmacologic spectrum of marrubium vulgare." **Comptes Rendus des Seances de la Societe de Biolgie et de ses Filiales (Paris)** 164(7), 1467-1472, 1970.

# HEART

**HERBS**

**Form:** Capsule.

**CONTENTS: HAWTHORN berries** *(Crataegus oxyacantha),* **MOTHERWORT** *(Leonurus cardiaca),* **Rosemary leaves** *(Rosmarinus officinalis),* **Kelp** *(Laminara, Macrocystis, Ascophyllum)* & **Cayenne** *(Capsicum annum).*

**PURPOSE: Nutritional tonic for the heart.**

**Other Applications:** The use of this blend may help prevent and/ or reduce the severity of and/or reduce the symptoms of many heart disease-related conditions, including atherosclerosis, angina, neuritis, neuralgia, rheumatism, liver problems, arteriosclerosis, coronary heart disease (prevention only), congestive heart disease, palpitations, etc. Consult your physician for any of these conditions. Use this blend as a tonic in long term health programs; **do not expect it to "cure" acute episodes.**

**USE:** 1. As Heart tonic: 2-4 capsules per day.
2. Examples of complete heart support programs:

## HEART SUPPORT PROGRAMS   *(# caps/day)*

|  | Heart Blend | Hi Blood Pressure | Diuretic Blend | Whole Body Tonic Blend | Cholesterol Reg. Blend | Circ. Blend | Fatigue Blend |
|---|---|---|---|---|---|---|---|
| Maintain Cardiac Health | 2-4 | 1-2 | --- | 2-3 | 2-4 | 0-2 | 0-3 |
| High Blood Pressure | 2-4 | 2-4 | 0-2 | 1-3 | 2-4 | 0-2 | 0-3 |
| Coronary Heart Disease | 2-4 | 0-3 | 0-4 | 0-3 | 1-3 | 2-4 | 1-3 |
| Edematous Conditions | 2-4 | 1-3 | Acute; 5-8 Chronic: 1-3 | 2-4 | 1-3 | 1-3 | 2-4 |
| Postoperative Recovery | 2-4 | 0-3 | 0-2 | 4-6 | 0-3 | 2-4 | 4-6 |

**Contraindications:**   None. This is an extremely safe preparation. But it may potentiate the action of digitalis. If you are under the care of a physician, keep him informed about your program so that doses of standard medications may be adjusted as necessary. For cardiac health, Rosemary and Motherwort are better used in a blend like this, than as single products. See Appendix A for a discussion of Cayenne.

Although the heart is perhaps the strongest muscle in the body, it takes remarkably little to put it out of commission. Block any main artery leading to it and the heart quits working, usually to the accompaniment of a great deal of agony. Blood clots and the gradual constricting of blood vessels are the most common means of killing the heart. Along the way to total heart failure, one can pick up any number of painful and dangerous diseases, including hypertension, angina and arteriosclerosis. This is an interesting blend of herbs designed as a genuine tonic, not just a momentary stimulant. The "heart" of this blend is the Hawthorn berry, boasting a century of effective application in cardiovascular disease, including angina, edema, dyspnea, hypertrophy, valvular problems, heart murmur, arrhythmia, brachycardia, mitral lesions resulting from rheumatism, hypertension, and so on. Motherwort and Rosemary have also been experimentally shown to possess mild cardiotonic and sedative activity, but are more effective when combined with other plants with similar pharmacological activity. Cayenne promotes general increased circulation and catalyzes the chemical reactions of the other herbs. The combining of powdered Cayenne and Hawthorn in a single capsule produces a special kind of synergism that augments the cardiotonic activity of both.

**HAWTHORN BERRY,** in the consensus of controlled laboratory and clinical experimentation of several countries (including Poland, Germany, Austria, Russia, Czechoslovakia, Bulgaria and the United States), functions by 1) peripheral vasodilation, i.e., by dilating the blood vessels away from the heart, thereby lowering the blood pressure and reducing the burden placed on the heart; 2) very mild dilation of coronary vessels; 3) increased enzyme metabolism in the heart muscle, leading to better coronary health, and 4) increased oxygen utilization by the heart (**1-6**). One study measured the effect of Hawthorn Berry on oxygen utilization by the heart during exercise. Using over 50 patients with coronary perfusion disorders who were receiving treatment in a sanatorium, the researcher found a 77% reduction in oxygen utilization with the herb, compared to a 25% reduction with standard forms of treatment (**1**). The study thereby confirmed the oxygen-saving effect of Hawthorn extract on the heart muscle under stress. In another study on human patients with primary heart disease, Hawthorn extract produced an improvement in almost all cases, as determined by a normalization of heart dynamics, i.e., the mechanical efficiency of the heart muscle. In patients with secondary heart disease the effect was not as great in terms of the number of cases helped, but significant effects were seen in those cases that were helped. The herb also helped patients whose heart disease was caused by hepatitis or other liver disease. The authors concluded that the enhancement and normalization of heart dynamics strongly suggested a positive effect of Hawthorn on the strength of heart contractions (**2**). Similar findings are reviewed by Ullsperger (**3**). Another property of Hawthorn was investigated by a Hungarian team that used dogs to demonstrate marked vasodilatory action and lowering of peripheral resistance to blood flow (**4**). Other experimentally verified properties of Hawthorn include the following: destruction of experimentally-induced blockade of anaerobic glycolysis, a condition that typifies some forms of heart disease caused by enzyme insufficiency (**7**); a quickening of the heart beat in patients with chronic cardiac insufficiency (**8,13**); and an increase in cardiac output and efficiency with an increase in heart rate and pulse amplitude (**9-12**). In spite of these facts, and its acceptance in other countries, and its well-known absence of side effects, Hawthorn has not received much attention by the modern medical establishment in the United States.

It is wise to understand the differences between Hawthorn Berry and digitalis. It used to be assumed that both belonged to the sams class of agents. But that hypothesis has been totally refuted by studies showing, for example, that Hawthorn may partly antagonize undesirable properties of digitalis (**13**). In addition, Hawthorn enhances pulse and positively potentiates the force of muscular contractions (**14**). It also enhances cardiac output or performance in rats as measured by stress swimming trials (**15-16**), and on isolated frog heart it has a tonic and normalizing action (**3**). Hawthorn differs from digitalis also in that it lowers the blood pressure through dilation of peripheral vessels not through a direct action on the heart (**17**). Hence, it preserves critical reflexive blood pressure regulation. In man, Hawthorn acts even on the healthy heart, to increase cardiac activity. However, in heart disease, especially cardiac insufficiency, Hawthorn appears to have a less immediate effect than digitalis. After longer periods of use, subjective betterment accompanied by objective measurable improvement in tonus and regulation of cardiac activity are observed with Hawthorn (**18**). Unlike digitalis, Hawthorn exhibits an absence of cumulative activity; it appears to assume a position somewhere between digitalis and adrenalin. Another important finding is the apparent synergism between Hawthorn Berry and digitalis, as suggested by the fact that heart tissue pretreated with either one becomes sensitized to the other, so that only about half the normal dose of the second is required to obtain normal results (**19**).

**MOTHERWORT** is one of those plants that has somehow found its way into native medical lore in every corner of the earth from Russia to Rumania, from America to Asia. The names given to it reveal that people everywhere recognize its principle uses. For where it isn't called Mother herb or Mother weed, etc., it is called Heart wort, Heart gold, Heart heal or Heart herb, etc. These names underscore the two main strengths of the herb: a uterine tonic (due to the alkaloid content) and a cardiac tonic (due to the glycoside content). In addition, the herb is often used to check diarrhea (due to the tannin content). As a cardiac tonic, Motherwort has been shown to be hypotensive (**20-22**), sedative (**23-25**) and antispasmodic. It calms palpitations and normalizes heart function in general. Recently, Motherwort extract was shown to inhibit myocardial cells, improve mesenteric circulation and increase coronary perfusion, in other words, to improve several aspects of coronary health (**26-27**).

**ROSEMARY LEAF** contains rosmaricine, the derivatives of which possess considerable smooth muscle stimulant activity (and some analgesic activity) (**28**). The herb possesses valuable aromatic essentials oils that calm and sooth irritated nerves and upset stomach, and extinguish strenuous anxiety. Rosemary is also very high in minerals, such as calcium, magnesium, phosphorus, sodium and potassium, that are required by nerves and cardiac muscle for proper functioning. *See Also PAIN*

**KELP** makes several contributions to this blend, but the three major effects of interest are nutritive (**29**), antibiotic (**30**) and hypotensive (**31**). In its own way, each of these properties enhances the cardiotonic effectiveness of the blend. The hypotensive principle is most important. The preparation "kombu", the blades of various *Laminaria* species, has been employed as a hypotensive agent in Japanese botanical medicine for many years. Research interest in this product picked up not too long ago when one investigator found that human hypertensive patients who drank "kombu" experienced significant improvement in blood pressure readings, subjective well-being, and cardiac efficiency, without any side effects (**32**). Following that study, other studies repeatedly documented the effect in humans (**33**), rabbits, rats and other animals (**34**). The active principles are believed to be laminine and histamine, though evidence exists that other cardiotonic principles may be present in various species of Kelp that find their way into the "kombu" preparation (**35-36**). With so much good evidence of hypotensive and cardiotonic benefit, it is lamentable that only a few proprietary herbal blends for the heart contain Kelp. *See Also CIRCULATION; FEVERS & INFECTIONS; WEIGHT LOSS; FATIGUE; BLOOD PURIFICATION/DETOXIFICATION; PAIN; INFERTILITY; MENTAL ALERTNESS/SENILITY; ENVIRONMENTAL POLLUTION; THYROID; DIABETES*

**CAYENNE** is the primary stimulant in the blend. Its presence assures the delivery of the other active principles to the vital systems of the body. In addition, it does contain important nutrients for the health of the circulatory system (**36**), such as alpha-tocopherols, vitamin C, minerals and other nutrients.

## OTHER NUTRIENTS

*The heart, like other muscle tissue, requires adequate nutrition in order to grow and function properly. The following recommendations for dietary supplementation are meant as guidelines only. Substantial individual differences will require departure from them.*

**VITAMINS**

*(Daily requirements unless otherwise noted)*

Vitamin A *25,000 I.U. minimum*
Vitamin B Complex
Vitamin B12 *25 mcg*
Vitamin B1 *25-100 mg*
Vitamin B2 *25-100 mg*
Vitamin B6 *25-100 mg*
Vitamin C *1,00-3,000 mg*
Vitamin D
Vitamin E *200-600 I.U.*
Bioflavanoids *300-600 mg*
Niacinamide *100 mg*
Choline *1,000 mg*
Inositol *1,000 mg*
PABA
Pantothenic acid

**MINERALS**

Iodine
Potassium
Calcium/Magnesium
Chromium
Zinc
Phosphorous

**MISCELLANEOUS**

Essential Fatty Acids
GLA
Lecithin
Brewer's Yeast

# REFERENCES

1. Kandziora, J. "Crataegutt-wirkung bei koronaren durchblutung-sstoerungen." **Muenchener Medizinischer Wochenschrift,** 6, 295-298, 1969.
2. Echte, W. "Die Einwirkung von Weissdorn-extrakten auf die dynamik des menschlichen herzens." (The effect of Hawthorn

extracts on the dynamics of the human heart). **Aerztliche Forshung,** 14(11), I/560-566, 1960.

3. Ullsperger, R. "Vorlaufige mitteilung ueber den coronargefaesse erweiternden wirkkoerper aus weissdorn." (Preliminary communication concerning a coronary vessel dilating principle from hawthorn). **Pharmazie,** 6(4), 141-144, 1951.
4. Hammerl, H., Kranzl, C., Pichler, O. & Studlar, M. "Klinisch experimentelle stoffwechseluntersuchungen mit einem crataegus extrakt." (Clinical and experimental investigations on metabolism with an extract of Crataegus). **Aerztliche Forshung,** 21(7), 261-270, 1967.
5. Kovach, A.G.B., Foldi, M. & Fedina, L. "Die Wirkung eines extraktes aus Crataegus oxyacantha auf die durchstromung der coronarien von hunden." (The effect of extracts from C. oxyacantha on the coronary circulation of dogs). **Arzneimittelforschung,** 9(6), 1959.
6. Mann, D. "Appropriate cardiovascular therapy: clinical and experimental study of the action of an injectable preparation of crataegus." **Zeitschrift fuer die Gesamte Innere Medizin und ihre Grenzgebiete,** 18(4), 145-151, 1963.
7. Koehler, U. **Cardiologia,** 31, 512, 1957.
8. Schittich, H. Mittl. Dr. W. Schwabe, "Aus unserer Arbeit", 2, 1957.
9. Koppermann, E. Aerztl. Forschg., 12, I/125, 1958.
10. Rewerksi, W., Tadeusz, P., Rylski, M. & Lewak, S. "Pharmacological properties of oligomeric procyanidin crataegus oxyacantha (hawthorn)." **Arzneimittel-Forschungen,** 21(6), 886-888, 1971.
11. Rewerksi, W. & Lewak, S. "Pharmacological properties of flavan polymers isolated from hawthorn (crataegus oxyacantha)." **Arzneimittel-Forschungen,** 17(4), 490-491, 1967.
12. Rewerksi, W. & Lewak, S. "Hypotonic and sedative polyphenol and procyanidin extracts from hawthorn." **Ger. Offen., 2, 145,211.** 1970.
13. Hockerts, T. & Muelke, G. "The coronary effect of aqueous extracts of Crataegus." **Arzneimittel-Forschungen,** 5, 755-757, 1955.
14. Wezler, **Arzneimittel-Forschungen,** 8, 175-177, 1958.
15. Boehm, K. "Results of investigation on crataegus. II. Animal experiments with total extracts and isolated active compounds." **Arzneimittel-Forschungen,** 6, 35-38, 1956.
16. Muth, H.W. "Studies on the vasoactive effects of Cratemon preparations." **Therapie Der Gegenwart,** 115(2), 242-255, 1976.

17. Boehm, K. **ArzticheForschgung,** 9, 442-445, 1955.
18. Fiedler, U. & Hildebrand, G. **Arzneimittel-Forschungen,** 3, 436-439, 1953.
19. Bersin, T., Mueller, A. & Schwarz, H. "Substances contained in crataegus oxyacantha. III. A heptahydroxyflavan glycoside." **Arzneimittel-Forschungen,** 5, 490-491, 1955.
20. Arustamova, F.A. "Hypotensive effect of leonaurus cardiaca on animals in experimental chronic hypertension." **Izvestiya Akademii Nauk Armyanski SSR, Biologicheski Nauki,** 16(7), 47-52, 1963.
21. Erspamer, L.V. "Pharmacology of leonurus cardiaca and leonurus marrubiastrum L." **Archives Internationales Pharmacodynamie et de Therapie,** 76, 132-152, 1948.
22. Isaev, I., & Bojadzieva, M. "Obtaining galenic and neogalenic preparations and experiments for the isolation of an active substance from leonurus cardiaca." **Nauchnye Trudy Visshiia Meditsinski Institut (Sofia),** 37(5), 145-152, 1960.
23. Kubota, S., & Nakashima, S. "The study of leonurus sibericus L. II. Pharmacological study of the alkaloid 'leonurin' isolated from leonurus sibericus L." **Folia Pharmacologica Japonica,** 11(2), 159-167, 1930.
24. Polyakov, N.G. "A study of the biological activity of infusions of valerian and motherwort and their mixtures." **Information of the first all Russian Session of Pharmacists,** Moscow, 319-324, 1964.
25. Schramm, G. **Planta Medica (Stuttgart),** 6, 39, 1958.
26. Xia, Y. X. "The inhibitory effect of Motherwort extract on pulsating myocardial cells in vitro." **Journal of Traditional Chinese Medicine,** 3(3), 185-188, 1983.
27. Zhang, C., et. al. "Studies on actions of extract of motherwort." **Journal of Traditional Chinese Medicine,** 2(4), 267, 1982.
28. Boido, A, Sparatore, F, Biniecka, M. "N-substituted derivatives of rosmaricine." **Studi Sassaresi, Sezione 2,** (Italian), 53(5-6), 383-393, 1975.
29. Binding, G.J. & Moyle, A. **About Kelp.** Thorsons Publishers Ltd. Wellingborough, England, 1974.
30. Biard, J.F., Verbist, J.F., Boterff, J., Rages, G. & Lecocq, M.M. "Seaweeds of French Atlantic coast with antibacterial and antifungal compounds." **Plant Medica,** Supplement , 136-151, 1980.
31. Funayama, S., & Hikino, H. "Hypotensive principle of laminaria and allied seaweeds." **Planta Medica,** 41, 29-33, 1981.
32. Kameda, J. "Medical studies on seaweeds. I." **Fukushima Igaku Zasshi,** 11, 289-309, 1961.

33. Ozawa, H., Gomi, Y. & Otsuki, I. "Pharmacological studies on laminine monocitrate." **Yakugaku Zasshi,** 87(8), 935-939, 1967.
34. Kameda, J. "Medical studies on seaweeds. II. Influence of tangle administration on experimental rabbit atherosclerosis produced by cholesterol feeding." **Fukushima Igaku Zasshi,** 10, 251, 1960.
35. Kosuge, T., Nukaya, H., Yamamoto, T. & Tsuji, K. "Isolation and identification of cardiac principles from laminaria." **Yakugaku Zasshi,** 103(6), 683-685, 1983.
36. Searl, P.B., Norton, T.R. * Lum, B.K.B. "Study of a cardiotonic fraction from an extract of the seaweed, Undaria pinnatifida. **Proceedings of the Western Pharmacology Society,** 24, 63-65, 1981.
37. Kanner, J., Harel, S. & Mendel, H. "Content and stability of alpha-tocopherol in fresh and dehydrated pepper fruits (Capsicum annum L.)." **Journal of Agriculture and Food Chemistry,** 27(6), 1979.

# HEMORRHOIDS/ASTRINGENT

## HERBS

**Form:** Capsule, Topical, Sitz Bath

**CONTENTS: SLIPPERY ELM** *(Ulmus vulva),* **WITCH HAZEL** *(Hamamelis virginiana),* **Mullein** *(Verbascum thapsus),* **Wild Alum** *(Geranium maculatum),* **Goldenseal root** *(Hydrastis canadensis).*

**PURPOSE: To soothe and heal hemorrhoids; and an effective general astringent for other purposes.**

**Other Applications:** Varicose veins; phlebitis.

**USE:** 1. Hemorrhoids, internal: 2-4 capsules per day.
2. Hemorrhoids, external: Mix with vasoline and apply directly to affected area.
3. Astringent, internal: 1-2 capsules as desired.
4. Astringent, external: Make strong tea or poultice and apply to desired area, except eyes.
5. To supplement the MENSTRUATION Blend: 1-2 capsules per day.
6. Supplement this blend with the LIVER PROBLEMS and DIGESTION blends when treating hemorrhoids.

**Contraindications:** None.

Hemorrhoids are enlarged veins in the mucous membrane in the rectal area caused by straining against hard, dry stools, by pressure on the veins from an enlarged uterus, by liver disorders, by heart disorders, or by tumors. Relief from the concomitant itching, bleeding, pain and general discomfort is obtained by compresses, sitz baths, analgesic ointments, and by ingesting capsules of herbs that attempt to tone up and remedy the situation from the inside out, by soothing inflamed and sore tissues, shrinking the swollen veins and toning up the body to remove the various causes of hemorrhoids. Each herb in this blend has a history of imparting hemorrhoidal relief. Some of the above herbs have found their way into modern ointments and medications, and this blend can certainly be used in any of the afore-mentioned sitz baths and compresses.

**SLIPPERY ELM BARK** is used both in poultices and internally to soothe irritated mucous membranes. One early American ethnobotanist described the various uses for Slippery Elm that he observed among the Indians and among the pioneers and settlers of the West as follows: urinary and bowel complaints, sore throat, scurvy, diarrhea, dysentery, cholera infantum, nutritious food, externally for ulcers, tumors, swellings, chillblains, burns and sores (**1**). In all of these uses, the demulcent property of the herb was the therapeutic agent. Slippery Elm was not highly recommended during the last century for hemorrhoids, for it was felt that this particular ailment should be treated primarily with astringents. One exception, a 19th century eclectic physician recommended an external application of Slippery Elm for hemorrhoids (**2**), but this is a rare reference. Modern works are more willing to include the treatment of hemorrhoids as within the realm of demulcents. Certainly, the mucilaginous property of the plant makes it an ideal application for hemorrhoids, both internally and externally. *See Also RESPIRATORY AILMENTS; BONE-FLESH-CARTILAGE*

**WITCH HAZEL LEAF** use began with the Indians, and was subsequently adopted by the white community. Now it is the premier treatment for hemorrhoids (**3-4**), finding its place in many currently available hemorrhoid preparations. Its effectiveness is due mainly to its very astringent nature, which, in turn has been attributed to its high content of tannic acid. However, a tannin free Witch Hazel water is also very astringent, so there must be other active principles in the plant. As usual, the whole is better than any of the parts. What laboratory tests have been done, show that Witch Hazel lowers blood pressure, decreases renal volume, accelerates respiration and inhibits peristalsis, indicating a primary effect on the venal system (**5**). This action would help explain why it works so well on hemorrhoids and other venous sicknesses like varicose veins and phlebitis (**6**). Witch Hazel leaf is also bacteriostatic to those surfaces that are washed by it, as has been demonstrated in controlled laboratory studies (**6a-7**). *See Also VAGINAL YEAST INFECTION*

**MULLEIN LEAF,** a demulcent, is used externally in poultices and internally in capsules to soothe irritated mucous membranes. The leaf yields a peculiar fatty matter that reduces swelling and pain. It was recommended by Dioscorides several hundred years ago, and the technique has survived ever since. Even though the plant was introduced to American soil from Europe, many North American Indian tribes used it extensively, including Catawbas, Choctaws, Creeks, Potawatomis and Menominees (**8**). In India, Mullein has enjoyed good popularity not only as a demulcent, but also as a bacteriostatic. In that country, and a few others, Mullein has been used to treat tuberculosis for centuries. That practice has found substantiation in laboratory tests wherein Mullein significantly inhibited *mycobacterium tuberculosis* (**9**). *See Also RESPIRATORY AILMENTS; ALLERGY*

**ALUM ROOT,** or Cranesbill root, a strong astringent, was introduced to medicine by the American Indians. Knowledgeable American physicians still use it to reduce inflammation of mucous membranes, curb irritation of hemorrhoidal tissue and to restore venous health. It is an especially powerful astringent for passive bleeding, as occurs in hematuria, hemoptysis and menorrhagia, and has a potent healing effect on the entire gastrointestinal tract. It came into use as a mouthwash for canker sores in the last century. Its use as a treatment for hemorrhoids was introduced to white physicians by the Meskwakis. An early ethnobotanist wrote, "This root is accounted a great medicine by the Meskwaki generally. It has many varied uses among them. It is used to cure sore gums and pyorrhoea, and to stop teeth from aching. It is also a cure for neuralgia. Its greatest use is in curing piles and hemorrhoids. A poultice of the pounded root is bound upon the anus to cause protruding piles to recede." (**10**) It was official in the USP from 1820-1916, and in the NF from 1916-1936. Like Mullein, it was found to be active against tuberculosis bacteria (**9**). *See Also MENSTRUATION*

**GOLDENSEAL ROOT** is, of course, used for many different complaints, hemorrhoids being just one of them. However, it is unclear just how Goldenseal alleviates this condition. One clue is provided by studies that found Goldenseal to constrict peripheral blood vessels (**5, 11-12**). A review of the other sections on Goldenseal in this book will reveal that the herb has profound effects on all parts of the gastrointestinal tract, as well as related systems. Whatever the mechanism, the herb has been successfully used for a couple of hundred years in the United States to reduce the inflammation and pain of hemorrhoidal tissue. *See Also STOMACH/INTESTINAL; INFLUENZA; EYES; VAGINAL YEAST INFECTION; FEVERS & INFECTIONS*

## OTHER NUTRIENTS

*Use the various nutrients listed below to provide the building blocks for tissue repair, the elimination of infection and reduction of discomfort. Individual needs may depart substantially from these general recommendations.*

### VITAMINS

*(Daily requirements unless otherwise noted)*

Vitamin A *25,000 I.U.*
Vitamin B Complex
Vitamin B1 *25-100 mg*
Vitamin B2 *25-100 mg*
Vitamin B6 *25-100 mg*
Vitamin C *1,000-3,000 mg*
Vitamin D *400 I.U.*
Vitamin E *600 I.U.*
Bioflavonoids

### MINERALS

Calcium/Magnesium
Zinc

### MISCELLANEOUS

Fluids

## REFERENCES

1. Rafinesque, C.S. **Medical fora or manual of medical botany of the United States,** Vol I., 1828, p. 15.

2. Felter, H. W. **The Eclectic Materia Medica, Pharmacology and Therapeutics.** Eclectic Medical Publications, Portland, Oregon, 1983 (first published 1922).
3. Trease, G.E. & Evans, W.C. **Pharmacognosy,** 11th Ed., Bailliere Tindall, London, 1978.
4. **The Dispensatory of the United States of America,** 23rd Ed., Lippincott, Philadelphia, 1943.
5. List, P.H. & Hoerhammer, L. **Hagers Handbuch der Pharmazeutischen Praxis.** Volumes 2-5, Springer-Verlag, Berlin.
6. Mockle, J.A. **Contributions a l'etude des plante medicinales du Canada.** Paris ed. Jouve, p. 63.
6a.D'Amico, M.L. "Ricerche sulla presenza di sostanze ad azione antibiotica nelle piante superiori." **Fitoterapia,** 21(1), 77-79, 1950.
7. Schaufelberger, D. & Hostettmann, K. "On the molluscicidal activity of tannin containing plants." **Planta Medica,** 48, 105-107, 1983.
8. Vogel, V.J. **American Indian Medicine.** Ballantine Books, New York, 1970.
9. Fitzpatrick, F.K. "Plant substances active against mycobacterium tuberculosis." **Antibiotics and Chemotherapy,** 4(5), 528-536, 1954.
10. Smith, H. **Ethnobotany of the Meskwaki.** Bulletin of Public Museum of Milwaukee 4, 189-274, 1928.
11. Genest, K. & Hughes, D.W. "Natural products in canadian pharmaceuticals." **Canadian Journal of Pharmaceutical Sciences,** 4(2), 41-45, 1969.
12. Ikram, M. "A review of the chemical and pharmacological aspects of genus berberis." **Planta Medica,** 28, 353-358, 1975.

# INFERTILITY

## HERBS

**Form:** Capsule, Tea

**CONTENTS: DAMIANA leaves** *(Turnera aphrodisiaca)*, **GIN-SENG (Siberian)** *(Eleutherococcus senticosus)*, **Sarsaparilla root** *(Smilax officinalis)*, **Saw Palmetto berries** *(Serenoa serrulata)*, **Licorice root** *(Glycyrrhiza glabra)*, & **Kelp** *(Laminara, Macrocystis, Asocphyllum)*.

**PURPOSE: To help assist fertility; To help ameliorate many forms of impotence and related problems.**

**Other Applications:** Hot flashes, vaginal-uterine infections, general tonic, arthritis, rheumatism, menstrual problems.

**USE:** 1. Infertility: 3-6 capsules per day. For best results use every day.
2. In conjunction with the WHOLE BODY TONIC blend, use 2 capsules of each per day.
3. For Hot Flashes: Take one capsule several times daily during critical periods. Supplement with 3-6 capsules per day of the FEMALE TONIC Blend.
4. If using blends VAGINAL YEAST INFECTION or FEMALE TONIC Blends for general female complaints, supplement with 2-3 capsules per day of this blend.
5. If using the PROSTATE PROBLEMS blend, additional support can be obtained by 1-2 capsules per day of this blend.

**Contraindications:**   None. For a discussion of Licorice root, see Appendix A. Avoid answering magazine ads for super formulas that sound like they are cure-alls. Damiana, the main ingredient in most of these, is best (and most safely) obtained from reputable herb manufacturers and dealers.

   While the search for the elusive perfect instantaneous aphrodisiac goes on, it is my contention that the solution to good sexual health lies in possessing and maintaining a sound reproductive system. Of the thousands of plants purported to have aphrodisiac properties, this blend contains only herbs with proven long-term effectiveness in regenerating good hormonal health. Because it enriches the entire genito-urinary and reproductive system, when used regularly, it diminishes the symptoms of arthritis, rheumatism, and especially menstrual problems. Evidence of the blend's effectiveness is provided by basic animal research, human research, clinical trials, cross-cultural verification, and pharmacological investigation. Though more work on the intricate and complex problems of impotence and infertility is needed, meanwhile, this blend provides the nutritive and metabolic support required by the body to sustain effective sexual activity and reproductive effectiveness.

**DAMIANA LEAF** has one of the strongest reputations for building enhanced sexual activity. This reputation extends over hundreds of years. Damiana's use as an aphrodisiac can be traced to the ancient Mayans (**1**), but in modern times it is also popularly used as a sexual stimulant (**2**). Damiana leaf contains beta-sitosterol and various aromatic oils that could have some stimulant effect on the sexual apparatus or could help build sexual health and reproductivity. Other uses for Damiana include its use to help treat coughs, kidney disease, and constipation. The best blends combine Saw Palmetto with Damiana.

**SIBERIAN GINSENG**'s centuries-old aphrodisiac use is known to almost everybody—indeed, highly controlled research has substantially verified that effect (**3-5**). The general tonic and anti-stress properties of Ginseng contribute to the overall health required of the body for proper sexual functioning (**6**). *See Also FATIGUE; WHOLE BODY; MENTAL ALERTNESS/SENILITY; BLOOD SUGAR*

**SAW PALMETTO BERRY** is often used in conjunction with Damiana to promote sexual health. Historically, Saw Palmetto berries were used in America to treat several related disorders of the genito-urinary system, including inflammation, rupture and blockage (**7-**

**9**). At least one authority from those years testified to its salving effect on gonorrhea (**8**). A primary application for this herb is to relieve congestion. *See Also RESPIRATORY AILMENTS, DIABETES, FEMALE TONIC, PROSTATE, NERVES & GLANDS, THYROID, DIGESTION*

**SARSAPARILLA ROOT** is used in the treatment of venereal disease and infertility in Honduras, Mexico, the United States, South America and China, and elsewhere, and by the North American Indians (**10**). The steroid saponins and genins of Sarsaparilla closely resemble, and are used in the synthesis of, steroid sex hormones. Preparations containing Sarsaparilla as the primary agent are commonly used in China in the treatment of syphilis with reported success rates as high as 90% (**11**). *See Also ARTHRITIS; BLOOD PURIFICATION/DETOXIFICATION; WHOLE BODY; DETOXIFY/NURTURE*

**LICORICE ROOT** contains an estrogenic activity that was first discovered in 1950 (**12**). Those researchers attributed this effect to the presence of estriol. Subsequently, the presence of beta-sitosterol was determined (**13**). In 1963, a report appeared revealing a very strong estrogenic activity in Egyptian Licorice Root (**14**). Nothing else happened along hese lines until 1970 when, with the aid of sophisticated techniques, beta-sitosterol and stigmasterol were isolated from the plant and found to be responsible for the estrogenic activity (**15**). This study was followed by another study conducted in Russia, in which researchers confirmed the presence of estrogenic material in the plant. They isolated the active material, glycestrone, and determined that the material was completely nontoxic (**16**). Two tests, one in 1975 (**17**) and one in 1979 (**18**), found contradictory evidence concerning the estrogenic properties of glycyrrhizin (a crude extract of Licorice Root). Those studies suggest that more work, utilizing *whole* herb should be done. Other studies have determined in Licorice Root the presence of other estrogens, including glizestrone, phytosterol, and 22,23-dihydrostigmasterol (**19**). In a very recent study on women experiencing infrequent menstruation, a Licorice Root preparation successfully induced normal ovulation (**20**). All of the above studies suggest that Licorice Root has good potential for maintaining and/or restoring good hormonal and reproductive health. As a whole body tonic, Licorice root contributes even further to adequate sexual health. *See Also ARTHRITIS; RESPIRATORY AILMENTS; SKIN; FEMALE TONIC; BLOOD PURIFICATION/DETOXIFICATION; CIRCULATION; FATIGUE; WEIGHT LOSS; ENVIRONMENTAL POLLUTION; FEVERS & INFECTIONS; THYROID; WHOLE BODY; DETOXIFY/NURTURE; MENTAL ALERTNESS/SENILITY*

**KELP** is used in Japan, China and Malaysia to treat uterine disorders, impotence and infertility, along with kidney problems, bladder weakness, cystitis, prostate gland enlargement, uterine disease and ovarian troubles (**21**). These uses are becoming more popular in Western countries as we begin to verify and extend those folk uses. Kelp's mode of action is probably derived from an extremely high content of trace minerals essential to proper hormone regulation by key glands and organs. In addition to its general tonic support of sexual capacity, Kelp has specific activity in a variety of illnesses. *See Also CIRCULATION; THYROID; ENVIRONMENTAL POLLUTION; MENTAL ALERTNESS/SENILITY; PAIN; HEART; BLOOD PURIFICATION/DETOXIFICATION; FATIGUE; WEIGHT LOSS; FEVERS & INFECTIONS*

# OTHER NUTRIENTS

*The health of the reproductive system, as well as good psychological health, requires the presence of adequate nutrition. Individual needs may depart substantially from these general recommendations.*

## VITAMINS

*(Daily Requirements unless otherwise noted)*

Vitamin A *25,000 I.U.*
Vitamin B Complex
Vitamin B1 *25-50 mg*
Vitamin C *1,000-3,000 mg*
Vitamin E *up to 1600 I.U.*
Pantothenic Acid *50-100 mg*
Choline *1,000 mg*
Inositol *1,000 mg*
PABA *100 mg*
Folic Acid *up to 400 mcg*
Niacinamide *50 mg*

## MINERALS

Iodine
Zinc
Calcium/Magnesium

## MISCELLANEOUS

Brewer's yeast
Wheat Germ (oil)
Lecithin
Cod Liver Oil

# REFERENCES

1. Roys, R.L. **The Ethno-Botany of the Maya,** Pub 2, Middle America Research Series, Tulane, University, New Orleans, 1931, p. 265.
2. Curtin, L.S.M. **Healing Herbs of the Upper Rio Grande.** Southwest Museum, Los Angeles, 1965.
3. Dardymov, I.V. "On the gonadotropic effect of eleutherococcus glycosides." **Lek. Srd. Dal'nego Vostoka,** 11, 60-65, 1972.
4. Lapustina, T.A., "The influence of liquid extract of thorny eleutherococcus root on the quality and quantity of bull's sperm." **Eleutherococcus in Livestock Breeding,** 88-95, 1967.
5. Maxisimov, J.L., "Thorny eleutherococcus: plant stimulator of the reproductive function of bulls."**Eleutherococcus in Livestock Breeding,** 96-102, 1967.
6. Brekhman, I.I., Dardymov, I.V., Bezdetko, G.N. & Khasina, E. "Moleuclar aspects in the mechanism of increasing nonspecific resistivity, caused by an eleutherococcus preparation." **5th International Congress Pharmacy.** San Francisco, 1972.
7. Culbreth, D.M.R. **A Manual of Materia Medica and Pharmacology.** Philadelphia, 1927, p. 99.
8. Potter, S.O.L. **Materia Medica, Pharmacy, and Therapeutics.** Philadelphia, 1906, 420.
9. Grieve, M. **A Modern Herbal.** New York, 1971, Vol 2, 720.
10. Leung, A.Y. **Encyclopedia of Common Natural Ingredients.** New York, 1980, 152.
11. Kiangsu Institute of Modern Medicine. **Encyclopedia of Chinese Drugs.** 2 Vols, Shanghai, Peoples Republic of China, 1977.
12. Costello, C.H. & Lynn, E.V. "Estrogenic substances from plants: I. Glycyrrhiza glabra." **Journal of the American Pharmaceutical Association,** 39, 177-180, 1950.

13. Pointet-Guillot, U. "Contribution a l'etude chimique et pharmacologique de la reglisse." Thesis, Paris, 1958.
14. Shiata, I. & Elghamry, M. "Estrogenic activity of glycyrrhiza glabra with its effect on uterine motility at various stages of the sex cycle." **Zentralblatt der Verterinarmedizin,** Ser. A, 10, 155-162, 1963.
15. Van Hulle, C. "Concerning the estrogenic activity of Licorice Root." **Pharmazie,** 25, 620-621, 1970.
16. Murave'ev, I.A., Kononikhina, N.F. "Estrogenic properties of glycyrrhiza glabra (licorice)." **Rast. Resur.,** 8(4), 490-497, 1972.

17. Sharaf, A., Gomaa, N. & El-Camal, M.H.A. "Glycyrrhetic acid as an active estrogenic substance separated from glycyrrhiza glabra (liquorice)." **Egyptian Journal of Pharmaceutical Sciences,** 16(2), 245-251, 1975.
18. Dekanski, J.B., Gottfried, S. & MacDonald, A. "Oestrogenic activity of enoxolone in rodents." **Journal of Pharmacy and Pharmacology,** 31, 62, 1979.
19. Lutomski, J. "Chemistry and therapeutic use of licorice (Glycyrrhiza glabra L.)" **Pharmazie in Unserer Zeit,** 12(2), 49-54, 1983.
20. Yaginuma, T., Izumi, R., Yasui, H., Arai, T. & Kawabata, M. "Effect of traditional herbal medicine on serum testosterone levels and its induction of regular ovulation in hyper-androgenic and oligomenorrheic women." **Nippon Sanka Fujinka Gakkai Zasshi,** 1982, 34(7), 939-944.
21. Binding, G.J. & Moyle, A. **About Kelp.** Thorsons Publishers Limited. Wellingborough, Northamptonshire, England, 1974.

# INFLUENZA

## HERBS

**Form:** Capsule.

**CONTENTS: COLDENSEAL** root *(Hydrastis canadensis),* **BAYBERRY** root bark *(Myrica cerifera), and* **Cayenne** *(Capsicum annum).*

**PURPOSE:** **To help the body rid itself of infectious conditions such as Influenza (flu), colds, Sore throat, and Congestion.**

**Other Applications:** None.

**USE:** 2-3 capsules, 4 times per day throughout illness and convalescence. Supplement with 2-3 capsules/day of FEVERS & INFECTIONS blend and 2-3 capsules/day of RESPIRATORY AILMENTS to promote freer breathing.

**Contraindications:** None. For a discussion of Cayenne, see Appendix A.

The main emphasis of this blend is on acute conditions. Prevention is best achieved with the FEVERS & INFECTIONS blend. As such, this blend is a little more concentrated in antibiotic principles than the other. Nevertheless, the two are sufficiently close in action to make the decision of which to use dependent to some degree on personal experimentation and experience. The choice will ultimately depend on your own body's innate abilities to handle bacterial and viral invasions. You may find that the more general and diffuse action of the FEVERS & INFECTIONS blend is more compatible with your physiology than the more specific and concentrated activity of this blend. This is the blend to be using while you're suffering from common flus, colds, sore throats and so forth. It combines the popular Goldenseal with a combination of herbs, Cayenne and Barberry Root Bark, that was extremely popular during the last century for stimulating the circulatory system during times of colds and chills. As mentioned, the antibiotic, antiseptic and antipyretic (anti-fever) properties of Goldenseal are somewhat stronger in this blend than in the FEVERS & INFECTIONS blend. Cayenne will increase capillary circulation and stimulate digestion, and bark of Bayberry root will provide nutritive, digestive, antipyretic and astringent properties. It is essential to use this blend daily throughout the convalescence period to insure rapid and complete recovery and to lessen the chances of recurrent problems.

**GOLDENSEAL ROOT** is the main constituent in this blend which means that its action predominates. In the FEVERS & INFECTIONS blend its action is synergistic (its effects are additive) with several other herbs. It is an important natural antibiotic, however, and you may wish to use more of it. The herb acts on the nervous system very much like Cinchona. It is especially well-suited for treating the mucous membranes, especially in cases of vaginal and uterine infections. Goldenseal has found effective use as a restorative medication following protracted fevers. The alkaloids of Goldenseal, especially berberine and hydrastine, have been used to combat a wide variety of infectious agents. For example, a study from India showed that berberine had protective effect in rats against amoebic infectious agents (**1**) and other Indian studies demonstrated a similar but even more pronounced protective effect against cholera (**2-4**). Goldenseal extract has been shown effective against gram positive bacteria, such as staph and strep, and against gram negative bacteria, such as Escherichia coli (**5-8**). In addition, these special alkaloids are effective against tuberculosis bacteria (**9-10**). A final note about Goldenseal constituents is that they have been found to cure giardiasis (**11**). This parasite is not well known to people of the United States, but it has been a major problem in Africa and Asia, and is beginning to surface more and more frequently in Western countries, including the United States, especially where drinking water supplies are contaminated by flooding. If this bug ever gains a foothold, there is not much that can be done chemically to remove it from the water, except distillation or reverse osmosis. It is generally conceded by health authorities that the

Rocky Mountain States have already had problems and are facing more. Three outbreaks, involving towns using small locally maintained reservoirs, have been recorded in Utah alone. Keep this blend in mind, just in case. *See Also VAGINAL YEAST INFECTION; NERVES & GLANDS; STOMACH/INTESTINAL; EYES; FEVERS & INFECTIONS; HEMORRHOIDS*

**BAYBERRY ROOT BARK** was one of the more consequential medicinal preparations of the previous century. The Thompsonians (Botanics) and the Eclectic physicians prescribed prodigious quantities of Bayberry bark and Cayenne, to treat hepatitis, stomatitis and pharyngitis. Recent research has revealed that Bayberry root bark contains antipyretic, antibiotic, and paramecicidal chemicals (**12**). It is an ingredient in Composition Powder used for colds and chills (**13**). Bayberry, an important nutritive supplement and digestive aid, helps insure that vital nutrients are absorbed into the blood stream. It is also astringent in nature. Bayberry root bark actually promotes healthy glandular activity throughout the entire body. As an astringent and tonic, the herb was official in the National Formulary until 1936. Despite its widespread occurrence, the Bayberry tree was used medicinally by just a few native American tribes. One group of Choctaws used it for fevers (**14**). This is an herb that deserves quite a bit more experimental attention. *See Also EYES*

**CAYENNE** increases the circulation of blood to peripheral tissues, ensuring that nutrients (including those obtained from this and other herbal preparations) are delivered to inflamed and infected areas. Though the practice is unsubstantiated scientifically, many people use Cayenne directly to treat sore throat and other cold symptoms, taking advantage of the herb's irritant property on the surface of exposed tissue. Others find this practice very painful, so exercise caution in applying the contents of these capsules directly to mucous membranes. *See Also CIRCULATION; FATIGUE; HIGH BLOOD PRESSURE; BLOOD PURIFICATION/DETOXIFICATION*

## OTHER NUTRIENTS

*Infectious diseases have a way of draining the body of its vitality very rapidly and very totally. These nutrients need replacing through the diet, or with the aid of dietary supplements. The following table is provided as a general guideline. Considerable individual departure from these recommendations may be expected.*

## VITAMINS

*(Daily requirements unless otherwise noted)*

Vitamin A *25,000-50,000 I.U.*
Vitamin B Complex
Vitamin B1 *25-100 mg*
Vitamin B2 *25-100 mg*
Vitamin B6 *25-100 mg*
Vitamin C *3,000-5,000 mg*
Vitamin D *400 I.U.*
Vitamin E *600 I.U.*
Pantothenic Acid *50 mg*
Niacinamide *50 mg*

## MINERALS

Calcium/Magnesium
Phosphorous
Potassium
Sodium

## MISCELLANEOUS

Cod Liver Oil
Essential Fatty Acid
GLA
HCl

## REFERENCES

1. Kulkarni, S.K., Dandiya, P.C. & Varandani, N.L. "Pharmacological investigations of berberine sulphate." **Japanese Journal of Pharmacology,** 22, 11-16, 1972.
2. Dutta, N.K. & Panse, M.V. "Usefulness of berberine in the treatment of cholera." **Indian Journal of Medical Research,** 50(5), 732-736, 1962.
3. Sharda, D.C. "Berberine in the treatment of diarrhea of infancy and childhood." **Journal of Indian Medical Association,** 54(1), 22-23, 1970.
4. Lahiri, S.C. & Dutta, N.K. "Berberine and chloramphenicol in the treatment of cholera and severe diarrhea." **Journal of the Indian Medical Association,** 48(1), 1-11, 1967.

5. D'Amico, M.L. "Ricerche sulla presenza di sostanze ad azione antibiotica nelle piante superiori." **Fitoterapia,** 21(1), 77-79, 1950.
6. Orzechowski, G. "Antibiotics from higher plants." **Pharmazie in unserer Zeit,** 10, 42-54, 1981.
7. Johnson, C.C., Johnson, G. & Poe, C.F. "Toxicity of alkaloids to certain bacteria. II. Berberine, physostigmine and sanguinarine." **Acta Pharmacologica et Toxicologica,** 8, 71-78, 1952.
8. Haginiwa, J. & Harada, M. "Pharmacological studies on crude drugs. V. Comparison of the pharmacological actions of berberine type alkaloid-containing plants and their components." **Yakugaku Zasshi,** 82, 726-731, 1962.
9. Fitzpatrick, F.K. "Plant substances active against mycobacterium tuberculosis." **Antibiotics and Chemotherapy,** 4(5), 528-536, 1954.
10. Wang, V.F.L. "In vitro antibacterial activity of some common chinese herbs on mycobacteria tuberculosis." **Chinese Medical Journal,** 68, 169-172, 1950.
11. Gupte, S. "Use of berberine in treatment of giardiasis." **American Journal of Diseases of Childhood,** 129, 866, 1975.
12. Paul, B.D., Rao, G.S. & Kapaida, G.J. "Isolation of myricadiol, myricitrin, taraxerol, and taraxerone from myrica cerifera root bark." **Journal of Pharmaceutical Science,** 63(6), 958-959, 1974.
13. Leung, A.Y. **Encyclopedia of Common Natural Ingredients.** New York, 1980.
14. Bushnell, D.I., Jr. **The Choctaw of Bayou Lacomb, St. Tammany Parish, Louisiana.** Bureau of American Ethnology Bulletin Nr. 48, Washington D.C., Government Printing Office, 1909.

# INSOMNIA

## HERBS

**Form:** Capsule.

**CONTENTS:** **VALERIAN** root *(Valeriana officinalis)*, **HOPS** *(Humulus lupulus)*, **Skullcap** *(Scutellaria lateriflora)*, & **Passion Flower** *(Passiflora incarnata)*.

**PURPOSE:** **To overcome common sleep disorders and nervous disorders; sedation.**

**Other Applications:** Anxiety, restlessness, hyperactivity, to relax, to aid meditation.

**USE:** 1. Insomnia: 2 capsules one hour before retiring; 2 capsules upon retiring.
2. Nervous disorders: 2 capsules, 3 times per day or as needed.
3. For relaxation or sedation: 2-4 capsules as needed.

**Contraindications:** None. Do not use while driving.

Although insomnia is not well understood, most experts agree that in 95% of the cases insomnia is a side effect or symptom rather than a primary disease in and of itself. Emotional stress, anxiety, and pain are common causes of insomnia. Vitamin B deficiencies comprise another class of causes. Serious nervous system disorders, that produce insomnia, are rare. One of my earliest research projects on herbs involved observing the effects of a blend containing Valerian root, Skullcap and Hops, on a woman who had suf-

163

fered, by her report, insomnia and other sleep disorders before she began using that blend and still suffered whenever she forgot to take it. To test that claim I put together an inert but similar appearing product to use as a "placebo". For the next six weeks she took two capsules each night before retiring but didn't know if they were real or fake. The next morning she filled out a questionnaire about how easily she fell asleep, how long she slept and how she felt upon awaking. The results confirmed her original report. She slept longer and got to sleep faster, and felt better in the morning when she took the "real" blend. In subsequent experiments I replicated and extended those results on the sedative nature of that blend. Passion Flower adds another proven sedative principle and enhances this products's overall effectiveness. Research from other countries, such as Russia, Japan and France further demonstrates the usefulness of these herbs in overcoming insomnia and generally calming the nerves.

**VALERIAN ROOT** is a primary sedative and is used when sleep disorders are the result of anxiety, nervousness, exhaustion, headache or hysteria. In addition, it has been especially effective in treating tachycardia that just precedes going to sleep (**1**). Since the sedative effects of Valerian root were discussed in the chapter on NERVOUS TENSION they will not be reviewed again here. But let me note that Valerian root has been used for these purposes since pre-Christian times and is cited in virtually every pharmacopoeia in the world. It is not surprising that modern science has confirmed its actions experimentally. What is disturbing is that Valium (no relationship to Valerian) continues to be the #1 most prescribed drug in the United States today, when a perfectly safe and effective natural product like this is readily available. *See Also HIGH BLOOD PRESSURE; NERVOUS TENSION*

**HOPS,** like Valerian root, also have pronounced sedative effects (**2-3**). But hops have a more direct relationship to the inducement of sleep. This fact has been known for many years. In the past, if not so much today, the 'hop-pillow' was a popular device for promoting the onset of sleep. It was used by King George III to cure his insomnia, and has worked for many other people since then. Some people claim to get headaches and become nauseated from laying their heads on such a great quantity of concentrated hops. I recall as a child getting faintly sick while driving by the huge Hop fields of Eastern Washington. Taken internally, remarkably large amounts of

Hops can be used without fear of any side effects. The active principle of Hops is normally assumed to be lupulin, but recent research suggests that other constituents may be even more important (**4**). *See Also NERVOUS TENSION*

**SKULLCAP** is another favorite remedy for sleep disorders and nervous complaints of all types. It occurs in this blend in greater concentration than in the NERVOUS TENSION blend, so that its ability to induce sleep is felt in greater measure. It is especially effective in reducing the severity of pain that sometimes accompanies sleep, and it numbs pains and aches that prevent some individuals from falling asleep easily. *See Also PAIN RELIEF; NERVOUS TENSION; NERVES & GLANDS*

**PASSION FLOWER** is an extremely popular herb in Europe where it is often used to induce relaxation and sleep (**5**), an effect first experimentally verified in 1920 (**6**). In that study, the researcher noticed that, unlike what happens with narcotics, sleep was induced normally, with easy, light breathing, with little or no neural or mental depression. Upon awakening the patients showed no signs of confusion or stupor or melancholy. In 1979, about 50 preparations on the market in Germany contained Passion Flower. Forty-two were sedatives and 6 were cardiotonics. These preparations were recommended for the following conditions: 1. Nervous or easily aroused children; 2. Cardiovascular neurosis; 3. Bronchial asthma; 4. Coronary diseases; 5. Weak circulation; 6. Sleep disorders; 7. Problems of concentration in school children; and 8. Geriatrics (**7**). Passion Flower was listed in the National Formulary from 1916-1936, and the following is written in the 1950 U.S. Dispensatory: "...Passion flower was formerly used as a nerve sedative to allay general restlessness, to relieve insomnia, and in the relief of certain types of convulsions and spasmodic disorders" (**8**). I believe the evidence shows that such uses are still legitimate. *See Also NERVOUS TENSION; FEMALE TONIC*

## OTHER NUTRIENTS

*Insomnia may or may not yield to a warm glass of milk, but the following schedule of nutrients should have a strong positive effect. Of course, individual needs may depart greatly from these general recommendations.*

## VITAMINS & MINERALS

*(Daily requirements unless otherwise noted)*

Vitamin B-1 *25-100 mg*
Vitamin B-2 *25-100 mg*
2Vitamin B-6 *25-100 mg*
Vitamin C *500 mg*
Vitamin D *400 mg*
Vitamin E *400-600 mg*
Niacinamide *100 mg*
Pantothenic Acid *150-200 mg*

## MINERALS

Calcium/Magnesium
Potassium

## REFERENCES

1. Straube, C. "The meaning of Valerian root in therapy." **Therapie der Gegenwart,** 107, 555-562, 1968.
2. Wohlfart, R., Haensel, R. & Schmidt, H. "The sedative-hypnotic principle of hops (4)." **Planta Medica,** 48, 120-123, 1983.
3. Haensel, R., Wohlfart, r. & Coper, H. "Narcotic action of 2-methyl-3-butene-2-ol contained in hops." **Zhurnal der Natuerforschungen,** 35 c, 1096-1097, 1980.
4. Wohlfart, R., Haensel, R. & Schmidt, H. "An investigation of sedative-hypnotic principles in Hops. Part 3." **Planta Medica,** 45, 224, 1982.
5. Lutomski, J. "Alkaloidy passiflora incarnata I." **Diss. Institut fuer Heilpflanzenforschung,** Poznan, 1960.
6. Leclerc, H. (cited in Lutomski, et al).
7. Lutomski, J., Segiet, E., Szpunar, K. & Grisse, K. "The meaning of Passion Flower in the healing arts." **Pharmazie in Unserer Zeit,** 10(2), 45-49, 1981.
8. Osol, A. & Farrar, G.E. **The Dispensatory of the United States of America,** 1950 edition. Philadelphia, J.B. Lippincott Co., 1947-1950.

# LAXATIVE

## HERBS

**Form:** Capsule.

**CONTENTS: BUTTERNUT root bark** *(Juglans cinera)*, **CASCARA Sagrada bark** *(Rhamnus purshiana)*, **Rhubarb root** *(Rheum palmatum)*, **Ginger root** *(Zingiber officinale)*, **Licorice root** *(Glycyrrhiza glabra)*, **Irish Moss** *(Chondrus crispus)*, & **Cayenne** *(Capsicum annum)*.

**PURPOSE: Laxative. Gentle but effective.**

**Other Applications:** To treat G.I. bleeding (1). As an adjunct in the treatment of liver disorders.

**USE:** Children under 5: Not recommended. Use bulk laxatives, such as Psyllium seed.
Children over 5: One capsule every 8 hours.
Youth, 13-17: 2-3 capsules every 8 hours.
Youth, 16-21: 2-3 capsules every 6 hours.
Adults under 60: 2-3 capsules every 4 hours.
Adults over 60: 1-2 capsules every 8 hours.
NOTE: One may expect considerable variation in these recommendations, depending upon general health, diet and medications being used.

**Contraindications:** None. For a discussion of Cayenne, see Appendix A.

During digestion, fluids and nutrients are absorbed in the small intestine, leaving a good deal of indigestible material to be disposed of by the large intestine, whose primary function it is to push that waste material along until it reaches the rectum, where reflexive actions result in evacuation. Peristalsis involves the contraction and relaxation of smooth muscles lining the walls of the intestines. In the small intestine, these muscular actions are slow and regular, but in the large intestine they are quite irregular, occurring at unpredictable intervals and lasting for unpredictable periods of time. Regularity of bowel movements is of utmost importance. There may be variation among people, but for any given person, bowel movements should normally occur at the same regular interval. Any variance from that pattern shouldn't be severe or prolonged, or it could result in constipation. Constipation is simply intestinal sluggishness, resulting in few or incomplete bowel movements. There are two general causal classes of constipation. One is organic in nature. Hypothyroidism and obstruction of the intestinal tract are examples. The second kind is generally attributed to poor dietary habits, lack of bulk-producing foods, and failure to heed the reflexive feelings signalling the need for proper evacuation. Constipation may be chronic, acute or simple diet-induced irregularity. Proper cathartic (an agent that promotes intestinal evacuation) treatment regimens for both chronic and acute constipation are built around the sensible use of several herbs. The proper treatment for diet-induced constipation is to include prunes, bran- and fiber-containing foods in the diet, and to cut out drugs such as caffeine and alcohol. It should be noted here that chronic constipation is often the result of the abuse of cathartics themselves. If you belong to the group of individuals who habitually use carthartics to induce bowel movements, you may be able to help your body regain control over this process by using only mild cathartics such as those in this blend, learning to relax and not worry about your condition, and by changing your dietary habits to include bran and fiber. Expect emotional strains and tensions as you begin to turn control of your bowel back to your body.

A few years ago I spent several months testing and retesting most of the various herbal laxatives and cathartics I could find, with the goal of developing **the** perfect herb laxative blend. The results of that research were never fully published (**2-3**), but years later, my attention was drawn to this particular combination of herbs. I was both pleased and surprised to find that it conformed almost precisely to the results of my research. In addition, it contained Butternut root bark, an herb I had ignored because it seemed to be out of vogue. This herb's claim on fame was and still is that it would produce the same laxative effect as the stronger laxatives **without any concomitant irritating side-effects.** Rising to the challenge, I carried out a preliminary series of clinical observations which verified that claim. **This blend is even superior to the one I developed through those arduous, painstaking years of laboratory and clinical research.** Its effectiveness is due not only to the Butternut, but in large measure also to that *sine qua non* of laxatives, Cascara Sagrada. I first learned of the properties of Cascara bark when, as a child, peeling and selling the bark for a little extra money, I would invariable lick my sore and tender fingers, and, shortly thereafter, I would suffer the 'drastic' consequences. However, the bark, being dried for at least a year before being used in laxative preparations, loses that "kick" we young bark peelers came to dread.

**BUTTERNUT ROOT BARK,** as alluded to above, went out of style sometime late in the 19th Century, mainly because laxative manufacturers seized upon other substances for marketing purposes. One of the most renowned botanists of the last century wrote in 1817 about this herb, as he observed its use among the early pioneers. He noted that it was one of the "most mild and efficacious laxatives" known (**4**). He observed that during the Revolutionary War, whenever patented medicines were scarce, army surgeons resorted to Butternut root bark. Another early observer, a medical doctor, also believed that Butternut was one of the "best and safest" laxatives to be found (**5**). Another example of its popularity is its use in Canada, as observed by a French pharmacist (**6**). It is good to see a renewal of interest in the cathartic properties of this herb in recent years, for it is good not only as a laxative but as a treatment for liver disorders (as practiced extensively in homeopathy) and intestinal sicknesses. An early American physician reports experiments in which it increased the manufacture and secretion of bile and increased the activity of glands in the walls of the intestinal tract (**7**). *See Also FEVERS & INFECTIONS*

**CASCARA SAGRADA** bark, dried and cured, is one of the most effective, gentle and non-habituating laxatives available. It is used very often not only by herbalists, but by doctors and the general public as well. Many proprietary laxatives are built around Cascara. Its effectiveness is mainly due to its high anthraquinone content (**8-11**). Anthraquinones, or A-factors, and their analogues act mainly on the large intestine where they arrive intact but are quickly hydrolyzed by colonic microflora to active agents. Cascara contains the mildest acting of all the A-factors. They produce a soft or formed stool in about six to eight hours with little or no griping. They have practically no effect on the small intestine, but cause vigorous peristalsis in the large intestine. These facts are verified in the writings of the Drug Evaluations of the American Medical Association, in Remington's standard reference book on drugs, and in several individual research papers (**e.g., 12-14**). The 1977 Formulary Service of the American Society of Hospital Pharmacists, Inc., emphasizes the mild action of Cascara and remarks further that the herb does not lose its efficiency with repeated use. The problem with many cathartics is that increased dosages often become necessary with prolonged use, indicating that habituation is occurring. Cascara does not possess this negative property. In fact, Cascara can be used to correct the habitual constipation incurred by the abuse of other laxatives. It operates not only as a non-habit-forming laxative, but as an aid in restoring the natural tone of the colon. Many over-the-counter laxatives contain Cascara, but you must be careful which one you pick, because some contain substances of questionable value. For instance, for some very ill-conceived reasons we don't have space to discuss here, some contain belladonna alkaloids (atropine and scopolamine). Stychnine is sometimes added to laxatives. It usually appears in the form of its parent source, *Nux vomica*. The amount of strychnine in a single tablet is harmless—as well as useless—but the total content of several tablets may be capable of causing fatal convulsions. Two other substances to avoid are podophyllum and aloin, both way too drastic in action for safe use. Summarizing the beneficial properties of Cascara, we noted that: 1) the cathartic action is mild; 2) it is unaccompanied by discomfort, griping or colic; 3) its action is limited to the large bowel; 4) its efficiency is not lost with repeated use; 5) it is not habit forming; and 6) it can correct habitual constipation by restoring intestinal tonus. The mode of action of A-factors is not clearly understood. They probably have a stimulant effect on important neural centers that regulate colonic muscular properties. One study of particular interest examined the action of Cascara in elderly patients. Compared to placebo control groups, Cascara showed good efficacy and good biological tolerance, promoted faster gastro-intestinal transit times, and, when supplemented with cianocobalamine and inositol, the treatment was marked by increased levels of vitamin B-12 (**15**). This latter finding showed that vitamin supplementation in conjunction with Cascara-based laxatives will help overcome vitamin deficiencies that the laxative may otherwise induce. It is interesting to note that the anthraquinones of Cascara, if extracted and used separately, even at high doses, will not produce the laxative effect. It is only when they are used in the raw form, as in the whole herb, that they produce the desired effect. *See Also DETOXIFY/NURTURE; LIVER DISORDERS*

**RHUBARB,** cultivated in China and Tibet, has an illustrious history of inclusion in many laxative preparations. It is generally considered a mild laxative that produces a soft stool 6-10 hours after ingestion (**17**), but should not be used by itself when the colon is totally evacuated, because the presence of astringent tannins may produce constipative feelings. On very rare occasions sensitive persons may experience mild colicky pains. The herb is an important part of this blend because the A-factors of the herb differ somewhat from those of Cascara. Only some of them reach the large intestines intact, while others are resorbed in the small intestine and are later released into the large intestine (**18**). The timing of the activity of Rhubarb is thus displaced to some degree from the other laxative agents in this blend, thereby promoting longer and smoother activity of the whole. Note again that chemicals under discussion here do not become active until, through fermentation from bacteria in the large intestine and intestinal wall, they undergo moderate chemical change (**19**). Then, and only then, they stimulate the secretion of mucous through the wall of the large intestine whereby the consistency of the intestinal contents is decreased. They also reflexively stimulate the musculature of the wall lining, whereby peristalsis and bowel emptying are increased (**20**). Were you to ingest the chemicals in active form, they would produce side effects like vomiting and nausea. Rhubarb is especially well suited for children since it is very mild in action. For chronic constipation, it may be used year-round, but should only be given when necessary, since prolonged use may lead to potassium deficiency. Rhubarb is, therefore, best used in a blend that respects the functioning of the whole organism. Rhubarb is useful for numerous other problems also. It has been shown to inhibit bacteria (**21-22**), cancer (**13**), liver, spleen and gallbladder problems, especially gallstones, jaundice and hemorrhoids (**23**), and upper digestive tract bleeding (**24**). It may be a historical value to note that Rhubarb was one of the plants used by the earliest colonists in America, being imported from Europe where its use as a laxative was the standard.

**GINGER ROOT** plays an important role in this blend; namely, it counterbalances the discomforting effects of colon reflex activity and imparts a pleasant degree of mildness to the blend's functioning. Ginger root also helps restore and normalize proper tone and reflex faculty to the gastro-intestinal tract (**25**). It is not only important that one use a proper laxative, but that one revitalize sick and flaccid muscles and glands. Ginger root helps do this (**17**). In addition, Ginger root has been shown to normalize peristalsis (**26**). *See Also DIGESTION; STOMACH/INTESTINAL; NAUSEA; FATIGUE; LOW BLOOD SUGAR; CIRCULATION*

**LICORICE ROOT,** besides being a mild aperient itself, helps to counterbalance the discomforting effects that may result from laxative use. It provides a mild boost to the adrenal system that may be stressed in certain debilitating conditions for which laxatives are often suggested. Most importantly Licorice root protects and heals distressed mucous membranes of the intestinal tract as confirmed by literally hundreds of studies (**27-30**). Some constituents of Licorice root (the sennosides) have been shown to be cathartic (**31**), but it is doubtful that this effect is prominent when the whole herb is ingested. However, in Germany, Licorice root is used for its mild laxative property. *See Also INFERTILITY; ARTHRITIS; RESPIRATORY AILMENTS; SKIN DISORDERS; FEMALE TONIC; BLOOD PURIFICATION/DETOXIFICATION; CIRCULATION; FATIGUE; WEIGHT LOSS; ENVIRONMENTAL POLLUTION; FEVERS & INFECTIONS; THYROID; WHOLE BODY; DETOXIFY/NURTURE; MENTAL ALERTNESS/ SENILITY*

**IRISH MOSS** is used as a stabilizer in such dairy products as ice creams, sherbets, chocolate milk, yogurt and whipped creams. It is used in syrups and toppings and provides both mouth feel and body to creamed soups and chowders. Since it is an unassimilated hydrocolloid it is used in raw form as a bulk laxative (**32**). It also coats and soothes the entire gastrointestinal tract. In various forms, it alleviates peptic and duodenal ulcers in humans while having no adverse effects on the colon (**33**). A recent patent claims a procedure for treating stomach and duodenal ulcers with an extract of Irish Moss (**34**). Irish Moss is not a recent herbal, having been used by the eary colonists in New England, and probably earlier. There has been some concern generated by articles showing various toxic properties of **carrageenan,** a processed extract of Irish Moss. Whole Irish Moss does not demonstrate any of the toxic properties of carrageenan because the digestive process is incapable of releasing carrageenan into the body. Irish Moss is neutral when it comes to cellular processes. *See Also STOMACH/INTESTINAL; THYROID*

**CAYENNE** provides just a little zip to the blend, acting as it does in so many cases, as an effective catalyst and augmenter of the other principles in the blend.

## OTHER NUTRIENTS

*The purpose of dietary supplementation when constipated is to provide dietary bulk and fiber, and the nutrients necessary to restore tonus to the large intestine. It is also meant to increase the efficiency of the digestive process in general. Individual needs may depart substantially from the following general recommendations.*

### VITAMINS

*(Daily requirements unless otherwise noted)*

Vitamin A *25,000 I.U.*
Vitamin B-1 *25-100 mg*
Vitamin B-2 *25-100 mg*
Vitamin B-6 *25-100 mg*
Vitamin C *500-1000 mg*
Vitamin D *400 I.U.*
Vitamin E *200 I.U.*
Niacinamide *50 mg*
Choline *300-500 mg*
Inositol *200-400 mg*

### MINERALS

Potassium
Calcium/Magnesium

### MISCELLANEOUS

Bran
Fiber
Prunes

## REFERENCES

1. List, P.H. & Hoerhammer, L. **Hagers Handbuch der Pharmazeutischen Praxis.** Volumes 2-5, Springer-Verlag, Berlin.
2. Mowrey, D.B. "Constipation, Part I." The Herbalist, June, 10-11, 1978.

3. Mowrey, D.B. "Constipation, Part II" Unpublished Manuscript, 1978, for personal reasons. This paper summarizes several months worth of work on herbal laxatives and various combinations thereof, and concludes with the author's own recommendations for an effective herbal blend.

4. Bigelow, J. **American Medical Botany, Being a Collection of the Native Medicinal Plants of the United States.** 3 vols. Cummings & Hilliard, Boston, 1817-1820.

5. Gunn, J.D. New **Domestic Physician or Home Book of Health.** Moore, Wilstach, Keys. 686, 1971. Cincinnati, 1st ed., 1857 and 1861 edition.

6. Mockle, J.A. **Contributions a l'Etude des Plantes Medicinales du Canada.** Paris ed. Jouve Pubs.

7. Felter, H. W. **The Eclectic Materia Medica, Pharmacology and Therapeutics.** Eclectic Medical Publications, Portland, Oregon, 1983 (first published 1922), p. 328.

8. Nelemans, F.A. **Pharmacology.** 14, suppl. I, 73-77, 1976.

9. Godding, E.W. **Pharmacology.** 14, Suppl. 1, 78-101, 1976.

10. van Os, F.H.L. **Pharmacology.** 14, Suppl. 1, 18-29, 1976.

11. Fairbairn, J.W., & Mahran, G.E.D.H. **Journal of Pharmacy and Pharmacology,** 5, 827-838, 1953.

12. Breimer, D.D. & Baars, A.J. "Pharmacokinetics and metabolism of anthrquinone laxatives." **Pharmacology,** 14, supple 1, 30-47, 1976.

13. Lemmens, L. **I.R.C.S.,** 2, 1094, 1974.

14. Fairbairn, J.W. & Moss, M.J.R., **Journal of Pharmacy and Pharmacology,** 22, 584, 1970.

15. Marchesi, M., Marcato, M. & Silvestrini, C. "Clinical experience with a preparation containing cascara sagrada and boldo in the therapy of simple constipation in the elderly" **Giornale di Clincia Medica (Bologna),** 63(11-12), 850-863, 1982.

16. Fairburn, J.W. "The active constituents of the vegetable purgatives containing anthracene derivatives. I. Glycosides and aglycones." **Journal of Pharmacy and Pharmacology,** 1, 683-692, 1949.

17. List, P.H. & Hoerhammer, L. **Hagers Handbuch der Pharmazeutischen Praxis.** Volumes 2-5, Springer-Verlag, Berlin.

18. Chirikdjian, J.J., Kopp, B. & Beran, H. "Laxative action of a new anthraquinone glycoside from rhubarb root." **Planta Medica,** 48(1), 34-37, 1983.

19. Cresseri, A., Peruto, A.I. & Longo, R. **Archiv der Pharmazie.,** 293, 615, 1966.

20. Fairburn, J.W. "The cathartic action of anthraquinones." **The Pharmacology of Plant Phenolics.** Ed. Academic Press, N.Y., 1959, 39-49.
21. Chen, C.H., Li, T.T., Su, H.L., Wang, C.I. "Chinese rhubarb. VII. Mechanism of antibiotic action of anthraquinone derivatives. Effect on the respiration of staphylococcus aureus." **Sheng Wu Hua Hsueh Yu Shen Wu Wu Li-sueh,** 3(4), 426-433, 1963.
22. Su, H.L., Chen, C.H. "Chinese Rhubarb. II. Paper chromatography of anthraquinones." **Yao Hsueh Hsueh Pao,** 10(12), 725-730, 1963.
23. Kiangsu Institute of Modern Medicine. **Encyclopedia of Chinese Drugs.** 2 Vols. Shanghai, Peoples Republic of China, 1977.
24. Dong-hai, J., Yu-hua, M., Shou-jing, C., Chuen-tang, L, Hung-nien, S. & Chang-min, C. "Resume of 400 cases of acute upper digestive tract bleeding treated by rhubarb alone." **Pharmacology,** 20 (Suppl 1), 128-130, 1980.
25. Glatzel, H. "Treatment of dyspeptic disorders with spice extracts." **Hippocrates,** 40(23), 916-919, 1969.
26. Glatzel, H. **Dtsh Apoth Ztg,** 110, 5, 1970.
27. Cooke, W.M. & Baron, J.H. "Metabolic studies of deglycyrrhizinised licorice in two patients with gastric ulcers." **Digestion,** 4, 264-268, 1971.
28. Aarsen, P.N. & Noordwijk, J. von. "Comparison of the spasmolytic activity of sucus liquiritiae in treated and untreated form." **Therapeutische Umschau,** 7, 302, 1963.
29. Andersson, S., Barany, F., Caboclo, J.L.F. & Mizuno, T. "Protective action of deglycyrrhizinized liquorice on the occurrence of stomach ulcers in pylorus ligated rats." **Scandinavian Journal of Gastroenterology,** 6, 683-686, 1971.
30. Cross, S., & Rhodes, J. "Carbenoxolone: its protective action against bile damage to gastric mucosa in canine pouches." **Gastroenterology,** 62, 737, 1972.
31. Hattori, M., Sakamoto, T., Kobashi, K. & Namba, T. "Metabolism of glycyrrhizin by human intestinal flora." **Planta Medica,** 48, 38-42, 1983.
32. Meer Technical Bulletin G-15, Meer Corporation, North Bergen, New Jersey.
33. **Martindale: The Extra Pharmacopoeia.** 1977. The Pharmaceutical Press. London.
34. U.S. Patent 4150123 issued to W. Szturma, April 17, 1979.

# LIVER
# DISORDERS

## HERBS

**Form:** Capsule.

**CONTENTS: DANDELION** root *(Taraxacum officinale),* **CASCARA Sagrada bark,** *(Rhamnus purshiana)* **Licorice root** *(Glycyrrhiza glabra),* **Celery seed** *(Apium graveolens),* **Cayenne** *(Capsicum annum),* **Wild Yam root** *(Dioscorea villosa).*

**PURPOSE:** **To assist the body remedy liver disorders (hepatitis, cirrhosis and jaundice); Also maintains healthy liver, gallbladder, pancreas, and spleen; Laxative.**

**Other Applications:** Colon stimulant, indigestion and heartburn, gastritis, gallstones, constipation.

**USE:** 1. Hepatitis, cirrhosis, jaundice: 4-6 capsules daily, plus 2-3 capsules of the FEVERS & INFECTIONS Blend.
2. For gallbladder problems: 2-4 capsules per day along with 2-4 capsules of the FEVERS & INFECTIONS blend.
3. For glandular maintenance: 4-5 capsules per day. May use along with the TONIC—NERVE & GLAND blend.
4. Supplement this blend with 2 capsules, 4 times per day, of BLOOD PURIFICATION/DETOXIFICATION Blend.
5. Laxative: Mild effect at any use level.
6. For nausea, use NAUSEA Blend.

**Contraindications:** Though no evidence exists to prove that the steroid precursors in Wild Yam are allergenic, persons with severe estrogenic sensitivity should exercise caution if exceeding 2-4 capsules per day.

The following major functions are performed by the liver on a continuous basis: store and filter blood to remove harmful infectious organisms; form and secrete bile; store glycogen; buffer blood glucose levels; convert amino acids to glucose; convert galactose and fructose to glucose; metabolize fat, including beta-oxidation; manufacture lipoproteins; form cholesterol and phospholipids and convert carbohydrates and proteins to fats; metabolize protein; form urea from ammonia; form plasma proteins; synthesize non-essential amino acids and other metabolically important compounds. In order to perform all of these functions, the liver processes an incredible amount of blood, about three pints every minute. When the liver is diseased, many of these functions do not operate correctly.

The liver is the body's main chemical processing plant. Most of the blood arrives at the liver direct from the intestines via the portal vein, heavily laden with nutrients, as well as dietary toxic substances. The rest of the liver's blood supply arrives via the hepatic artery. Liver cells have the capacity to regenerate following many forms of illness, but not cirrhosis, which is technically scar tissue. The scar tissue permanently disrupts the liver's structure, resulting in more or less permanent loss of function. Alcohol is the main enemy of the liver and is the most common cause of cirrhosis. The next most harmful condition results from the infection of hepatitis viruses. A damaged liver (and a healthy one, under certain conditions) may fail to do its job properly. When that happens, toxins are no longer filtered out efficiently and may build up in the body, as will the by-products of protein metabolism such as ammonia. Sugar levels fall. Infection is common, and the kidneys may fail. Severe, uncontrollable bleeding is also common, with coma and death likely. But checked in time, a diseased or failed liver stands a good chance of healing very well.

You may notice a strong similarity between this blend and the DIABETES blend. Dandelion heads up the list of ingredients in both blends; however, the primary purpose of this product is to aid the body in combating various liver-related problems. The blend contains some herbs with extremely effective principles and should prove to be one of the most effective blends in this book.

**DANDELION ROOT** heads the list of excellent medicinal foods for the liver and related organs and glands. This high position is supported by available research. In studies with rats, it stimulates the flow of bile to the same degree that an injection of bile into the liver does (**1**). Bile injections are a standard way to stimulate bile flow in the rat. The rat is used because it does not have a gallbladder; therefore the increase in bile, after the administration of Dandelion must result from a direct influence on the liver. For organisms with gallbladders, Dandelion causes contraction of that organ thereby promoting the flow of bile (**2**). One researcher, using dogs, observed a three to four times increase in the rate of bile secretion following Dandelion administration (**3**). Clinical observations in humans have shown that Dandelion enhances the flow of bile as well as dramatically improves such conditions as bile duct inflammation, liver congestion and gall stones (**2**). Elsewhere, Dandelion has been used to treat chronic hepatitis, swelling of the liver, jaundice and dyspepsia with deficient bile secretion (**4**). Around the world, the herb is used as a cholagogue and diuretic. Clinical studies with a German over-the-counter preparation "Hepatichol", containing Dandelion and a few other herbs, on several cases of gallstones, acute and chronic bile duct and gallbladder inflammation, jaundice, dyskinesia of the bile duct and jaundice caused by complete obstruction by gallstones, showed more or less complete recovery within several days depending on the severity of symptoms (**5**). With the aid of sophisticated probes, this preparation was further tested on healthy and sick subjects and shown to significantly enhance both the concentration and the secretion of bilirubin in the duodenum. Dandelion is choleretic, i.e., it stimulates bile production and leads to an increased cleansing of the bile duct. It is cholekinetic, i.e., it increases the movement of the bile, especially such that it leads to an evacuation of the gallbladder. Substances that are both choleretic and cholekinetic are true cholagogues. Finally, in case of edematous complications due to liver disorders, it has a diuretic action (**6**). *See Also DIABETES; BLOOD PURIFICATION/DETOXIFICATION; SKIN DISORDERS; NERVES & GLANDS*

**CASCARA SAGRADA,** normally a great laxative, is used in smaller amounts in folk medicine to treat liver disorders and gallstones. Its use to remedy hepatic disease has been confirmed by modern research (**7-8**). We owe the discovery of this property to the early American eclectic physicians, who were unanimous in their praise for the herb to treat jaundice and other hepatic conditions (**6,9-10**). It was first fully described in about 1805, but did not enter into official medical use as a laxative until 1877. After that, its popularity as a laxative gradually came to overshadow its remedial use in liver disorders, especially in the practice of orthodox medicine. *See Also DETOXIFY/NURTURE; LAXATIVE*

**LICORICE ROOT** as a treatment for hepatitis is thought to have originated in China. Licorice is, of course, one of the most pre-scribed herbs in China, second only to Ginseng in Chinese herbal-ism (**11**). It is called the "Great Detoxifier" and is used especially for the spleen, kidneys, liver and stomach, as well as for many other ailments (**12**). In Europe, Licorice root, because of its diuretic prop-erty, is used to treat urinary and kidney problems (**13**). Modern research provides evidence for the use of Licorice root in treating liver disorders, especially as these are connected with the cortico-steroid metabolism (**14**). In one study, carried out by the Research Group of Liver Disease at China's Shanxi Medical College, it was found that Licorice root decreased the accumulation of triglyceride in the liver, increased glycogen levels, prevented the development of experimental cirrhosis and prevented the occurrence of ex-perimentally induced lesions in the liver (**15**). In Japan, a popular preparation composed of glycyrrhizin (an active constituent of Licor-ice root) has been extensively used to treat hepatitis with a great deal of success (**16-18**). While nobody is certain how it works, a recent study found that Licorice root induces the production of interferon, a substance produced by the body that is successfully used to treat victims of hepatitis B (**16**). *See Also INFERTILITY; ARTHRITIS; THYROID; WHOLE BODY; SKIN DISORDERS; RESPIRATORY AILMENTS; FEMALE TONIC; CIRCULATION; WEIGHT LOSS; ENVIRONMENTAL POLLUTION; MENTAL ALERTNESS/SENILITY; DETOXIFY/NURTURE; FEVERS & INFECTIONS*

**CELERY SEED** has not been subjected to the same amount of research investigation as many other herbs. Nevertheless, in addi-tion to its diuretic activity, it has been shown to possess other definite medicinal properties, including a blood pressure lowering property (**19**), antioxidative principle (**20**), and sedative activity (**21-22**). Of immediate importance to this chapter, it has been shown to possess insulin-like activity (**23**) and to suppress adrenaline hyper-glycemia (**24**). These findings, taken together, suggest that this lowly herb, if eaten regularly, can promote a certain degree of health, especially in the vital organs of the body, including the glands, heart and nerves. *See Also ARTHRITIS*

**CAYENNE** again acts as the catalyst and reaction promoter in this blend, enhancing its overall effectiveness.

**WILD YAM ROOT** preparations were used to treat bilious colic by American physicians long before the herb's steroid properties be-came known. It sometimes rapidly and effectively reduced the pain of biliary colic, caused by gallstones; and eased the passage of small stones (**9**). Some writers noted that the treatment did not always work, but that it was nevertheless one of the best anti-spasmotic treatments known, applicable for all forms of colicky and paroxysmal pain, ovarian neuralgia, spasmotic dysmenorrhea and indigestion (**6**). Part of the therapeutic action of Wild Yam root on overall liver health is due to its ability to lower blood cholesterol levels and lower blood pressure. These properties would indirectly help the liver by increasing its efficiency and reducing stress (**25-27**). *See Also FEMALE TONIC*

## OTHER NUTRIENTS

*The liver benefits directly, almost before any other organ of the body, from the continuous supply of dietary nutrients. Its incredible tasks are made that much easier if dietary habits include only those substances which impart good health. Avoid alcohol, sugar, food additives and other toxic substances that put great strain on the liver. The following recommendations are meant as guidelines only. Individual requirements may vary.*

### VITAMINS

*(Daily requirements unless otherwise noted)*

Vitamin A *25,000-50,000 I.U.*
Vitamin B1 *25-100 mg*
Vitamin B2 *25-100 mg*
Vitamin B6 *25-100 mg*
Vitamin C *1,000-10,000 mg*
Vitamin D *400 I.U.*
Vitamin E *400-600 I.U.*
Choline *2-3 g*
Inositol *2-3 g*
Folic acid *40 mcg*

### MISCELLANEOUS

Brewer's Yeast
Lecithin
Yogurt
Liver
Protein

# REFERENCES

1. Buesemaker, "Concerning the choleretic activity of Dandelion," **Naunyn-Schmiederbergs Archiv fuer Experimentelle Pharmakology und Pathologie,** 181, 512, 1936.
2. Leclerc, H. **Phytotherapie,** Paris, 1927, cited by Ripperger, W. "Pflanzliche laxantien und cholagogue wirkungen." **Medizinische Welt,** 9, 1463-1467, 1935.
3. Chabrot, E. & Charonnat, R. "Therapeutic agents in bile secretion." **Ann. Med.,** 37, 131-142, 1935.
4. Bentely, R. & Trimen, H. **Medicinal Plants,** J & A Churchill, London, 1880, Vol 3, 159.
5. Faber, K. "The dandelion—*Taraxacum officinale* Weber." **Pharmazie,** 13(7), 423-435, 1958.
6. Felter, H. W. **The Eclectic Materia Medica, Pharmacology and Therapeutics.** Eclectic Medical Publications, Portland, Oregon, 1983 (first published 1922).
7. Kerharo, J. & Bouquet, A. **Plantes Medicinales et Toxiques de la Cole d'Ivoire,** Haute-Vota, Vigot, Paris, 1950.
8. Dalziel, J.M. "The useful plants of west tropical africa." In Dalziel and Hutchinson's appendix to **The Flora of West Tropical Africa,** London, 1937.
9. Ellingwood, F. **American Materia Medica, Therapeutics and Pharmacognosy.** Eclectic Medical Publications, Portland, Oregon, 1983.
10. Culbreth, D.M.R. **A Manual of Materia Medica and Pharmacology.** Philadelphia, 1927, p. 99.
11. Teeguarden, R. **Chinese Tonic Herbs,** Japan Publications, Inc., Tokyo & New York, 1984.
12. Leung, A.Y. **Chinese Herbal Remedies,** Universe Books, New York, 1984.
13. Lutomski, J. "Chemistry and therapeutic uses of licorice root." **Pharmazie in Unserer Zeit,** 12(2), 49-54, 1983.
14. Tamura, Y., Nishikawa, T., Yamada, K., Yamamoto, M. & Kumagai, A. "Effects of glycyrrhetinic acid and its derivatives on delta four-five alpha- and 5 beta-reductase in rate liver." **Arzneimittel-Forschungen,** 29(4), 647-649, 1979.
15. Zhao, M., Han, D., Ma, X., Zhao, Y., Yin, L. & Li, C. "The preventive and therapeutic actions of glycyrrhizin, glycyrrhetic acid and crude saikosides on experimental cirrhosis in rats." **Yao Hsueh Hsueh Pao,** 18(5), 325-331, 1983.

16. Fujisawa, K., Watanabe, Y. & Kimura, K. "Therapeutic approach to chronic active hepatitis with glycyrrhizin." **Asian Medical Journal,** 23, 745-756, 1980.

17. Iwamura, K. "Ergebnisse der therapie mit dem medikament strong neo-minophagen C der chronischaggressiven hepatitis in Japan." **Therapeiwoche,** 30, 5431-5445, 1980.

18. Yamamoto, S., Maekawa, Y., Imamura, M. & Hisajima, T. "Therapeutic effects of stronger neo-minophagen C on chronic hepatitis." **Clinical Medicine and Pediatrics,** 13, 73-75, 1958.

19. Kiangsu Institute of Modern Medicine. **Encyclopedia of Chinese Drugs.** 2 Vols. Shanghai, Peoples Republic of China, 1977.

20. Courtin, J. "Product aiding the sun-tanning of the skin." **Fr. Demande 2,295,735,** 23 July 1976.

21. Bjeldanes, L.F. & Kim, I. "Phthalide components of celery essential oil." **Journal of Organic Chemistry,** 42(13), 2333-2335, 1977.

22. Bjeldanes, L.F. & Kim, I. "Sedative activity of celery oil constituents." **Journal of Food Science,** 43(1), 143-144, 1978.

23. Best, C.H. & Scott, D.A. "Possible sources of insulin." **Journal of Metabolic Research,** 3, 177-179, 1923.

24. Sharaf, A.A., Hussein, A.M. & Mansour, M.Y. "Studies on the antidiabetic effect of some plants." **Planta Medica,** 2, 159-168, 1963.

25. Sokolova, L.H. "Effect of saponins on the development of experimental atherosclerosis." **Farmakologia i Toxikologia,** 21(6), 85-90, 1958.

26. Lesskov, A.I., Martinova, R.G. & Sokolov, S.Y. "Polysponin--a new drug with antisclerotic action." **Khimiko Farmatsevtiches-kii Zhurnal,** 2, 147-150, 1975.

27. Sokolova, L.N., Kichenk, V.I., Rostozkii, B.K. & Gubina, G.P. "Diosponine—a new drug for treatment of patients with atherosclerosis." **Meditsinskaya Promyshlennost SSSR,** 7, 43-48, 1961.

# MENSTRUATION

## HERBS

**Form:** Capsule, Douche, Enema, Tea, Gargle

**CONTENTS: CRANESBILL** root *(Geranium maculatum)*, **RASPBERRY** leaves *(Rubus idaeus)*, **Witch Hazel leaves** *(Hamamelis virginiana)*, **Uva-Ursi leaves** *(Arctostaphylos uva-ursi)*, **Papaya leaves** *(Carica papaya)*, **Shepherd's Purse** *(Capsella bursa-pastoris)*, **Black Haw bark** *(Viburnum prunifolium)*.

**PURPOSE: To decrease excessive flow during menstruation. Astringent.**

**Other Applications:** To be used externally or internally, wherever there is a need for a powerful astringent: Hemorrhage; sore throat and mouth; rectum; internal bleeding caused by ulcers; diarrhea; hemorrhoids; to regulate blood pressure; false labor pains; threatened miscarriage; to prevent abortions; chronic mucous discharges.

**USE:** 1. Menorrhagia (excessive menstrual flow): 4-6 capsules per day. Tea: 4 capsules; Douche: From cool tea; Enema: From warm tea.
2. Diarrhea: 2-3 capsules every 4-5 hours as needed. Supplement with the NAUSEA Blend: 2-3 capsules every hour as needed.
3. Hemorrhoids: Use in conjunction with the HEMORRHOIDS/ASTRINGENT Blend: 3 of each blend per day.

185

4. To supplement the VAGINAL YEAST INFECTION Blend: 2-3 capsules per day, or 2 capsules per meal.

**Contraindications:**    None.

Excessive menstrual flow may signal the presence of mild to severe underlying disease, even cancer, and must be brought to your physician's attention. Meanwhile, you should be aware that iron is being lost and must be replaced. Iodine and Vitamin C must also be replenished regularly. This blend can and should be used by anybody in need of astringent medication. It extends and amplifies the astringent principle found in the VAGINAL YEAST INFECTION blend. Its purpose is to rapidly correct many forms of diarrhea, and to ameliorate symptoms of slow, steady menorrhagia. The gastro-intestinal (G.I.) tract will improve in function and tonus. Although designed for use by women experiencing the discomforts of periodic diarrhea and menorrhagia, the blend can be used by anyone with diarrhea. Four of seven herbs in this blend are high in tannic acid, a primary astringent.

**CRANESBILL ROOT** was relied upon by early American Indians to treat diarrhea (**1**), dysentery (**2**), leukorrhea (**3**), and hemorrhoids (**4**), among other conditions. These people passed this knowledge on to the early settlers, and thus into the black bag of many early physicians, who discovered it would also reduce chronic menorrhagia (**5**), especially in cases of prolonged, but slow bleeding. One early physician remarked, "I . . . esteem geranium (cranesbill) more highly than any other vegetable astringent, where a simple tonic astringent action is needed. It is palatable, prompt, efficient, and invariable in its effects, and entirely devoid of unpleasant influences," (**6**).

**RASPBERRY LEAF** provides adjunctive support for the anti-diarrheal aspect of this blend. That effect is primarily due to the astringent nature of the leaves. In addition, Raspberry leaves are important to some of the secondary applications of this product. One scientific study showed that a principle in the leaf is responsible for relaxing the smooth muscles of the uterus and intestine when they are in tone, and that same principle causes contraction of the uterus when it is not in tone (**7**). The relaxation effect probably accounts for the traditional therapeutic value of Raspberry leaves in aiding parturition. The contracting effect may explain the ability of the leaves to remedy extreme laxity of the bowels. *See Also FEMALE TONIC; DIABETES; EYES*

**WITCH HAZEL LEAF** appears in this blend, as well as VAGINAL YEAST INFECTION, because of its reliable astringent property. The reader is referred to the V.Y.I. blend for a discussion, and to the HEMORRHOIDS/ASTRINGENT blend for a discussion of Witch Hazel's involvement in hemorrhoid treatment.

**UVA-URSI LEAF** is a confirmed astringent with urinary antiseptic properties (**8-9**). This action is due to the high concentration of a known antiseptic, arbutin, in the herb. Arbutin, in passing through the system, yields hydroquinone, which may turn the urine dark or brownish-green, a harmless condition. Hydroquinone is a urinary disinfectant. Uva-ursi leaves also contain anesthetic principles capable of numbing pain in the urinary system. Crude extracts of Uva-Ursi also possess some anti-cancer property (**10**). Finally, this herb has been shown to have good antibiotic activity (**11-12**). *See Also DIURETIC; DIABETES*

**PAPAYA LEAF** is best known as a digestive aid, but is included in this blend on the strength of recent research findings that indicate that it also possesses an antihemolytic property, i.e., it should reduce the severity of bleeding and hemorrhage throughout the body (**13**). In this regard, it will inhibit menorrhagia. It is also an emmenagogue, that is, it will promote menstruation in women who have trouble menstruating, or who menstruate only with pain. Of importance to some individuals is the possibility that Papaya leaf may counteract the hemolytic effect (and jaundice) of glucose-6-phosphate dehydrogenase deficiency produced when certain drugs are ingested (especially the antimalarial primaquine). Members of the black races are especially vulnerable to this problem. *See Also DIGESTION; STOMACH/INTESTINAL*

**SHEPHERD'S PURSE** possesses mild astringency. It also contains several substances which could help female physiological processes. Among those substances are saponins, choline, acetylcholine (ACh), and tyramine. Choline and ACh stimulate the cholinergic elements of the autonomic nervous system, which are particularly important for proper neuro-muscular function. It is effective in treating menorrhagia characterized by lengthy and frequent almost colorless flow (**6**). Basic chemical analysis has determined that the principles of Shepherd's Purse coagulate blood (**14**). The herb also reduces urinary tract irritation and atony. It will clear up blood in the urine, and may eliminate mild forms of hemorrhage (**15**). Shepherd's purse is an example of an herb used around the world, throughout the ages, by many different peoples, all for the same or similar purposes. Interestingly, in that light, there is little record of the American Indians having used it for anything but its nutritive value. Other modern studies have found uterine contracting and blood pressure lowering effects in Shepherd's Purse (**16-17**). And the herb has also been found to enhance uterine tonus (**9**).

**BLACK HAW BARK** was a discovery of the early American physician, who used it more than any other herb for practically all female problems, believing it would relax the uterus, relieve painful menstruation, fight diarrhea, and generally tone up the whole female reproductive system (**18**). Black Haw was official in most pharmacopoeias during the 19th century, for treatment of dysmenorrhea, threatened abortion and asthma (**19**). Use of the herb tapered off during the 1st half of this century, but the herb is now enjoying a comeback. Recently, chemists discovered several uterine muscle relaxants in the herb (**20**). These significant findings have helped to validate earlier uses of the herb.

## OTHER NUTRIENTS

*Menstrual problems can have very complex causes, and severe problems should be treated under the care of a trained physician. Nutritional support of the genital-urinary system will help the body repair itself and may lead to proper functioning. Individual requirements may differ significantly from the following nutritional guidelines.*

### VITAMINS

*(Daily requirements unless otherwise noted)*

Vitamin A  *25,000 I.U.*
Vitamin B1  *25-50 mg*
Vitamin B2  *25-50mg*
Vitamin B6  *25-50mg*
Vitamin B12  *up to 50 mcg*
Vitamin C  *1000 mg*
Vitamin D  *400 I.U.*
Vitamin E  *600 I.U.*
Folic Acid  *400 mcg*

## MINERALS

Iron
Iodine
Calcium/Magnesium

# REFERENCES

1. Barton, B.J. **Collections for an Essay towards a Materia Medica of the United States.** 3rd ed., with additions. Philadelphia, printed for Edward Earle and Co. 1810.
2. Lewis, W.H. & Elvin-Lewis, M.P.F. **Medical Botany. Plants Affecting Man's Health.** Wiley-Interscience Series. New York 1977.
3. Winder, W. "On Indian Diseases and Remedies." **Boston Medical And Surgical Journal,** Vol. XXXIV(1), Feb 4, 1846, 10-13.
4. Smith, H.H. **Ethnobotany of the Meskwaki Indians.** Bulletin of the Public Museum, Vol. IV, No. 2, Milwaukee, 1928.
5. Felter, H.W. **The Eclectic Materia Medica, Pharmacology and Therapeutics.** Eclectic Medical Pubs, Portland, 1983. 391. (1st published, 1922).
6. Ellingwood, R. **American Materia Medica, Therapeutics and Pharmacognosy.** Eclectic Medical Pub., Portland, 1983. 347.
7. Burn, J.H. & Withell, E.R. "A principle in raspberry leaves which relaxes uterine muscles." **Lancet,** 2(6149), 1-3, 1941.
8. List, P.H. & Hoerhammer, L. **Hagers Handbuch der Pharmazeutischen Praxis.** vols 2-5. Springer-Verlag. Berlin. 1969-1976.
9. Trease, G.E. & Evans, W.C. **Pharmacognosy.** 1978. 11th ed. Bailliere Tindall. London.
10. Hartwell, J.L. "Plant remedies for cancer." **Cancer Chemotherapy Reports,** 1960, July, 19-24.
11. Benigni, R. "The presence of antibiotic substances in the higher plants." **Fitoterapia,** 19(3), 1-2, 1948.
12. Danilowski, U. **Arch. Exp. Path. Pharmacol.,** 35, 105, 1895.
13. Pousset, J.L. "Antihemolytic action of an extract of Carica papaya bark. Possibilities of use in glucose-6-phosphate dehydrogenase deficiencies." **Dakar Med,** 1979, 24(3), 255-262.
14. Kuroda, K. & Takagi, K. "Physiologically active substances in capsella bursa pastoris." **Nature,** 220(5168), 707-708, 1968.

15. Kochman, M. "Zur wirkung des hirtentaischels, Capsella bursa pastoris, auf den uterus." **Muenchener Medizinische Wochenschrift,** 67, 1284, 1920.
16. Kuroda, K. & Kaku, T. "Pharmacological and chemical studies on the alcohol extract of capsella bursa pastoris." **Life Sciences,** 8(3), 151-155, 1969.
17. Shipochliev, I. "Extracts from a group of medicinal plants enhancing the uterine tonus." **Veterinary Sciences,** 18(4), 94-98, 1981.
18. Hale, E.M. **The Special Symptomatology of the New Remedies.** Philadelphia, 1877.
19. Youngken, H.W. **Textbook of Pharmacognosy.** 5th ed. Blakiston. Philadelphia, 1943.
20. Jarboe, C.H., Schmidt, C.M. & Nicholson, J.A. & Zirvi, K.A. "Uterine relaxant properties of viburnum." **Nature,** 212, 837, 1966.

# MENTAL ALERTNESS/SENILITY

## HERBS

**Form:** Capsule, Tea

**CONTENTS: PEPPERMINT** *(Mentha piperita),* **SIBERIAN GINSENG** *(Eleutherococcus senticosus),* **Skullcap** *(Scutellaria lateriflora),* **Wood Betony** *(Stachys officinalis),* **Gotu Kola** *(Hydrocotyle asiatica),* & **Kelp** *(Laminaria, Macrocystis, Ascophyllum).*

**PURPOSE: To improve poor memory; To increase concentration capability and mental stamina; To overcome the effects of aging on mental attributes.**

**Other Applications:** Poor circulation, irritability, anxiety, insomnia, hyperactivity, depression.

**USE:** 1. Adults, general use: As desired, up to 12 capsules per day.
2. Adults, acute conditions: 3-4 capsules, 3 times per day.
3. Hyperactive children: 2-3 capsules in morning; 1-2 capsules at dinner. Use 3-4 capsules of Ginger root per day.
4. To supplement the FATIGUE blend: 2-3 capsules per day.
5. To supplement the LOW BLOOD SUGAR blend: 1-4 capsules per day.

**Contraindications:** None.

With growing age, the blood supply to the brain usually decreases and brings on the death of cerebral neurons. Nerve death is also caused by alcoholism, smoking, Vitamin B-Complex deficiency and so on. Decreased mental function invariably results. Similar conditions can result from genetic lesions, biochemical deficits, trauma and maternal pre-natal health. Neural cell damage cannot easily be reversed. As a general rule, brain cells do not replace themselves. Sometimes, however, remaining live brain cells can take over the functions of their dead neighbors. Therefore, there is always hope for continued healthy functioning. Mental dysfunction, including poor memory and the inability to concentrate also result from unnecessary restlessness, irritability, hypersensitivity and nervous excitability. The goals of this blend are to help younger, healthy individuals improve the efficiency of their mental faculties, to prevent the onset of senile brain damage, to arrest any degeneration in progress, or delay its onset as long as possible, to help healthy tissue compensate for deficiencies, and secondarily, to curb irritability, hypersensitivity, etc. To accomplish these ends the blend must increase healthy arterial and venous circulation, and improve the general health of the nervous system and the rest of the body, especially the adrenal system. These herbs provide circulation to the cells of the brain, nurture nerves, calm irritability, impart restfulness and clarity of mind, and generally increase mental capabilities. They probably will not reverse any neural damage already sustained, but the increased mental capacity experienced may make you think they have.

**PEPPERMINT LEAF,** due to the presence of several essential oils, prevents congestion of the blood supply to the brain, helps to clear up any circulatory congestion that exists, stimulates circulation, and strengthens and calms nerves. It is this last effect which has been noted so often by clinicians treating deficiencies in the ability to concentrate. The calming effect produced by Peppermint allows the patient to apply himself directly to the task at hand. University students have benefited greatly through participation in loosely controlled experiments assessing the effects of Peppermint tea on test-taking skills and examination scores (**1**). *See Also FATIGUE; DIGESTION*

**SIBERIAN GINSENG** is, of course, the famous Asiatic tonic, that has been shown in numerous studies to affect mental and physical behavior (**2-3**). In geriatric use, Ginseng has been proven beneficial in restoring mental abilities (**4-5**). Ginseng helps by directly affecting the adrenal-pituitary axis (**6**), which effect is most often manifested as increased resistance to the effects of stress (**7**). The herb also aids mental function by improving circulation (**8**). Studies have also demonstrated the ability of Ginseng to help learning (**9-10**). Other studies show that Ginseng is a direct central nervous system stimulant (**11-13**). All of these effects, and others discussed more fully in chapters on LOW BLOOD SUGAR, FATIGUE and WHOLE BODY TONIC blends, contribute to the pronounced beneficial effects of Ginseng on mental health, the prevention of senility, and the remedy of lost mental powers. *See Also FATIGUE; WHOLE BODY; INFERTILITY; LOW BLOOD SUGAR*

**SKULLCAP** is one of the best nervines in the plant kingdom. Read about this herb in the chapters on INSOMNIA, NERVOUS TENSION, NERVES & GLANDS and PAIN RELIEF. We note here only that the herb probably affects mental abilities by removing the nervous tension that often interferes with learning, recall, logical thinking and memory formation. In this regard, it very much resembles a muscle relaxant (**14**).

**WOOD BETONY** is also a good nervine with known hypotensive properties (**15**). It is used primarily to reduce nervousness through a mild sedative action. *See Also INSOMNIA; NERVOUS TENSION; PAIN RELIEF*

**GOTU KOLA,** being a naturally excellent neural tonic, slowly builds mental stamina and neural health. It is an excellent treatment for nervous breakdown. In addition, Gotu Kola, according to Asian and European practice, is an excellent blood purifier, glandular tonic and diuretic. It is used around the world for diseases of the skin, blood and nervous system, for leprosy and syphilis, psoriasis, cervicitis, vaginitis, blisters and so forth (**16**). India is the country in which Gotu Kola is perhaps most popular. There the plant has enjoyed a long history of folk use, and like our Goldenseal, its potential uses have been well explored. The people of India use the plant specifically to improve memory and longevity (**17**). *See Also FATIGUE; WHOLE BODY TONIC*

**KELP** is included in this blend to provide nutritional support to the nervous system and heart, in the form of vitamins, minerals and cell salts. In addition, it supplies a hypotensive principle. This property is likely to have a sparing effect on cardiac and neural tissues, i.e., it saves them from unnecessary stress, prolongs their effective lifetime, and increases their efficiency during daily use. Japanese researchers found that Laminaria exhibits definite hypotensive and blood cholesterol lowering activity when given to rabbits and humans (**18-20**). This effect is probably due to histamine content (**21**), but could also be a property of the iodine, the amino acid laminine (**22**), or some combination of minerals or other nutrients. *See Also* FEVERS & INFECTIONS; CIRCULATION; THYROID; ENVIRONMENTAL POLLUTION; PAIN; INFERTILITY; HEART; FATIGUE; BLOOD PURIFICATION/DETOXIFICATION; WEIGHT LOSS

# OTHER NUTRIENTS

*Mental capacities are very much a function of nutritional chemistry. The entire functioning of the nervous system depends upon the adequate supply of essential nutrients. The following recommendations are meant as guidelines only. One should determine his or her own requirements and stick with them.*

## VITAMINS

*(Daily requirements unless otherwise noted)*

Vitamin B Complex
Vitamin B1 *25-300 mg*
Vitamin B2 *25-300 mg*
Vitamin B6 *25-300 mg*
Vitamin C *1,000-3,000 mg*
Vitamin E *400 I.U.*
Choline *1,000 mg.*
Inositol *1,000 mg*
Folic Acid *400 mcg*
Niacinamide *100 mg*

## MINERALS

Calcium/Magnesium
Phosphorous
Zinc

## MISCELLANEOUS

HCl
Brewer's yeast

# REFERENCES

1. Mowrey, D.B. Informal study conducted among graduate students at Brigham Young University, 1978. Was not double-blind, but did include a placebo control group.
2. Blohkin, B.N., "The influence of eleutherococcus root extracts and leaves on human work capacity with statistical and dynamic loadings." **Eleutherococcus and Other Adaptogenic Plants of the Far East,** 7th se., 191-194, 1966.
3. Berdyshev, V.V. "The influence of eleutherococcus and physical stress on the organism of sailors in the tropics." **Led. Sred. D'nego Vostoka,** 10, 64-66, 1970.
4. Zhou, D.H. "preventive geriatics: an overview from traditional chinese medicine." **American Journal of Chinese Medicine,** 10(1-4), 32-39, 1982.
5. Turkevich, O.M., et. A., "Using eleutherococcus to treat patients with senile and arteriosclerotic psychoses." **24th Session of the Committee to Study Ginseng and Other Medicinal Plants of the Far East.** VBaldivostok, 96 pages.
6. Kirilov, O.I. "The effect of fluid extract of eleutherococcus root on the pituitary-adrenocortical system." **Slb. Otd. Acad. Nauk S.S.S.R.,** 23, 3-5, 1964.
7. Golotin, G.F. & Bojko, S. N., "Research on the increased resistance of organisms treated with eleutherococcus and other medicines." **Material for Study of Ginseng and Other Medicinal Plants of the Far East,** 5, 257-259.
8. Dardymov, I.V., Khasina, E.I. & Melnikov, V.N. "On eleutherococcus glycosides regulatory influence upon stress regulation." **Stress & Adaptation,** "Shtiintsa", Kishenev, 168, undtd.
9. Golikov, P.P. "Influence of aqueous extracts of roots, stems and leaves of eleutherococcus and ginseng on the mental abilities of working humans." **Mater. K. Izuch. Zhen-shenya i Drug. Lek. Dal'nego Vostoka,** 5, 233-235, 1963.
10. Hyuchenok, R.Y. "Eleutherococcus medicines' effects on rates' memory." **Medicines of the Far East,** U.S.S.R. Acad of Sciences, Vladivostok, 83-85, 1972.
11. Saratikov, A.S., "Some results of the search for and study of stimulants of the central nervous system of plant origin." **Stim. CNS.** Tomsk U. Press, 1, 3-23, 1966.
12. Brekhman, I.I., "Toxicity and general action of eleutherococcus." In **Eleutherococcus root—new stimulating and toning remedy.** VI Lenin Inst. Of Phys. Culture., Leningrad, U.S.S.R., p. 6-21, 1960.

13. Kucherenki, T.M. "Changes in the conditioned reflexes of dogs under the influence of eleutherococcus." In **Papers on the Study of Ginseng etc.,** Valdivostok, 237-240, 1963.
14. Usow, V. **Farmakologiia I Toksikologiia,** 21(2), 31-34, 1958.
15. Zinchenko, T.V. & Fefer, I.M. "Investigation of glycosides from betonica officinalis." **Farmatsevt. Zhurnal,** 17(3), 35-38, 1962.
16. List, P.H. & Hoerhammer, L. **Hagers Handbuch der Pharmazeutischen Praxis.** Volumes 2-5, Springer-Verlag, Berlin.
17. Chopra, R.N. **Indigenous Drugs of India.** Arts Press, Calcutta, 2nd Ed., Chopra, R.N., Chopra, I.C.,et al., Calcutta, India, 1933.
18. Kameda, J. "Medical studies on seaweeds. I." **Fukushima Igaku Zasshi,** 10, 251-269, 1960.
19. Kameda, J. "Medical studies on seaweeds. II." **Fukushima Igaku Zasshi,** 11, 289-309, 1961.
20. Ozawa, H., Gomi, Y. & Otsuki, I. "Pharmacological studies on laminine monocitrate." **Yakugaku Zasshi,** 87(8), 935-939, 1967.
21. Funayama, S. & Hikino, H. "Hypotensive principle of laminaria and allied seaweeds." **Planta Medica,** 41, 29-33, 1981.
22. Takemoto, T., Daigo, K. & Takagi, N. "Hypotensive constituents of marine algae. I. A new basic amino acid (laminine) and the other basic constituents isolated from laminaria augustata." **Yakugaku Zasshi,** 84(12), 1176-1179, 1964.

# NAUSEA

## HERBS

**Form:** Capsule

**CONTENTS:** **GINGER** root *(Zingiber officinale)*, **Licorice root** *(Glycyrrhiza glabra)*, & **Cayenne,** *(Capsicum annuum).*

**PURPOSE:** **To help diminish the symptoms of nausea that result from motion sickness, morning sickness, or stomach disorders; to ameliorate symptoms of vertigo and dizziness.**

**Other Applications:** Headaches; Learning disabilities that result from inner ear disturbances.

**USE:** 1. Nausea: The use of this blend to treat nausea is somewhat unique among herbal preparations. The basic rule of thumb, developed over hundreds of case studies and experiments, is "Use enough that you experience a Ginger aftertaste like a mild burning sensation in the throat and/or stomach." That might be two capsules, like before a road, plane or boat trip, or a dozen capsules, as during a case of stomach flu. The following are rough guides:

Motion Sickness: 2-4 capsules 1/2 hour ahead of time;
2-4 capsules whenever symptoms first begin to occur
Morning Sickness: 3-8 capsules before arising;
3-5 capsules as needed
Dizziness, Vertigo: 2 capsules every 1/2 hour

Stomach Flu: 4-6 capsules at first indication;
As many as needed every 1/2 hour from then on.
Headache: 2-4 capsules as needed.

**Contraindications:** None. Only minute amounts of Licorice and Cayenne should be in this blend. Their influence should only be felt when large quantities of the blend are being ingested, and then the influence will only be mild. See Appendix A for complete discussions of these two herbs.

Nausea is a symptom that arises from many physiological conditions, some of which are the result of stomach and digestive problems, such as the flu, gallstones, indigestion and poisoning. Conditions like ear infections, vertigo, motion sickness, headache, fever and inflammations, psychological stimuli, and dizziness cause nausea indirectly, taking advantage of rich neural connections between the stomach and certain brain centers. Certain nutritional states, such as pantothenic acid and vitamin B6 deficiencies, can make a person more susceptible than usual to nausea-causing events. Most medicines for nausea attempt to curb it either through the nervous system, or through neutralization of the nauseating toxins in the stomach. This blend appears to work at both levels, a determination that was verified only after years of research. The primary effects of this blend are due to the Ginger root. **Licorice root** is added for its gastrointestinal healing properties. A minute amount of **Cayenne** is present for its pleasantly stimulating effect. In earlier versions of this blend, I combined the Ginger root with other carminatives, such as fennel, catnip and peppermint, all good herbs in their own right. However, none of them were as good as Ginger root; they only served to dilute the Ginger root. Licorice root and Cayenne, however, provide properties that Ginger root does not possess, and actually potentiate the activity and effectiveness of the Ginger root.

**GINGER ROOT** has been the subject of my intense interest, both professional and avocational, for several years. This relationship began when I discovered that a powdered, encapsulated version of the herb kept me from throwing up during a bout with the "24-hour" flu. I subsequently passed the capsules out to anyone who had the slightest tendency toward being nauseated, or having diarrhea. It worked wonders. Eventually, a colleague and I published a paper on the effects of Ginger root on motion sickness (**1**). We chose motion sickness because it was the easiest form of nausea to bring under experimental control. Compared to dimenhydrinate, the most common over-the-counter drug, Ginger root was significantly better. But that's just one kind of nausea. Briefly, here is a summary of my findings on the effects of Ginger root on various types of nausea, involving the participation of literally hundreds of people, over a period of eight years.

**1. Motion Sickness.** The herb worked for over 90% of the people who tried it, if they used it correctly. It was most effective when 2-4 capsules were ingested prior to travel. Two more capsules were ingested about every hour or so, or immediately upon feeling the least sign of upset stomach. Often, the amount used decreased over the duration of the trip, probably at least partly because anxiety decreased as the person learned to trust the herb, and he or she could then relax. Ginger root was equally effective for car, boat, train or plane rides, with boat rides requiring the closest attention to proper maintenance.

**2. Morning Sickness.** Ginger root was effective in reducing or eliminating morning sickness in just over 75% of the cases. Some cases were dramatic, such as the woman who had tried everything else during two extremely sick pregnancies. Nothing worked. On the third pregnancy, she tried Ginger root, and it worked extremely well. Generally, the women who had the most success used about the same regimen. They took anywhere from 3-8 capsules before getting out of bed in the morning, then stayed in bed and kept taking the herb (up to the 8-10 capsule range) until any nausea they felt upon waking was gone. Throughout the day, they took 3-5 capsules at the slightest hint of nausea, and then relaxed quietly until the nausea went away.

**3. Dizziness and Vertigo.** Not only did Ginger root prevent nausea, but it eliminated dizziness as well in 40-50% of the cases I observed. About half a dozen cases involved people who were unable to leave their homes, ride in a car or train for years. If they did they got hopelessly dizzy and then terribly sick. They took Ginger root to help subdue the nausea, and were amazed to have the vertigo disappear also. Compared to doses required for other conditions, very little Ginger root was required, usually 2-4 capsules periodically during the day.

**4. Stomach Flu.** Here's where people have needed the largest doses. Effective treatment regimens have gone like this: At the *very first* sign of nausea, or even sooner, if the patients suspected they were in line for a contagious virus, they took a "handful" (probably anywhere from 6 to 10) of capsules, and then 2-4 every half hour or hour, until they were certain the danger period had passed. How did they know? Well, in my case, I just gradually backed off until I quit feeling even faintly nauseated. Of course, the problem with *preventing* illness is, without sophisticated tests, you're never certain you would have become ill anyway. But if you and whoever else took the Ginger root were the *only* ones in the family or neighborhood who didn't get sick, even though you took care of and cleaned up after those who were ill, that's good evidence of effective preventive treatment. I have seen that happen on several occasions. Those people who used Ginger root to treat stomach flu *after* they had the illness, and were feeling nauseated, took 10-12 capsules all at once and hoped they weren't too late. If they were too late, they vomited up the Ginger along with the rest of their stomach contents. And sometimes, due to the pungent nature of the herb, that was not pleasant. If the capsules stayed down, then the nausea would dissipate. The motto, if any, is: Catch it early and don't skimp on the dosage. Remember, 12 capsules equals only a tablespoon full, and we're dealing with a whole herb, not an extract.

**5. Other Conditions.** In my observations and studies, Ginger Root has effectively eliminated headaches, remedied certain learning disabilities, and been as effective in eliminating diarrhea as it is in preventing nausea. Studies by other individuals have shown that Ginger root has a slight stimulating effect on the heart, vasomotor and respiratory centers (**2**), something most of us can use. It prevents a rise in serum and hepatic cholesterol levels that could occur from cholesterol-rich diets (**3**), and it promotes digestion (**4**).

**Toxicity.** One could legitimately wonder what side effects are going to arise if people all across the land are ingesting large quantities of Ginger root. After performing toxicity tests in scores of rats and mice, I did not observe even slight toxic symptoms at doses 10 times those that a human would normally ingest. To my knowledge, no other study exists that shows toxicity. Lethal dosage levels have been established, but are so high that the herb has been accepted as completely safe by the FDA. Out of the hundreds of human trials I have observed, no toxic effects have been manifested. I know people who use this blend on a daily basis, to treat chronic problems, without the slightest indication of a side effect. They tell me, "Take away my Ginger root only at the risk of your life." So I let them keep it.

## OTHER NUTRIENTS

*Maintaining adequate metabolic health can reduce the tendency toward chronic nausea that afflicts many people, and can help you recover from nauseating illnesses much faster. Individual needs may vary widely. Use the following table as a guideline only.*

### VITAMINS

*(Daily requirements unless otherwise noted)*

Pantothenic Acid *100-200 mg*
Vitamin B1 *25 mg*
Vitamin B2 *25 mg*
Vitamin B6 *100 mg*
Niacinamide *100 mg*

### MINERALS

Potassium
Calcium/Magnesium
Phosphorous

### MISCELLANEOUS

Liver

## REFERENCES

1. Mowrey, D.B. & Clayson, D.E. "Motion sickness, ginger and psychophysics." **The Lancet,** March 20, 655-657, 1982.
2. Ally, M.M. "The pharmacological action of zingiber officinale." **Proceedings of the Pan Indian Ocean Scientific Congress,** 4th, Karachi, Pakistan, Section G, 11-12, 1960.
3. Gujral, S., Bhumra, H. & Swaroop, M. "Effect of ginger (zingiber officinale roscoe) oleoresin on serum and hepatic cholesterol levels in cholesterol fed rats." **Nutrition Reports International,** 17(2), 183-189, 1978.
4. Glatzel, H. "Treatment of dyspeptic disorders with spice extracts." **Hippokrates,** 40(23), 916-919, 1969.

# NERVES & GLANDS

## HERBS

**Form:** Capsule, Tea

**CONTENTS: GOLDENSEAL** root *(Hydrastis canadensis)*, **GENTIAN** root *(Gentiana lutea)*, **Chamomile flowers** *(Matricaria chamomilla)*, **Blue Vervain** *(Verbena hastata)*, **Dandelion root** *(Taraxacum officinale)*, **Yellow Dock root** *(Rumex crispus)*, **Skullcap** *(Scutellaria lateriflora)*, **Wood Betony** *(Stachys officinalis)*, **Kelp** *(Laminaria, Macrocystis, Ascophyllum)*, **Cayenne** *(Capsicum annum)*, **Saw Palmetto berries** *(Serenoa repens-sabal)*.

**PURPOSE: Nerve and gland tonic.**

**Other Applications:** Infections, Fevers, Anxiety, Insomnia, Inflammations, Anorexia, Indigestion.

**USE:** 2-4 capsules per day.

**Contraindications:** None. For discussion of Cayenne, see Appendix A.

This blend is meant to be a general dietary supplement, to be used on a daily basis, by virtually anyone engaged in the process of toning up the body's general functions, improving the overall health of the nerves and glands, or recovering from illness. The blend contains several clinically and scientifically verified tonics for the glands and nerves. Heading the list is that grand tonic, **Goldenseal.** The Cherokees were probably the first group to discover a variety of applications for this plant. It eventually became a standard part of

American herbal medicine. **Dandelion** is used as a tonic in America, Europe and China; **Yellow Dock** in America, Europe, Japan, & India; **Chamomile** in America, Russia, Europe and Mexico; **Skullcap** and **Wood Betony** in America, Europe and India; **Gentian,** in America & Europe; **Kelp** in America, Europe, and all over Asia; Cayenne, in America, Mexico, Europe, Asia and Africa; and **Saw Palmetto** in America.

**NOTE:**  For an herb to qualify as a culture-wide tonic, it must be accessible and freely in use by that culture for scores or even hundreds of years. It must benefit the majority of those who use it, and those beneficial effects must be fairly general, gentle and enduring. Toxic side effects must be very low or absent, even with prolonged use, and it can't be too nasty in flavor. Though many candidate herbs can be found in manuals under the heading "tonic", only a few ever attain the status of a major tonic. Generally, science does not investigate a product to determine if it is a tonic; science needs to be more specific. But, in how many specific ways does a plant need to be shown effective, in order to qualify as a general tonic? That is probably an impossible question to answer. The qualification of a tonic must, in the last analysis, rest upon the manner in which it is used by the people. This herbal blend contains herbs that have met the qualifications but, except for the more generally active Goldenseal and Kelp, are still somewhat specific to the glands and nerves. The WHOLE BODY TONIC blend contains other great tonics for the body. The following discussions emphasize the cultural use of the plants, and scientific studies are cited only where I have felt the need to validate a plant's general mode of action. The specific actions of the herbs of this blend can be found, in most cases, in the discussions of the other blends in which they occur.

**GOLDENSEAL** is a plant originally of pure North American use, to which have been ascribed practically every medicinal trait a plant could possess. It has been called a cure-all, a panacea, and God's gift to mankind. Whether it deserves all of these accolades may be disputed. Indisputably, however, when consumed in small quantities, on a regular basis, it is an effective neural and glandular tonic. Its active principles include hydrastine and berberine, which are both potent antibiotics, vasoconstrictors and uterine tonics. These alkaloids occur in dozens of pharmaceutical preparations in the United States and Canada, which are usually over-the-counter products: elixirs, tablets, capsules, teas, suppositories, etc. They are used as tonics, stomachics, antacids, antispasmodics, to fight gastritis, colitis, varicose veins, menstrual problems, rheumatism, muscle aches, diarrhea and piles, ulcers, jaundice, and so on. Goldenseal has acquired an international reputation, occurring in over a dozen foreign pharmacopoeias. *See Also VAGINAL YEAST INFECTION, STOMACH/INTESTINAL, FEVERS & INFECTIONS, INFLUENZA, EYES, HEMORRHOIDS.*

**GENTIAN ROOT** is an example of one of those herbs with an incredible reputation in one country, but largely overlooked by the rest of the world. The Germans have been using this herb as a tonic for centuries. Other European nations have too, but to a much lesser degree. Gentian is a simple bitter. All bitters reflexively stimulate the activity of the glands, but each in its own way. Gentian is one of the best understood, acting on the whole digestive process, to stimulate appetite and increase digestion by stimulating the flow of bile. Simple dyspepsia, or severe anorexia, can be effectively treated by this herb. German scientists have been intensively studying Gentian root for decades. Their findings confirm the herb's tonic qualities (**1-2**). *See Also DIABETES, CIRCULATION, THYROID, STOMACH/INTESTINAL.*

**CHAMOMILE** is a favorite of women and children in Europe (and in some parts of the United States), and is part of the daily diet of many of these people. It is the best-known European "cure-all." Like Gentian and Dandelion, it is also a bitter tonic. Proven properties of Chamomile are many. Leading the list is an antispasmodic effect (**3**), which has been shown to be comparable to papaverine (**4**). One of the longest known and most firmly established properties of this herb is its anti-inflammatory effect (**5**). Internally or externally applied, it will reduce inflammation caused by infections, wounds, metabolic disorders and so forth. Used on the teeth it relieves swelling and pain very effectively. Related to the above properties is Chamomile's sedative property (**6**). Other proven actions of the herb include anti-ulcer (**7**), antibacterial (against both staph and strep) and antimycotic effects (**8**), as well as its usefulness in treating dermatological ailments (**9**). The traditional roles of a bitter, including a stimulating effect on the liver (**10**), have also been firmly established. Off and on, researchers have investigated the anti-tumor or anti-cancer properties of Chamomile, always with positive results (e.g., **11**). In his classic study of agents against cancer, Hartwell found Chamomile had been used against benign as well as malignant tumors and carcinomas of the liver, stomach, mouth, skin and brain, internally as well as externally (**12**). He also found it had been used against sclerosis of the liver and other organs, swelling nodes, Scirrhus (hard cancerous swelling), and breast and anal abscesses (**12**). The active principles of Chamomile include essential oils (chamazulen and bisabolol), flavanoids, glycosides, and a very important dicylic ether. The numerous known effective properties of this plant underscore its centuries-old use as a tonic for both adults and children. Cultures as divergent as Western Europe, Russia, and India have all used Chamomile for very similar tonic purposes down through the centuries. *See Also FEMALE TONIC*

**BLUE VERVAIN** has been used in folk medicine as a diuretic for edema, as an antidiarrhetic, a vulnerary, stimulant, sudorific, emmenagogue, diaphoretic, expectorant, for chronic bronchitis, rheumatism, as a stimulant for weakened conditions, nervous pains, sleeplessness, tiredness and anemia. The active principles are glycosides (verbenaline and verbenine), substances with weak parasympathetic mimicking activity, which probably accounts for most of the traditionally observed effects. In animal studies, it has been shown to contract smooth muscles of the uterus and gastro-intestinal tract, with very little toxicity (**13**). Vervain has also been proven to be anti-inflammatory and analgesic (pain killer) (**14**). Various Native American groups used Blue Vervain in their medicine, including the Menominees (to clear up cloudy urine), the Dakotas (for stomachache) and the Omahas (as a tonic). The herb was listed in the National Formulary from 1916 to 1926. Vervain, in one of its more than 300 subspecies, has been a popular medicinal plant in cultures all over the world for thousands of years, but has attracted very little attention from the scientific community, probably because it is mild acting. As part of a tonic blend, expect it to help restore vitality, gradually and mildly. *See Also FEVERS & INFECTIONS*

**DANDELION ROOT** is another effective bitter that has been used as a tonic and blood cleanser for hundreds of years, especially in Europe and China. All of the glands involved in any way with the digestive system respond rapidly and effectively to Dandelion. American science has never known quite what to make of or do with Dandelion. Because of the herb's high inulin content, its potential usefulness in the treatment of diabetes makes it a prime candidate for experimental investigation, but the political and economic constraints in this country simply do not reinforce the medicinal study of yard weeds. In Europe and Asia, where these constraints are absent or greatly reduced, medical science has fully incorporated the herb into its medical arsenal. But in reviewing the writings of American physicians over the last two centuries, and especially this century, one discovers a cyclical waxing and waning of interest in the plant that always falls just short of the decision to commit research money to its scientific investigation. Routine U.S.D.A. analyses have, however, provided some very interesting data, like the fact that Dandelion greens are richer in Vitamin A than even carrots, and exceed the Vitamin B, C and D content of most other traditional vegetables. *See Also SKIN; DIABETES; BLOOD PURIFICATION/DETOXIFICATION; LIVER DISORDERS*

**YELLOW DOCK ROOT** achieves its tonic properties through the astringent purification of the blood supply to the glands. Like other herbs in this blend, it is often used in seasonal cleanses and other blood detoxification programs. Among all herbs, it has one of the strongest reputations for clearing up skin problems, liver and gall bladder ailments, and glandular inflammation and swelling. High in iron, Yellow Dock is an effective tonic treatment for anemia. Docks of all kinds were used by Native American tribes for a host of conditions, and many of these treatments were trade secrets, closely guarded by medicine men. When Yellow Dock was introduced to America from Europe, it was quickly included in the medicine man's pouch, being more effective than most native species. Some Indian doctors, in fact, became more proficient than their European counterparts in using Yellow Dock to treat jaundice. *See Also SKIN; BLOOD PURIFICATION & DETOXIFICATION*

**SKULLCAP** is a favorite herb among those who have discovered its effectiveness in treating numerous ailments. Its use as a tonic is derived from its bitter principles, although its calmative property is probably due to the presence of a volatile oil, scutellarin. Skullcap was used by several American Indian tribes and was listed in the National Formulary and U.S. Pharmacopoeia for a while. However, it has never achieved the level of recognition it deserves, mainly because of a series of events that took place almost 200 years ago. A New England physician reported having prevented several cases of hydrophobia with the plant, and several other "doctors" got on the bandwagon, making exaggerated claims along those lines. As a result the herb lost all credibility, and fell into disrepute. Interestingly, as far as I know, nobody has ever attempted to experimentally verify the original claims for its use against rabies. Nor have many of the other purported uses for Scullcap been systematically investigated. The use of Skullcap as a tonic is shared by Americans, Europeans and Asians. *See Also NERVOUS TENSION; INSOMNIA; PAIN*

**WOOD BETONY** was used in medieval England to cure "monstrous nocturnal visions, devils, despair and lunacy". Among these early peoples, Wood Betony was one of the most highly prized of herbs, for it could be used to keep the world sane and safe. This basic principle persisted through the ages, being adapted to fit whatever current theories of behavior, sane and insane, prevailed at the time. Today, we believe that man's inner peace, ability to sleep at night, and ability to deal with the pressures of everyday life, are more or less functions of his physical health. We have also discovered the hypotensive properties of Wood Betony. So, today we use the herb to calm the nerves, encourage relaxing sleep, and tone up glandular functioning. We are, after all, civilized and intelligent people.... *See Also PAIN; NERVOUS TENSION*

**KELP** is an important general nutritive tonic for the peoples of essentially every land in which it grows. Until recent years it was, however, eaten almost exclusively and universally by the Japanese. Cultural studies have been undertaken to determine what differences the Japanese intake of Kelp has made. Heading the list is a dramatically lower breast cancer rate. Also on the list are: less obesity, less heart disease, less respiratory disease, less rheumatism and arthritis, less high blood pressure, less thyroid deficiency, less constipation and gastro-intestinal ailments, and less infectious disease. The Japanese consume between 5 and 7.5 grams of Kelp per capita per day. It is used in almost every meal, as garnish, in soup, as a vegetable, in cakes, jellies and jams, sauces, salads and flour. The flour is used to make noodles, one the most common Japanese foods. Interestingly, among those Japanese social-economic groups most heavily Westernized—the rich and urban—Kelp consumption has been decreasing and all of the above diseases have been increasing. Among the the poor and the rural people, Kelp consumption has been increasing and the disease rates have been decreasing. That's why Kelp occurs in so many of the blends in this book. *See Also DIABETES; PROSTATE; FEVERS & INFECTIONS; WEIGHT LOSS; FATIGUE; BLOOD PURIFICATION/DETOXIFICATION; HEART; PAIN; INFERTILITY; MENTAL ALERTNESS/SENILITY; ENVIRONMENTAL POLLUTION*

**CAYENNE** has positive effects on circulation, the heart, the stomach and all other systems of the body. But it is not usually thought of as a tonic. It is generally considered a carminative and a stimulant. The stimulant property, however, is so prevalent that increased tonus of nerves and glands is a major end result of its action. Cayenne will insure the rapid and even distribution of the active principles of the rest of the herbs to critical functional centers of the body, including those involved in cellular respiration, metabolism, data transmission, and neural-hormonal activation. Cayenne is included in several other blends for this reason: In extremely small quantities it can dramatically increase the efficiency of most other herbs. *See Also FATIGUE; CIRCULATION; HIGH BLOOD PRESSURE*

**SAW PALMETTO BERRY** is an old American tonic, dating at least as far back as the Maya. John Lloyd, a famous early American medicinal botanist, observed that animals fed on these berries grew sleek and fat. When the word got around, many settlers began feeding them to their stock with the same remarkable results. Soon, medical researchers were investigating the berries and verifying the claims. Especially in the 1870's, many articles were published reporting experimental verification of Saw Palmetto berry's effects on body weight, general health and disposition, tranquilization, appetite stimulation, and reproductive health. Eventually, pressure from proponents of the herb from within the medical establishment lead to the inclusion of Saw Palmetto in the National Formualry and U.S. Pharmacopoeia. It was dropped from the USP in 1916 and the NF in 1950 as the enthusiasm of the medical profession for natural agents dwindled in this century. Nobody expressed doubt about the herb's effectiveness, but nobody was able to extract any active principle that would perform all the functions of the whole plant. At that point its future as an officially recognized drug was doomed. As a tonic, and as a food source, however, we can continue to enjoy these thoroughly American berries by ingesting them in blends like this one. *See Also INFERTILITY; RESPIRATORY AILMENTS; DIABETES; FEMALE TONIC; PROSTATE; THYROID; DIGESTION*

## OTHER NUTRIENTS

*Nutritional supplementation of nature's tonics can enhance and prolong their activity. Individual needs may depart substantially from the following general recommendations.*

### VITAMINS

*(Daily requirements unless otherwise noted)*

Vitamin B-1 *25-100 mg*

Vitamin B-2 *25-100 mg*
Vitamin B-6 *25-100 mg*
Vitamin C *500-1,000 mg*
Vitamin D *400 I.U.*
Vitamin E *400-600 I.U.*
Niacinamide *100 mg*
Folic acid *400 mcg*
Pantothenic Acid *100 mg*

## MINERALS

Calcium/Magnesium
Phosphorus
Zinc

# REFERENCES

1. Glatzel, H. "Treatment of dyspeptic disorders with spice extracts." **Hippokrates,** 40(23), 916-919, 1969.
2. Deininger, R. "Amarum-bitter herbs. Common bitter principle remedies and their action." **Krankenplege,** 29(3), 99-100, 1975.
3. Verzarne, P.G., Szegi, J. & Marczal, G. "Effect of certain chamomile compounds." **Acta Pharmaceutica Hungarica,** 49(1), 13-20, 1979.
4. Yakolev, V. & von Schlichtegroll, A. "Antiinflammatory activity of (-)-alpha-bisabolol, an essential component of chamomile oil." **Arzneimittel-Forschung,** 19(4), 615-616, 1969.
5. Jakovlev, V., Isacc, O., Thiemer, K. & Kunde, R. "Pharmacological investigations with compounds of chamomile. II. New investigations on the antiphlogistic effects of (-)-alpha-bisabolols and bisabolol oxides." **Planta Medica,** 35(2), 125-140, 1979.
6. Loggia, R.D., Traversa, U., Scarcia, V. & Tubaro, A. "Depressive effects of chamomilla recutita (l.) rausch, tubular flowers, on central nervous system in mice." **Pharmacological Research Communications,** 14(2), 153-162, 1982.
7. Szelenyi, I., Isaac, O. & Thiemer, K. "Pharmacological experiments with compounds of chamomile. III. Experimental studies of the ulcerprotective effect of chamomile." **Plant Medica,** 35(3), 218-227, 1979.
8. Shipochliev, T. "Extracts from a group of medicinal plants enhancing the uterine tonus." **Veterinary Sciences** (Sofia), 18(4), 94-98, 1981.

9. Isaac, O, & Kristen, G. "Old and new methods of chamomile therapy. Chamomile as example for modern research of medicinal plants." **Medizinische Welt,** 31(31-32), 1145-1149, 1980.

10. Pasechnik, I.K. "Cholertic action of matricaria officinalis." **Farmakilogiia i Toksikologiia,** 468-469, 1969.

11. Kraul, M.A. & Schmidt, F. "The growth-inhibiting effect of certain extracts from flores chamomilae and of a synthetic azulene derivative on experimental mice tumors." **Archive der Pharmazie (Weinheim),** 290, 66-75, 1957.

12. Hartwell, J.L. "Plants used against cancer: a survey." **Lloydia,** 31, 71, 1968.

13. List, P.H. & Hoerhammer, L. **Hagers Handbuch der Pharmazeutischen Praxis.** Volumes 2-5, Springer-Verlag, Berlin.

14. Sakai, S. "Pharmacological actions of verbena officinalis extracts." **Gifu Ika Daigaku Kiyo,** 11(1), 6-17, 1963.

# NERVOUS TENSION

## HERBS

**Form:** Capsule.

**CONTENTS:** **VALERIAN** root *(Valeriana officinalis)*, **Passion Flower** *(Passiflora incarnata)*, **Wood Betony** *(Stachys officinalis)*, **Black Cohosh root** *(Cimicifuga racemosa)*, **Skullcap** *(Scutellaria lateriflora)*, **Hops** *(Humulus lupulus)*, & **Ginger root** *(Zingiber officinale)*.

**PURPOSE:** **Nervine and calmative for anxiety, fear, being over-worked, hysteria and other problems aggravated by emotional disturbances. An essential product for the "modern man."**

**Other Applications:** Insomnia, childhood hyperactivity, psycho-somatic problems, hives, shingles, ery-sipelas, restlessness.

**USE:** 1. For most conditions: 2-3 capsules every four hours as needed.
2. Insomnia: 2 capsules 2 hours before retiring; 2 capsules upon retiring. Or use INSOMNIA blend.
3. Hyperactivity: 2 capsules at breakfast and lunch. Use with TONIC—NERVE & GLAND blend.
4. To supplement HEART blend: 2 capsules per day.
5. To supplement HIGH BLOOD PRESSURE blend: 2-3 capsules per day.
6. To supplement PAIN RELIEF blend: 1-2 capsules as desired.

**Contraindications:**   None. Used alone or in conjunction with other blends and medications, this blend is completely safe.

The nervous system is designed to not only translate your wishes into actions through control over the muscles, but to receive, transmit, store, organize and retrieve information. That information reflects the status of the world about you, the internal state of your body and your expectations about what the world and your body will be like a moment from now. The nervous system is usually divided into subsystems for the purpose of clarification of function and anatomy. For example, there are the central and peripheral nervous systems, or the autonomic and voluntary nervous systems, or the sympathetic and parasympathetic divisions of the autonomic nervous system. For our purposes, the distinction between the cholinergic and adrenergic nervous systems is of most value. The adrenergic nervous system is so named because all nerves involved depend on the presence of adrenalin (and related compounds) for proper function. The cholinergic system depends on the presence of acetylcholine (ACh). The two systems work in opposition at times, and complement one another at other times. Generally, when you are aroused, ready for action, your body produces adrenalin-type chemicals so that the adrenergic system can operate correctly. At times of rest and relaxation, the cholinergic system takes over, allowing you to digest food, sleep, recover from stress, etc. If you stay in a prolonged state of arousal, the constant presence of adrenalin-related chemicals and their metabolites will do damage ranging from ulcers to hypertension to insomnia. You need to relax often. Commercial sedatives, tranquilizers and anti-anxiety drugs help you accomplish that but their side-effects usually outweigh their value. The world of medicinal foods provides many potent but safe calming and relaxing agents.

This blend contains such a group of safe herbs whose sedative properties are known throughout the world. Only in an encapsulated product such as this could they all be so easily combined. Of these herbs, Valerian root has been experimentally investigated most often, particularly in the Soviet Union, where for mysterious reasons it has become politically expedient to propagandize the herb's benefits to the people. Much of their research is therefore questionable, but much of it also appears sound and reliable. This blend can be expected to provide mild sedation and tranquilization at the recommended usage. Although some of the herbs in this blend are significant relaxants and sedatives by themselves, most of these herbs work best in combination.

**VALERIAN ROOT,** as well as its valepotriate constituents, are tranquilizing on the nervous system. For centuries man has used this plant to calm upset nerves, treat psychological disorders, pain and headache. In 1966, the active ingredients were finally discovered (**1**). In a remarkable series of animal experiments that followed, the herb was proven to be sedative, to improve coordination, and to antagonize the hypnotic effects of alcohol (**2**). Meanwhile, clinical evidence obtained by careful testing by trained medical practitioners was accumulating. This evidence showed that in humans, Valerian root was strongly sedative. It also had a marked tendency to increase concentration ability, as well as energy level (**3**). The laboratory and clinical sources therefore merged into one overwhelming mass of documentation. To review all studies done to date, would fill several pages, but here are some examples of the kind of work being done with Valerian root and preparations made from it. Valmane, a German drug containing pure substances from Valerian root, has been frequently studied. It has been shown to suppress and regulate the autonomic nervous system in patients with control disorders, to be mildly sedative, to help regulate psychosomatic disorders, and relieve tension and restlessness (**4**). In another study, hypertensive men were given a glass of water containing extract of Valerian root. After a given period of time an examination revealed a general tranquilizing effect and EEG readings that indicated an elective neurotropic action on higher brain centers, thereby fulfilling criterion for being labeled a tranquilizer (**5**). One of the more interesting studies was performed on childhood behavior disorders. One hundred twenty children exhibiting various kinds of psychosomatic disturbances and behavioral disorders such as learning disability, hyperactivity and anxiety were treated for several weeks with Valmane. During that period over 75% experienced significant progress or complete recovery (**6**). Many other studies similar to that have been performed (e.g. **7-10**), but space does not permit their review here. *See Also HIGH BLOOD PRESSURE; INSOMNIA*

**PASSION FLOWER** was first discovered, in Peru, by the Spanish doctor Monardes in 1569. According to him the herb was highly treasured among the mountain people. So he and other explorers took it back to the Old World where it quickly became a favorite herb tea. Later, the herb came back to America with the early settlers. In many countries in Europe, and in the U.S. and Canada, the use of Passion Flower to tranquilize and settle edgy nerves has been firmly entrenched for 200 years or more. Not until the last 100 years, however, have researchers been able to verify the unique medicinal properties of this plant. In 1897, the analgesic property was proven, followed in 1904 by the discovery of principles that prevented, without side effects, sleeplessness caused by brain inflammation (**11**). Passion flower contains two major groups of chemicals, glycosides and flavanoids. The glycosides contain the very active harman and its derivatives. These substances when isolated from the plant can cause just the opposite reactions for which the whole is commonly used. The flavanoids do not by themselves yield the proper results either. Only when the two are combined, as in whole herb, do researchers observe the herb's main effect, a sedative property (**12**). The sedative effect of Passion flower has been firmly established in many studies (**13-14**). *See Also INSOMNIA; FEMALE TONIC*

**WOOD BETONY** is mentioned in European herbals as far back as 1600's. It is one of Europe's and America's favorite relaxants and headache remedies. As near as I can determine, the plant was popular among early American eclectic physicians who probably learned of its value in herbals from the Old World, and its use persists because of the value placed on it by the eclectics. The Indians did not use it except to reduce swellings, but the eclectics used it as a tonic, sedative, astringent and vulnerary (wound healer) (**15**). Almost all modern herbals, published in the United States, list Wood Betony (e.g.**16-17**) and extol its virtues along these lines: "Unsurpassed for headache, insanity, neuralgia, all pains in the head or face, heartburn...palsy, convulsions...nervous complaints" (**18**). Scientific verification is minimal. In fact, experimental work of any sort is hard to find. One study, however, did demonstrate that the glycosides of Wood Betony have observable hypotensive activity (**19**). This effect would explain most of the clinically observed properties, since a substance that is hypotensive would tend to relax nervous tension as well as loosen up constrictive blood vessels that are producing headaches, etc. *See Also PAIN; NERVES & GLANDS*

**BLACK COHOSH** has hypotensive and vasodilatory properties which are firmly supported by basic research. One investigator found that the plant had a general hypotensive effect due to the presence of active, water soluble resin (**20**). He hypothesized that the active principle influences the circulation directly through the central nervous system and indirectly through an inhibition of vasomotor centers involved in the handling of some forms of vertigo and auditory problems (interestingly, one of the few remaining medically recognized uses of Cimicifuga extract is to relieve auditory tinnitus). Other researchers have also found hypotensive properties as well as vasodilatory effects (**21**). Such experimental verification follows hundreds of years of using Black Cohosh for exactly the purposes finally substantiated. Black Cohosh is a primary nerve and smooth muscle relaxant and works great in cases of irritated nerves and general restlessness. The Russians have recently approved Black Cohosh extract for use as a central nervous system tonic and a treatment for high blood pressure (**22**). *See Also FEMALE TONIC; HIGH BLOOD PRESSURE; CHOLESTEROL REGULATION*

**SKULLCAP** is another good tonic and nervine, effective for insomnia, excitability, restlessness and other nervous complaints. Most research on this plant has been carried out in Russia at most of her major universities. A typical study finds that Skullcap is hypotensive or relaxing (**23**). Some major Russian medical books discuss the scientific findings in great detail. Therein, experiments are reviewed which have proven Skullcap to be a tonic (**24**), a sedative (**25**), an anti-epileptic (**26**), and so on. American experience with Skullcap dates from the last century, where one doctor wrote, "Scull-cap is a valuable tonic nervine and antispasmodic. It is especially useful in...neuralgia, convulsions, delirium tremens...nervous excitability, restlessness, and inability to sleep, and indeed in all nervous affections" (**27**). From that time to the present, natural health experts have recognized the value of Skullcap for these kinds of problems. *See Also INSOMNIA; NERVES & GLANDS; PAIN*

**HOPS** are one of the traditional nervine, sedative type agents employed in folk medicine throughout the Western world. Suggestions for use are all very similar: "Hops are most commonly used for their calming effect on the nervous system. Hop tea is recommended for nervous diarrhea, insomnia and restlessness" (**28**). Hops have also been the fortunate subject of a great deal of modern scientific investigation. One recent study showed that Hops are truly sedative, as opposed to merely muscle-relaxing (**29-30**). They are also fast acting. A soothing, relaxing calm will be experienced within 20-40 minutes after ingesting the herb (**31-32**). The earliest demonstration of sedative action in Hops was made in 1966, after other investigators had tried unsuccessfully for many years (**33**). Some later studies were also unsuccessful, because the active principles are somewhat elusive. In fact, the most industrious group of researchers admitted that, after several unsuccessful trials, they kept at it simply because they knew the herb worked. Lupulin is accepted as the active ingredient, but one other successful study found another unidentified antispasmotic principle in Hops (**34**). *See Also INSOMNIA*

**GINGER ROOT** is usually used as a carminative to soothe upset stomach. Its action is not fully understood, but at least one bit of research indicates that it has cholinergic action (**35**). This finding would make sense in the context of the known physiological properties of Ginger root, and it would indicate further that the herb antagonizes the effects of adrenergic stimulation. This last term refers to that part of the nervous system that comes into play when you are under stress. The adrenergic nervous system subserves the body's needs during such times. However, when stress passes, the cholinergic nervous system cuts in and attempts to restore equilibrium to the body, including the nerves, glands and muscles. Ginger root used in times of stress would therefore tend to offset the nerve-wracking effects of that stress, helping to calm the system and inhibit that "pins and needles" feeling. *See Also FATIGUE; CIRCULATION; LAXATIVE; NAUSEA; STOMACH/INTESTINAL; DIGESTION; LOW BLOOD SUGAR*

## OTHER NUTRIENTS

*Good nutritional and dietary practices are rare among the hurry, scurry, uptight group. Yet, in order for the nervous system to function properly, to support that kind of lifestyle, it must receive adequate nutritional support. Individual needs may depart substantially from the following general recommendations.*

### VITAMINS

*(Daily requirements unless otherwise noted)*

Vitamin B-1 *25-100 mg*
Vitamin B-2 *25-100 mg*
Vitamin B-6 *25-100 mg*
Vitamin C *500-1000 mg*
Vitamin D *400 I.U.*
Vitamin E *400-600 I.U.*
Niacinamide *100 mg*
Folic acid *400 mcg*
Pantothenic Acid *100 mg*
Choline *1-2 g*

## MINERALS

Calcium/Magnesium
Phosphorus
Zinc
Potassium

## MISCELLANEOUS

Lecithin
Brewer's Yeast
Essential Fatty Acid
GLA

# REFERENCES

1. Thies, P.W. & Funke, S. "Concerning the active principles of Valerian." **Tetrahedron Letters,** 1155-1162, 1966.
2. v. Eickstedt, K.S., et.al., **Arzneimittel-Forschungen,** 19, 316, 1969; and 19, 993, 1969.
3. Schaette, R. **Dissertation Muenchen,** 1971. and Schaette, R. "Stable valerian preparations." **Ger. Offen. 2,230,626,** 10 Jan. 1974.
4. Boeters, U. "Treatment of autonomic dysregulatioin with valepotriates (Valmane)." **Muenchener Medizinische Wochenschrift,** 37, 1873-1876, 1969.
5. Kempinskas, V. "On the action valerian." **Famakologiia i Toksikologiia,** 4(3), 305-309, 1964.
6. Klich, R. & Gladbach, B. "Childhood behavior disorders and their treatment." **Medizinishce Welt,** 26(25), 1251-1254, 1975.
7. Straube, G. "The meaning of Valerian root in therapy." **Therapie der Gegenwart,** 107, 555-562, 1968.
8. Hoenke, E. "Concerning psychic-vegetative effects of a supposed antihistaminic." **Nervenarzt,** 37, 448-453, 1953.
9. Ruecker, G. "Concerning the active principles of Valerian." **Pharmazie in Unserer Zeit,** 8(3), 78-86, 1979.
10. Szafran, H., Szmal, Z. & Sobotka-Wierzbowicz, J. "Evaluation of rhizomes and roots of Valeriana officinalis: Pharmacological investigations." **Herba Polska,** 18(1), 11-17, 1972.
11. Lutomski, J. "Alkaloidy Pasiflora incarnata L." **Dissertation , Institut for Medicinal Plant Research,** Poznan, 1960.
12. Ambuehl, H. "Anatomical and chemical investigations on Passiflora coerula L. und Passiflor incarnata L." **Diss. Nr. 3830 ETH,** Zurich, 1966.

13. Lutomski, J., Malek, B., Rybacka, L. "Pharmacological investigation of the raw materials from passiflora genus. 2. pharmacochemical estimation of juices from the fruits of passiflora edulis and passiflora edulis forma flavicarpa." **Planta Medica,** 27, 112, 1975.
14. Lutomski, J., Segiet, E., Szpunar, K. & Grisse, K. "The meaning of Passion flower in the medicine." **Pharmazie in Unserer Zeit,** 10(2), 45-48, 1981.
15. Smith, H. H. "Ethnobotany of the Potawatomi." **Bulletin of the Public Museum,** 7, 32-127, 1933.
16. Lust, J. **The Herb Book,** Benedict Lust Pubs., 1974.
17. Grieve, M. **A Modern Herbal,** 2 vols., Dover Pubs., New York, 1971 (original edition—1931).
18. Kloss, J. **Back to Eden,** Woodbridge Press Pubs., Santa Barbara CA, 1939. p. 331.
19. Zinchenko, T.V. & Fefer, I.M. "Investigation of glycosides from betonica officinalis." **Farmatsevt. Zhurnal,** 17(3), 35-38, 1962.
20. Salerno, G.L. **Minerva otorinolaringologica,** 155, 5.
21. Genazzani, E. & Sorrentino, L. "Vascular action of acteina: active constituent of actaea racemosa L." **Nature,** 194(4828), 544-545, 1962.
22. Hutchens, A.R. **Indian Herbology of North America,** Merco, Ontario, Canada, 1973.
23. Usow, V. **Farmakologiia i Toksikologiia,** 21(2), 31-34, 1958.
24. Meshkovsky, M.D. **Ekarstvennye Sredstva,** (Medical Preparations), Medicina Pubs, Moscow, 1967.
25. Gammerman, A.F., Yourkevitch, I.D., Eds. **Wild Medical Plants.** Bello-Russ Pubs, Academy of Science, Institute of Experimental Botanics and Microbiology, Minsk, Bello-Russia, 1965.
26. Daraban, E.V. **Medical Preparations,** Zdorovie Pubs, Kiev, 1966.
27. Gunn, J.D. **New Domestic Physician or Home Book of Health.** Moore, Wilstach, Keys Cinncinnati. 1861.
28. Lust
29. Wohlfart, R., Haensel, R. & Schmidt, H. "An investigation of sedative-hypnotic principles in Hops. Part 4." **Planta Medica,** 48, 120-123, 1983.
30. Leclerc, H. "Pharmacology of humulus lupulus L." **Presse Medicale (Paris),** 42, 1652, 1934.
31. Wohlfart, R., Haensel, R. & Schmidt, H. "An investigation of sedative-hypnotic principles in Hops, Part 3." **Planta Medica,** 45, 224, 1982.

32. Stocker, H. **Schweizer Brauerei Rundschau.** 78, 80, 1967.
33. Berndt, G. **Deutsche Apotheker Zietung,** 106, 158, 1966.
34. Caujolle, F., Pham-Huu-Chanh, Duch-Kan, P. & Bravo-Diaz, L. "Spasmolytic action of hop (humulus lupulus)." **Agressologie,** 10(5), 405-410, 1969.
35. Suzuki, Y., Kajiyama, K., Taguchi, K., Hagiwara, Y. & Imada, Y. "Pharmacological studies on Zingiber mioga (1) General pharmacological effects of water extracts." **Folia Pharmacologia Japonia,** 75, 669-682, 1979.

# PAIN
# RELIEF

## HERBS

**Form:** Capsule.

**CONTENTS: WHITE WILLOW** bark *(Salix alba)*, **Wood Betony** *(Stachys officinalis)*, **Skullcap** *(Scutellaria lateriflora)*, **Rosemary leaves** *(Rosmarinus officinalis)*, **Raspberry leaves** *(Rubus idaeus)*, **Blue Vervain** *(Verbena hastata)*, & **Kelp** *(Laminaria, Macrocystis, Ascophyllum)*.

**PURPOSE: To provide relief from minor pain (analgesic).**

**Other Applications:** Headache (migraine and tension), neuralgia, neuritis, rheumatism, gout, to reduce fever, anxiety.

**USE:** 4-12 capsules per day, as needed (see text below).

**Contraindications:** None.

Pain is perhaps the most important and complex sense we have. We don't like it, but without it we would die a lot sooner. It's the body's early warning system. It warns us to withdraw our finger from the stove as soon as possible. It also informs us when we are sick, or need a change of diet, or even when to get out of the sun. Pain is a symptom, not a disease. So, while you are trying to relieve the pain, you should determine and attend to the cause. This blend contains the best analgesics the plant kingdom has to offer, short of habituating alkaloids like morphine. But for every ten people, there are ten kinds of pain. The treatments of pain reflect the causes of pain. Play around with the dosage if you don't get immediate results (but never take more than 12-15 capsules/day). While all the herbs in this blend contribute in their own way to the relief of pain, White Willow bark has the most immediate effect.

**WHITE WILLOW BARK** is the original source of salicin—the forerunner of aspirin, though weaker in activity. Down through the ages, well before the discovery of salicin, White Willow bark was used to combat pain of many different sorts, including rheumatism, headache, fever, arthritis, gout, and angina. It is mentioned in ancient Egyptian, Assyrian and Greek manuscripts, and was used to combat pain and fevers by Galen, Hippocrates and Dioscorides. Many native American tribes used it for headache, fever, sore muscles, rheumatism and chills. In the middle 1700's it was used to treat malaria. Extracts of the bark were first tested between 1821 and 1829 during which time salicin was identified, but it wasn't until 1874 that it was conclusively shown to reduce the aches and soreness of rheumatism. In 1838, salicylic acid was produced through the oxidation and hydrolysis of salicin. A couple of years later, this product was proven effective against rheumatic fever. First in 1853, and later in 1893, independent researchers produced acetylsalicylic acid from salicylic acid. This new product became known as aspirin. Aspirin was subsequently shown to be effective against general pain, as well as the pain of rheumatism, gout and neuralgia. Other derivatives of salicylic acid have likewise been proven effective. Interestingly, salicin, the original constituent of White Willow bark is converted through oxidation to salicylic acid **within the body.** The concentration of salicin in the bark is rather small, and different individuals will require different amounts to ease aches and pains, but the chemical is there, and we can take advantage of it in its natural state. Incidentally, used in the raw form, the bark yields other decomposition products of salicin that may enhance the analgesic, antipyretic, disinfectant and antiseptic properties of the product. Laboratory tests show that the bark can relieve minor pains associated with headache, rheumatism and related conditions. Augmented in its activity by the other herbs in the blend, White Willow bark should provide relief to many people whose pain is susceptible to aspirin-like compounds (General references for White Willow: **1-4**).

**WOOD BETONY** has had many folk uses over the past 400 years, including those of antidiarrhetic, carminative, astringent, and sedative. It has been used for heartburn, gout, nervousness, catarrh, bladder and kidney stones, asthma and fatigue. Among the eclectic physicians of the last century it was a much used medicinal plant.

These doctors, more than any other group of men in history, were able to utilize the healing potential of plants. But with the advent of modern medicine, the lore of Wood Betony along with many other valuable plants became scarce. Fortunately, today's herbalists continue to sing its praises, but not many researchers have investigated the many claims. One existing piece of work demonstrated significant hypotensive activity in the glycoside constituents of Wood Betony (**5**). Another study discovered that Wood Betony is active against tuberculosis bacteria (**6**). Since we know there are active principles in the herb, it would seem to deserve more active research attention. *See Also NERVOUS TENSION; NERVES & GLANDS*

**SKULLCAP** has a checkered history for pain relief. Some cultures strongly recommend it for the relief of headache and related pain, while other cultures overlook this application entirely. For a period of time, it was officially listed in the United States Pharmacopoeia. During the late 1700's a certain Dr. Vandesveer discovered that he could prevent hydrophobia, and is said to have prevented 400 persons and 1000 cattle from getting rabies after being bitten by mad dogs. The herb's effectiveness in this regard was scorned by medical science, and indeed, by almost everybody, but on the balance, no one has ever tried putting it to a good controlled test. . . . At any rate, many physicians of the 19th Century used Skullcap with great success, to treat nervous diseases, convulsions, neuralgia, insomnia, restlessness and even tetanus. These uses have persisted till the present day, but again little scientific research has been carried out. In one study, it was found to stabilize and normalize blood pressure (**7**). This may explain why it is usually recommended for pain associated with nervous conditions. It may best be considered a minor neural sedative, whose main purpose is to induce sleep without pain by sedating a restless and excitable body (**8**). Twitching, tremulous pain may also be quieted by Skullcap (**9**). Of related interest, though of uncertain pertinence to the control of pain, is a finding that Skullcap can prevent rises in serum cholesterol in animals on a high-cholesterol diet (**10**). This property does explain the folklore use of Skullcap to remedy atherosclerosis. *See Also INSOMNIA; NERVOUS TENSION; NERVES & GLANDS*

**ROSEMARY LEAF** has been effectively used in Europe and China to treat headaches and stomach pains. A few years ago, Italian researchers demonstrated moderate analgesic activity in this herb (**11**). Additionally, inclusion in this blend takes advantage of the herb's essential oil in moderating the activity of the other herbs and imparting to the body the essence of that oil. The oil contributes substantially to the calming and soothing of tense nerves and muscles. In China, Rosemary leaf is used as an analgesic, smooth muscle stimulant, headache remedy, and antimalarial.

**BLUE VERVAIN** was shown in 1964 to have definite analgesic and antiinflammatory activity (**12**). The demonstration of these properties confirmed folk uses of the herb that dated back hundreds of years. Verbenalin, one of the active principles of Vervain, has moderate parasympathetic properties, i.e., it has a calming, restorative effect on the nervous system (**2,13**). *See Also NERVES & GLANDS; FEVERS & INFECTIONS*

**KELP** is useful in this blend as a provider of iodine, vitamins and minerals. The prevention of painful conditions such as rheumatism and arthritis can sometimes be accomplished through nutrition. We know, for example, that an excess of acid-forming foods can precipitate painful episodes, as in the case of uric acid contribution to rheumatic pain. Acidity and lack of essential nutrients that insure the health of the nerves and their insulating sheaths can lead to inflammation and neuritis. Iodine, acting as a tranquilizer, can interrupt the physical chain that goes disease-to-pain-to-aggravation-more disease-more pain, etc. Kelp also supplies essential vitamins and mineral salts that nourish nerves (**14**).

## OTHER NUTRIENTS

*Pain is related to nutrition in a very complex manner. It appears that certain "natural" pain killers are produced by the body. Diets high in choline and other nutrients may supply the substrates for these chemicals. Individual requirements may depart substantially from the following general recommendations.*

### VITAMINS

*(Daily requirements unless otherwise noted)*

Vitamin B Complex
Vitamin B1 *25 mg*
Vitamin B2 *25 mg*
Vitamin B6 *25 mg*
Vitamin E *400 I.U.*

Pantothenic Acid *100 mg*
Niacinamide *25 mg*

**MINERALS**

Calcium/Magnesium
Phosphorous

# REFERENCES

1. Thomson, W.R. **Herbs That Heal.** Charles Scribner's Sons. New York, 1976, pp. 81-82.
2. List, P.H. & Hoerhammer, L. **Hagers Handbuch der Pharmazeutischen Praxis.** Volumes 2-5, Springer-Verlag, Berlin.
3. Lewis, W.H. & Elvin-Lewis, M.P.F. **Medical Botany,** John Wiley & Sons, Inc., New York, 1977.
4. Thomson, W.A.R. **Medicines from the Earth,** McGraw Hill Book Co. Limited, Maidenhead, England, 1978.
5. Zinchenko, T.C., & Fefer, I.M. "Investigation of glcosides from Betonica officinalis." **Farmatsevt. Zhurnal,** 17(3), 35-38, 1962.
6. Fitzpatrick, F.K. "Plant substances active against Mycobacterium tuberculosis" **Antibiotics and Chemotherapy,** 4(5), 528-536, 1954.
7. Usow, T. **Farmakologiia i Toxikologiia,** 21(2), 31-34, 1958.
8. Kurnakov, B.A. "Pharmacology of skullcap." **Farmakologiia i Toksikologiia,** 20(6), 79-80, 1957.
9. Shibata, S., Harada, M. & Budidarmo, W. "Constituents of Japanese and Chinese crude drugs. III. Antispasmodic action of flavanoids and anthraquinones." **Yakugaku Zasshi,** 80, 620-624, 1960.
10. Aonuma, S., Minuma, T. & Tarutani, M. "Effects of coptis, scutellaria, rhubarb and bupleurum on serum cholesterol and phospholipids in rabbits." **Yakugaku Zasshi,** 77, 1303-1307, 1957.
11. Boido, A., Sparatore, F., Biniecka, M. "N-substituted derivatives of rosmaricine." **Studi Sassar,** Sez 2, 53(5-6), 383-93, 1975.
12. Sakai, S. "Pharmacological actions of verbena officinalis extracts." **Gifu Ika Daigaku Kiyo,** 11(1), 6-17, 1963.
13. Thomson, *op.cit.,* p. 156-157.
14. Binding, G.J. & Moyle,A. **About Kelp,** Thorson's Publisher's Limited, Wellingborough, Northamptonshire, England, 1974.

# PARASITES & WORMS

## HERBS

**Form:** Capsule

**CONTENTS: GARLIC** *(Allium sativum)*, **BLACK WALNUT** *(Juglans nigra)*, & **Butternut bark of root** *(Juglans cinera)*.

**PURPOSE: To rid the body of parasites and worms (not intended for external application).**

**Other Applications:** Snakebites, trauma, shock.

**USE:** 3 capsules, four times per day until problem is eliminated.

**Contraindications:** None.

Parasitic infections arise from the intrusion of roundworms, tapeworms, protozoa and flukes into the body. They enter via the mouth or the skin. They are found in contaminated soil, vegetables, meat, water, watercress, and feces. Symptoms include colicky pains, diarrhea, anemia, cardiac insufficiency, nausea, perianal & perineal pruritis, dysentery, amebic hepatitis, weight loss, intestinal toxemia, colic and cirrhosis. There are many pharmaceutical preparations available for dealing with parasites, but the plant kingdom provides some agents that are safer to use, and just as effective. All three herbs in this blend have at one time or another been used in medical practice to kill and/or expel worms from the G.I. tract. There are many other vermifuges (parasite killers) and anthelmintics (parasite expellers) in the plant kingdom; most are caustic, toxic or simply too noxious to use. This blend was chosen for both the sureness and the mildness of its total action.

**GARLIC** is used by Eastern and Western cultures to kill and expel parasites and worms (**1**). Many American Indians benefited from this property of Garlic, as the Greeks and Romans did on the other side of the world. And some of the early American physicians successfully destroyed worms with Garlic. Japanese, European, Russian, and American research has shown that the presence of allicin, the odoriferous principle, and allyl sulfide is responsible for this and many other beneficial properties (e.g., **2-4**). Roundworms, pinworms, tapeworms and hookworms all succumb to the volatile powers of Garlic (**5-6**). You may on occasion even find this herb in an ointment for external application against ringworm. *See Also FEVERS & INFECTIONS; HIGH BLOOD PRESSURE*

**BLACK WALNUT BARK,** including the kernel and green hull, have been used to expel various kinds of worms by the Asians, as well as by some American Indian tribes. External applications have been known to kill ringworm (**7**). The Chinese use it to kill tapeworm with extremely good success (**8**). The high tannin content is primarily responsible for its anthelmintic property, although other constituents such as juglandin, juglone and juglandic acid may also be involved. Since this is the only chapter in which Black Walnut appears in this book, a discussion of ellagic acid is included here, even though it probably has little to do with the anthelmintic effect. There are stories going around about the ability of Black Walnut to protect people from electrocution because it contains ellagic acid. These tales may be misleading. In the late 1960's, as part of a doctoral dissertation project by one of its members, a team of scientists investigated the pharmacological properties of this chemical, small amounts of which are found in Black Walnut. Using relatively large doses they found that it could both lower blood pressure, and, paradoxically, block the lowering of blood pressure by other agents (**9-11**). In addition, if injected intravenously, ellagic acid produced sedation and protected mice from death after a normally lethal degree of electroconvulsive shock (**12**). Due to the method of administration and dosage, it is extremely doubtful that any of these effects would show up in humans ingesting whole herb material. It is more likely that the minute amount of ellagic acid in the whole herb would be metabolically neutralized long before it was absorbed by the tissues of the body. More important than these studies was another carried out by the same team in which they found that *several* constituents of Black Walnut, including ellagic acid, juglone, several strong and weak acids, and alkaloids, had anti-cancer properties (**13**). More work in this latter area could have been most fruitful. Unfortunately, the team of scientists (from the University of Missouri) ended their studies of Black Walnut and its constituents before some of the really interesting questions were answered.

**BUTTERNUT BARK OF ROOT,** or White walnut, is used to expel, rather than kill, worms (vermifuge) during the normal course of laxative-induced cleansing. When combined with anthelmintics, Butternut bark of root provides the means to eliminate the parasitic mass from the body. These properties were known in America in the early 1800's and probably even earlier (**14**). Mode of action is not known. *See Also LAXATIVE; FEVERS & INFECTIONS*

## *OTHER NUTRIENTS*

*Intestinal worms are especially nasty about increasing the difficulty with which your body can obtain nutrients from food. It is important, while attempting to rid the body of the parasites, that you continue to ingest needed nutritional substances. The following table is meant as a simple checklist of materials that may be especially necessary, or that may help balance out your dietary intake.*

**VITAMINS**

*(Daily requirements unless otherwise noted)*

Vitamin A *25,000 I.U.*
Vitamin B Complex
Vitamin B1 *25-100 mg*
Vitamin B2 *25-100 mg*
Vitamin B6 *25-100 mg*
Vitamin B12 *5 mcg*
Vitamin D *1,000 I.U.*
Pantothenic Acid *100 mg*

**MINERALS**

Calcium/Magnesium
Iron
Potassium

**MISCELLANEOUS**

GLA
Essential Fatty Acid

Cod Liver Oil
Brewer's yeast

## REFERENCES

1. Leung, **Chinese Herbal Remedies,** p. 68.
2. Stoll, A. & Seebeck, E. "Chemical investigations of alliin, the specific principle of garlic." **Advances in Enzymology,** 11, 377, 1951.
3. Jezpwa, L, Rafinski, T., Wrocinski, T. "Investigations on the antibiotic activity of allium sativum L." **Herba Polonica,** 12, 3, 1966.
4. Yamada, Y. & Azuma, K. "Evaluation of the in vitro antifungal activity of allicin." **Antimicrobial Agents Chemotherapy,** 11, 743, 1977.
5. Rico, **Comptes. Rend. Soc. Biol.,** 95, 1597, 1926.
6. Rao, RR., Rao, S.S. & Venkatoraman, P.R. **Journal Scient. Ind. Res.,** 5, 31, 1946.
7. Harris, W.R. **Practice of medicine and surgery by the Canadian tribes in Champlain's time.** 27th ann. Archeol. Rep. Min. Educ., Ontario, 1915 (written in 1900).
8. Leung, A.Y. **Chinese Herbal Remedies,** Universe Books, New York, 1984.
9. Bhargava, U.C. "Pharmacology of ellagic acid from black walnut." From **Dissertation Abstracts B,** 29(1), 294-295, 1967.
10. Bhargava, U.C. & Westfall, B.A. "Antagonistic effect of ellagic acid on histamine liberators." **Proceedings of the Society of Experimental Biology and Medicine,** 131(4), 1342-1345, 1969.
11. Bhargava, U.C., & Westfall, B.A. "Mechanism of blood pressure depression by ellagic acid." **Proceedings of the Society of Experimental Biology and Medicine,** 132(2), 754-756, 1969.
12. Bhargava, U.C., Westfall, B.A. & Siehr, D.J. "Preliminary pharmacology of ellagic acid from juglans nigra (black walnut)." **Journal of Pharmaceutical Sciences,** 57(10), 1728-1732, 1968.
13. Bhargava, U.C. & Westfall, B.A. "Antitumor activity of juglans nigra (black walnut) extractives." **Journal of Pharmaceutical Sciences,** 57(10), 1674-1677, 1968.
14. Rafinesque, C.S. **Medical Flora or Manual of Medical Botany of the United States."** Vol 2., Atkinson & Alexander, Philadelphia, 1830.

# PROSTATE PROBLEMS

## HERBS

**Form:** Capsule.

**CONTENTS: PARSLEY** *(Petroselinum sativum)*, **SAW PALMETTO** berries *(Serenoa repens-sabal)*, **Cornsilk** *(Stigmata maydis)*, **Buchu leaves** *(Barosma crenata)*, **Cayenne** *(Capsicum annum)*, **Kelp** *(Laminaria, Macrocystis, Ascophyllum)*, & **Pumpkin seeds** *(Curcurbita pepo)*.

**PURPOSE:** **To help provide symptomatic relief of prostate problems: To help the body overcome the effects of enlarged and/or inflamed prostate.**

**Other Applications:** Diuretic.

**USE:** 1. Inflamed prostate: 4-8 capsules per day.
2. Enlarged prostate: 3-6 capsules per day.

**Contraindications:** None. Exercise care when using any diuretic type preparation as it can cause serum potassium depletion if used in large amounts for an extended period of time. For discussion of Cayenne, see Appendix A.

Bacterial infection in other parts of the body may occasionally migrate to a man's prostate gland, resulting in an acute and very painful inflammation called prostatitis. Prostatic hypertrophy, or enlargement, is another common prostate ailment that usually causes severe distress in males. This blend helps fight prostatitis and prostatic hypertrophy in at least four ways. First, it acts to stimulate

233

urine flow when an enlarged prostate is inhibiting such flow. Second, it helps reduce inflammation and infection. Third, it helps decrease the size of the enlarged prostate. Fourth, it helps prevent these conditions. When the enlarged prostate clamps so tightly around the urethra that complete urinary relief is never experienced, **CORNSILK, PARSLEY,** and **BUCHU** will promote urination, soothe irritated tissues and provide that "Ahh" feeling. The **SAW PALMET-TO** has a more direct influence on the enlarged prostate, reducing inflammation, pain and that dull aching throb.

**PARSLEY** is the foremost diuretic to be recommended when urination is painful and incomplete due to an enlarged prostate squeezing the urethra so tightly that urination is difficult. The presence of apiol and myristicin as well as other flavanoids in Parsley will stimulate urination and provide relief. There is much talk of overdoses of pure apiol being harmful to the kidneys and liver. One need not fear poisoning from the plant itself (**1**). The leaves of Parsley are very nutritive, containing up to 25% protein (**2**). The plant is also high in vitamin B and potassium (**3**) as well as vitamin C and provitamin A (**4**). Parsley works best in blends with other herbs, such as Buchu and Cornsilk. *See Also DIABETES; DIURETIC; BONE-FLESH-CARTILAGE*

**SAW PALMETTO BERRY** acts directly on the enlarged prostate to reduce inflammation, pain and throb (**5**). In sub-hypertrophied cases, it may also reduce swelling to some degree, but in case of true hypertrophy it is not known whether the herb brings relief by decreasing gland size or by reducing pain and irritation. It also increases the bladder's ability to contract and expel its contents (**6**). Credit for the discovery of these principles goes to the early American Eclectic physicians who so effectively transformed native American flora into a medicinal storehouse. *See Also INFERTILITY; RESPIRATORY AILMENTS; DIABETES; FEMALE PROBLEMS; NERVES & GLANDS; THYROID; DIGESTION*

**CORNSILK** is a diuretic and acts much like Parsley. The gumlike substance is the active principle, but the herb also contains a surprisingly large number of other substances, including fatty acids, menthol, glycosides, thymol, saponins, sugar, steroids, vitamins C & K, and so forth. Cornsilk is contained in several over-the-counter type diuretic products in Europe and America (where it used to be an officially recognized medicinal agent), and is popular in China also. What little solid research there is on Cornsilk has been done by Japanese and Chinese investigators. None of that research deals directly with prostate problems, but it does demonstrate the remarkable diuretic properties of the herb (**7**). Most herbalists around the world agree that Cornsilk directly reduces painful symptoms and swelling due to several inflammatory conditions, including cystitis, pyelitis, oligouria, hepatitis, and all edematous conditions. *See Also DIURETIC*

**BUCHU LEAF** is provided as a urinary disinfectant, one of the important secondary considerations when treating prostate problems. The leaves are also mildly diuretic in their own right. By themselves, Buchu leaves are seldom used for acute prostate problems, but they lend just the right antiseptic property to preparations used for acute as well as chronic prostate problems. While Buchu is familiar to very few Americans and Europeans, it is practically a household item in South Africa where it was introduced to the rest of the world by the Hottentots (Buchu or BooKoo is a Hottentot word). The South Africans prize the herb mainly for diseases of the kidney, urinary tract and prostate (**8**). Buchu works because its volatile oil stimulates urination and is excreted virtually unchanged by the kidneys, rendering the urine slightly antiseptic (**9**). Proprietary drugs are available in South Africa and the United States that still employ Buchu leaves as a urinary antiseptic (**10**). *See Also DIURETIC; VAGINAL YEAST INFECTION*

**CAYENNE** is included in this blend once again as a mild systemic stimulant to insure the diffusion of the active principles of other herbs throughout the body via the vascular system.

**KELP** has been used for scores of years by Asian peoples to treat disorders of the genital-urinary tract, including kidney, bladder, prostate and uterine problems. Of concern to us here are its normalizing and remedial effects on the enlarged prostate. Clinical documentation is available to show that Kelp ingestion on a daily basis gradually reduces the prostate in older men to the point that urination becomes painless, even though it is not certain how that occurs (**11**). An educated guess would be that healing is achieved through Kelp's general cleansing effect on the bloodstream (**12**), its antibiotic properties (**13**) and the fact that it supplies so many essential elements (**14**). Thus Kelp maintains a healthy interchange of body fluids, thereby diminishing prostate ailments that may be due to stagnation and congestion of glandular tissues. *See Also THYROID; CIRCULATION; ENVIRONMENTAL POLLUTION; FEVERS & INFECTIONS; WEIGHT LOSS; FATIGUE; BLOOD PURIFICATION/DETOXIFICATION; HEART; INFERTILITY; PAIN; MENTAL ALERTNESS/SENILITY; DIABETES*

**PUMPKIN SEED** has a reputation of being a non-irritating diuretic. This property makes the seed especially well suited to treat the enlarged prostate. Native American Indians used it successfully for this purpose long before the settlers adopted it for their own purposes **(15)**. Today, it is universally accepted for this specific purpose (though its main use continues to be as an anthelmintic). However, in spite of a good deal of clinical work, I am not aware of any published laboratory or experimental work on Pumpkin seeds.

## OTHER NUTRIENTS

*Like the other glands of the body, the prostate requires a healthy supply of dietary nutrients for efficient operation. The following general recommendations may vary widely from individual to individual.*

### VITAMINS & MINERALS

*(daily requirements unless otherwise noted)*

Vitamin A *25,000 I.U.*
Vitamin B-1 *25-100 mg*
Vitamin B-2 *25-100 mg*
Vitamin B-6 *25-100 mg*
Vitamin C *1,000-5,000 mg*
Vitamin E *600 I.U.*

### MINERALS

Zinc

## REFERENCES

1. List, P.H. & Hoerhammer, L. **Hagers Handbuch der Pharmazeutischen Praxis.** Volumes 2-5, Springer-Verlag, Berlin.
2. Murphy, E., Marsh, A.C. & Willis, B.W. "Nutrient content of spices and herbs." **Journal of the American Dietetic Association,** 72, 174-176, 1978.
3. Hutchens, A.R. **Indian Herbalogy of North America,** Merco, Ontario, Canada, 1973.
4. Schauenberg, P. & Paris, F. **Guide to Medicinal Plants,** Keats Pubs., New Canaan, Connecticut, 1977.

5. Felter, H. W. **The Eclectic Materia Medica, Pharmacology and Therapeutics.** Eclectic Medical Publications, Portland, Oregon, 1983 (first published 1922).
6. Ellingwood, F. **American Materia Medica, Therapeutics and Pharmacognosy.** Eclectic Medical Publications, Portland, Oregon, 1983.
7. Leung, A.Y. **Chinese Herbal Remedies,** Universe Books, New York, 1984, 47-49.
8. Matt, J.M. & Breyer-Brandwijk, M.G. **The Medicinal and Poisonous Plants of Southern and Eastern Africa.** E. & S. Livingstone, LTd., Edinburgh & London, England, 1962.
9. Tyler, V.E., Brady, L.R. & Robbers, J.E. **Pharmacognosy,** 7th ed., Lea & Febiger, Philadelphia, 1976.
10. Parke-Davis Labs, tech notes.
11. Personal communication from Dr. H. Tamamoto, Tokyo, Japan, 1983.
12. Kimura, A. & Kuramoto, M. "Influences of seaweeds on metabolism of cholesterol and anticoagulant actions of seaweed." **Tokushima Journal of Experimental Medicine,** 21, 79-80, 1974.
13. Mautner, H.G., Gardner, G.M. & Pratt, R. "Antibiotic activity of seaweed extracts." **Journal of the American Pharmaceutical Association,** 42(5), 294-295, 1953.
14. Newberne, P.M., & McConnell, R.G. "Nutrient deficiencies in cancer causation." **Journal of Environmental Pathology and Toxicology,** 3, 323-356, 1980.
15. Vogel, V.J. **American Indian Medicine.** Ballantine Books, New York, 1970.

# RESPIRATORY
# AILMENTS

## HERBS

**Form:** Capsule, Gargle, Tea, Mouthwash

**CONTENTS: PLEURISY ROOT** *(Asclepias tuberosa)*, **Wild Cherry bark** *(Prunus virginiana)*, **Slippery Elm bark** *(Ulmus fulva)*, **Plantain** *(Plantago ovata)*, **Mullein leaves** *(Verbascum thapsus)*, **Chickweed** *(Stellaria media)*, **Horehound** *(Marrubium vulgare)*, **Licorice root** *(Glycyrrhiza glabra)*, **Kelp** *(Laminaria, Macrocystes, Ascophyllum)*, **Cayenne** *(Capsicum annuum)*, & **Saw Palmetto** *(Serenoa serrulata)*.

**PURPOSE:** **To relieve the distress of respiratory ailments, such as pneumonia, asthma, bronchitis, croup, tuberculosis, colds, flu, hayfever, emphysema (acts to soothe, tone, and relieve irritation).**

**Other Applications:** Allergies, fevers, colitis, cancer; as a diuretic.

**USE:** 1. To relieve general respiratory distress: 4-6 capsules per day.
2. As a tea: 2-4 capsules per cup.
3. As a gargle: 2 capsules per cup.

**Contraindications:** None. For a discussion of Licorice root and Cayenne, see Appendix A. Due to mild diuretic action, consider potassium supplementation.

Respiratory ailments encompass a wide variety of conditions, varying both in intensity and cause. Some involve inflammation, edema and destruction of the tiny air sacs of the lungs; others are caused by simple infections or allergies. They all share the common feature of respiratory irritation and distress. This blend is meant primarily as a treatment for the symptoms. However, some of the herbs have been shown to remedy and/or prevent some forms of respiratory disease itself. Virtually every herb in this blend has been shown to help relieve distress due to cough, infection or inflammation. Some, such as Wild Cherry bark and Horehound, are major constituents in many commercial cough medicines. Slippery Elm bark, Cayenne, Licorice root and Mullein leaves can also be found in over-the-counter cough medications. Simply swallowing the capsules is perhaps the least effective method of using this blend. Teas and gargles are the best methods. A bit of honey, saturated with the contents of one or two capsules is also recommended.

**PLEURISY ROOT,** with a reputation extending back several centuries, is a much used treatment for colds, flu, bronchitis, tuberculosis, pleurisy, and so on (**1**). In America, it was the primary expectorant for several decades. One early practitioner, after twenty-five years of continuous study and use, stated that the herb possessed "...an almost specific quality of acting on the organs of respiration, powerfully promoting...expectoration," and that it "...proved equally efficacious...in pneumonic fevers, colds, catarrhs, and diseases of the breast in general" (**2**). His enthusiasm was shared by the majority of early medical practitioners. Today, the herb has been rediscovered, and the testimonials of hundreds of people affirm its usefulness.

**WILD CHERRY BARK**'s use for reducing the symptoms of respiratory distress is without equal in the herb kingdom. Its widespread inclusion in over-the-counter cough medications testifies to its acceptance by the pharmaceutical and medical industries (many such preparations, however, on the mistaken assumption that the herb is just for taste, only use cherry flavoring). The real thing, the actual bark, is much more effective than most cough drop or throat lozenge-type preparations. The American Indians and early settlers were aware of this property of the bark of North America's unique Wild Cherry tree (**3-5**), and it is still included in the USP (**6**). *See Also HAYFEVER & ALLERGIES*

**SLIPPERY ELM BARK,** due to its high and peculiar mucilage content, is remarkably effective, both internally and externally, against sore and inflamed mucous membranes, and is one of the best agents for combating coughs. Indian uses for this herb were, and still are, many and varied. The Mohegans used it with great success to treat coughs (**7**). And the Pillager Ojibwas used it to treat sore throat (**8**). In fact, the American Indians obtained more mileage from this herb than practically any other medication, using it variously to ease childbirth and reduce the pain of labor, for toothaches, dysentery, diarrhea, leprosy, ulcers, rheumatism, eye lotions, and all forms of external sores and wounds (**9**). One early frontiersman remarked that he felt that a person could subsist for a great length of time on the nutritive value of the bark alone (**10**). *See Also BONE-FLESH-CARTILAGE; HEMORRHOIDS/ASTRINGENT*

**PLANTAIN,** one of the most underrated of all herbs, is included on the basis of its similarities to the other mucilaginous herbs in this blend, and on the strength of modern research. For example, scientists recently treated a number of cases of chronic bronchitis with Plantain and found that the herb provided very good symptomatic relief of pain, coughing, wheezing and irritation (**11**). These findings concur with research carried out in India which demonstrated beneficial effects from Plantain seeds on coughs and colds (**12**). *See Also BONE-FLESH-CARTILAGE; VAGINAL YEAST INFECTION; WEIGHT LOSS; CHOLESTEROL REGULATION*

**MULLEIN LEAF** is also used in India for upper respiratory problems (**12**). A high content of mucilage and saponins renders this herb ideal for the treatment of respiratory ailments, from coughs and colds to emphysema, asthma and whooping cough. In addition to the soothing effect imparted by the mucilage, Mullein possesses good antibiotic properties (**13-15**). During the Civil War, the Confederates relied on Mullein for treatment of respiratory problems whenever their medical supplies ran out (**16**). Several different and unrelated Indian tribes used Mullein for similar purposes (**9**).

**CHICKWEED** was another plant well-liked by the American Indians for the relief it gave for such respiratory problems as bronchitis, whooping cough, colds, sore throat and flu (**16**). It achieved near panacea status in some cases. In European folklore, the herb was used for very similar purposes, including tuberculosis. Modern research on Chickweed, though scanty, has at least demonstrated the presence of antibiotic properties which are effective against certain respiratory pathogens (**1**). Chickweed is also used to treat rheumatism, gout, joint disease, blood disease, eye inflammation and hemorrhoids. The effectiveness of these assorted uses probably depends on the herb's high nutritive content, which includes vitamin A, several B vitamins, vitamin C, phosphorous, zinc and calcium.

**HOREHOUND**'s popularity as a cough remedy can hardly be disputed. Not so well known is the fact that Horehound and/or its derivatives are used in virtually thousands of bronchial medications around the world (**17**). Its activity is no doubt due to a high content of volatile oil. This oil has vasodilatory, as well as expectorant properties (**18**). The water extracts have biological activity that could affect brain respiratory centers in a positive manner (**19**). *See Also HAYFEVER & ALLERGIES*

**LICORICE ROOT** has been the subject of numerous scientific studies involving anti-inflammatory and antitussive properties. A typical study shows that it curbs inflammations throughout the body, including the lungs and throat (**20-22**). Licorice root derivatives have been shown to be as effective as codeine in terms of suppressing coughs (**22**). Sugars, glycosides and other constituents with adrenocortical-like activity are probably responsible for its effectiveness.

**SAW PALMETTO BERRY** also contains anti-inflammatory principles, as well as being a strong expectorant. Its primary purpose in this blend is to remove catarrh from the mucous membranes. Saw Palmetto is best known for its effects on sexual function. *See Also INFERTILITY; DIABETES; FEMALE TONIC; PROSTATE; NERVES & GLANDS; THYROID; DIGESTION*

**KELP** and **CAYENNE** provide nutritive support and stimulate circulation, thereby increasing the oxygen exchange capacity of the lungs. The nature of Cayenne is to break up mucous, promoting the expectorant nature of other herbs in the blend.

## OTHER NUTRIENTS

*Many respiratory problems can be nipped in the bud, so to speak, through the proper use of nutrient supplementation. Because individual differences are so great, your needs may depart substantially from the following recommendations.*

## VITAMINS

*(Daily requirements unless otherwise noted)*

Vitamin A *25,000 I.U.*
Vitamin B Complex
Vitamin B1 *25-50 mg*
Vitamin B2 *25-50 mg*
Vitamin B6 *25-100 mg*
Vitamin B12 *10 mcg*
Vitamin C *1,000-3,000 mg*
Vitamin D *600-2,000 I.U.*
Vitamin E *400-800 I.U.*
Choline *1,000 mg*
Inositol *1,000 mg*
Pantothenic Acid *150-200 mg*
Niacinamide *50 mg*

## MINERALS

Manganese
Calcium/Magnesium
Phosphorous
Potassium
Sodium

## MISCELLANEOUS

Bee Pollen
HCl
Liver
Lecithin
Yogurt

## REFERENCES

1. Fitzpatrick, F.K. "Plant substances active against mycobacterium tuberculosis." **Antibiotics and Chemotherapy,** 4(5), 528-536, 1954.
2. Millspaugh, C.F. **American Medicinal Plants.** Dover Publications, Inc. New York, 1974 (originally published 1892), 540-541.

3. Brendle, T.R. & Unger, C.W. "Folk Medicine of the Pennsylvania Germans: The Non-Occult Cures." In **Proceedings of the Pennsylvania German Society,** Vol XLV, Pt II, 1-303, Norristown, Pennsylvania German Society, 1935.
4. Landes, R. "Potawatomi Medicine," **Transactions, Kansas Academy of Science,** Vol LXVI, No. 4 (Winter, 1963), 553-99.
5. Smith, H.H. **Ethnobotany of the Ojibwe Indians.** Bulletin of the Public Museum, Vol IV, No. 3. Milwaukee, 1932.
6. **The Pharmacopoeia of the United States of America.** Various publishers from 1820 till present.
7. Tantaquidgeon, G. "Mohegan medicinal practices, weather-lore, and superstition," **Forty-third Annual Report of the Bureau of American Ethnology,** 1925-26. Washington, D.C., Government Printing Office, 1928, 265-267.
8. Smith, H.H. **Ethnobotany of the Ojibwe Indians.** Bulletin of the Public Museum, Vol IV, No. 3, Milwaukee, 1932.
9. Vogel, V.J. **American Indian Medicine.** Ballantine Books, New York, 1970.
10. Hunter, John D. **Manners and Customs of Several Indian Tribes Located West of the Mississippi...** Reprint of Philadelphia, 1823, Minneapolis, Ross & Haines, 1957.
11. Matev, M., Angelova, I., Koichev, A., Leseva, M. & Stefanov, G. "Clinical trial of a Plantago major preparation in the treatment of chronic bronchitis." **Vutreshni Bolesti (Sofia),** 21(2), 133-137, 1982.
12. Chopra, R.N., Nayar, S.L. & Chopra, I.C. **Glossary of Indian Medicinal Plants.** Council of Scientific & Industrial Research, New Delhi, India, 1956.
13. Fitzpatrick, F.K. "Plant substances active against mycobacterium tuberculosis." **Antibiotics and Chemotherapy,** 4(5), 528-536, 1954.
14. Benoit, P.S., Fung, H.H.S., Svoboda, G.H. & Farnsworth, N.R. "Biological and phytochemical evaluation of plants. XIV. Antiinflammatory evaluation of 163 species of plant." **Lloydia,** 39(2-3), 160-171.
15. **Indian Journal of Experimental Biology,** 7, 250, 1969.
16. Scully, V. **A Treasury of American Indian Herbs.** Bonanza Books, New York, 1960, 212-213.
17. Bartarelli, M. "Marrubium vulgare and its pharmaceutical uses, Part I." **Bollettino Chimico-Farmaceutico,** 1966, 105(11), 787-798.

18. Karryev, M.O., Bairyev, C.B. & Ataeva, A.S. "Some therapeutic properties and phytochemistry of common horehound." **Izvestiia Akademii Nauk Turkm. SSSR, Seriia Biologicheskaia,** 3, 86-88, (1976);

19. Cahen, R. "Pharmacolgic spectrum of marrubium vulgare." **Comptes Rendus des Seances de la Societe de Biologie et de ses Filiales,** 164(7), 1467-1472, 1970.

20. Nasyrov, K.M. & Lazareva, D.N. "Anti-inflammatory activity of glycyrrhizic acid derivatives." **Farmakologiia i Toksikologiia,** 1980, 43(4), 399-404.

21. Lutomski, J. "Chemistry and therapeutic use of licorice (Glycyrrhiza glabra L.)" **Pharmazie in Unserer Zeit,** 1983, 1(8339), 1442.

22. Anderson, D.M. & Smith, W.G., "The antitussive activity of glycyrrhetinic acid and its derivatives." **Journal of Pharmacy and Pharmacology,** 13, 1961, 396-404.

# SKIN
# DISORDERS

## HERBS

**Form:**   Capsule, Poultice, Compress

**CONTENTS:** **CHAPARRAL** *(Larrea divaricata)*, **DANDE-LION root** *(Taraxacum officinale)*, **Burdock root** *(Arctium lappa)*, **Licorice root** *(Glycyrrhiza glabra)*, **Echinacea** *(Echinacea augustifo-lia)*, **Yellow Dock root** *(Rumex crispus)*, **Kelp** *(Laminaria, Macrocystes, Ascophyllum)*, & **Cayenne** *(Capsicum annuum)*.

**PURPOSE:   For skin disorders; Rash; Itch; Psoriasis; General cleansing; Eczema; Acne Vulgaris; Dry and scaly skin.**

**Other Applications:**   All other conditions of the skin that constitute wasting, from the most minor forms of scale and rash to such perverse conditions as leprosy and cancer.

**USE:**   1. Daily Maintenance: 2-6 capsules per day.
2. General Cleansing: 2-3 capsules, 3-4 times per day.
3. For serious skin conditions: 6-8 capsules per day, supplemented by additional Chaparral, Dandelion and Echinacea.
4. An excellent blood purification program is 3-4 capsules per day of this blend, and the same amount of the ARTHRITIS and BLOOD PURIFICATION/DETOXIFICATION blends.
5. If used in conjunction with the LIVER DISORDERS and

FEVERS & INFECTIONS blends, use 3-4 per day of this blend.

6. To supplement the BONE-FLESH-CARTILAGE Blend: 3 capsules per day.

**Contraindications:** None. Chaparral, though often called creosote bush, contains no creosote. More on Licorice root and Cayenne is found in Appendix A.

Skin is often viewed as simply the external covering or shell of the body. Overlooked is the fact that it is inextricably connected to deeper tissues by millions of capillaries, veins, nerves and other structures with which the skin interacts continuously, and from which it derives life. The condition of the skin reflects the relative health of many of those underlying systems. The skin also has functions which are strictly its own, such as breathing, perspiring, sensory information processing, and oil production. Any surface indication of malfunction is repeated over and over again in the underlying supportive tissues, glands, blood and nerves. This blend attacks external skin disorders from within, purifying the blood, carrying away waste, reinforcing the blood's ability to ward off infectious agents. Several of the herbs in this blend constituted the fundamental treatment for diseases like typhoid, diptheria, cholera, syphilis and malignant skin conditions during the last century. Widespread use resulted in the documentation of a number of other uses. The assumption was that "bad blood", blood poisoning, and tissue alteration due to infectious diseases are the culprits in many of man's problems. Purify the blood, and you've eliminated much of the problem. There is considerable evidence that other cultures developed the same uses for these herbs. Enough scientific evidence exists to justify the blend's place in modern man's medicine cabinet.

**CHAPARRAL** caused quite a stir in the early '70's, as it appeared that its anti-cancer properties were at last becoming scientifically proven (**1**). Further human trials failed to establish the Chaparral connection. However, close analysis of those trials revealed gross deficiencies in procedure (**2**), and so the effectiveness of the herb remains *un-disproven,* awaiting further clinical trials. Animal studies, meanwhile, strongly suggest that Chaparral or its main constituent, NDGA (nordihydroguaiaretic acid), is toxic against cancer cells (not normal cells). It produces almost complete inhibition of aerobic and anaerobic glycolysis and respiration in some kinds of cancer cells (**3**). The herb's effectiveness against other forms of skin diseases may be attributed to its anti-microbial properties (**4**), its ability to increase ascorbic acid levels in the adrenals (**5**), its tonic quality which allows it to increase life-span (**6**), or to some other, as yet undiscovered mechanism. For a further discussion of cancer research, see DETOXIFY/NURTURE. *See Also ARTHRITIS; BONE-FLESH-CARTILAGE*

**DANDELION ROOT,** besides having some potential for fighting cancer (**7**), has a reputation dating at least to the ancient Greek physician, Theophrastus. After being introduced to America, it became a plant of almost obsessive desire among early Indian tribes (**8**). The Chinese have also derived benefits from Dandelion over the ages, using it to treat infections, pneumonia, liver disease and cancer of the breast (**9**). In general, the plant stimulates liver activity, thereby encouraging the elimination of toxins in the blood. It stimulates the flow of bile and the excretion of urea (**10**). More about its liver activity is discussed in LIVER DISORDERS. A marked hypoglycemic effect is discussed under DIABETES. *See Also BLOOD PURIFICATION/ DETOXIFICATION; NERVES & GLANDS*

**BURDOCK ROOT** is your all around blood purifier, its action being simple but profound. Documented effects include treatment of scrofula, scurvy, venereal eruptions, leprosy, and other cankerous skin conditions (**8, 11**). In addition to its alterative (blood building) property, it is strongly diuretic and diaphoretic. Priddy Meeks, an early American herbalist is credited with removing "a bunch" growing on the upper lip of a young girl, with a treatment consisting of equal parts of Burdock and two other herbs in this blend, Dandelion and Yellow Dock (**12**). This case is just one of thousands that testify to the herb's effectiveness. *See Also BLOOD PURIFICATION/DETOXIFICATION; DETOXIFY/NURTURE; BONE-FLESH-CARTILAGE*

**LICORICE ROOT,** until this century, was overlooked by Western cultures as a cure or treatment for skin conditions. But the Chinese have relied on its alterative properties for centuries (**13**). Modern Western research has firmly established the effectiveness of Licorice Root along these lines, beginning with ulcers, and extending to cancer (**14**). The effectiveness of Licorice Root, taken internally, may be due to its antimicrobial activity (**15**), its ability to induce interferon production (**16**) or to its effect on the adreno-cortical system. This latter effect has been firmly linked to an ability to erase symptoms of dermatological problems (**17**). Topical preparations based on Licorice Root derivatives have been shown to be effective against a wide variety of skin problems, including eczematous dermatoses (**18-22**), contact dermatitis (**23**), anal piles (**23**), inflammatory eye conditions (**23**), pruritis (**21**), all manner of itchy inflammatory conditions (24), neurodermatitis (**25**), atopic eczema (**25**), lichen simplex (**25**), and infantile eczema (**25**). Combined with neomycin, these preparations have cured impetigo. Topical preparations of Licorice root derivatives worked best on chronic conditions (**25**). Overall, their activity compares favorably with hydrocortisone (**26**). *See Also ARTHRITIS; RE-SPIRATORY AILMENTS; FEMALE TONIC; CIRCULATION; FATIGUE; BLOOD PURI-FICATION/DETOXIFICATION; WEIGHT LOSS; THYROID; ENVIRONMENTAL POLLU-TION; FEVERS & INFECTIONS; WHOLE BODY; MENTAL ALERTNESS/SENILITY; DE-TOXIFY/NURTURE*

**ECHINACEA** alone accounts for hundreds of cases of reportedly cured boils, gangrene, ulcerations, animal, reptile and insect bites, abscesses and so on. Perhaps no other herb was loved and used more than this one by early American eclectic physicians. Their description of the herb's properties and case histories fill page after page in medical books that might devote one or two pages on today's better known herbs such as Lobelia. Laboratory studies show that the herb increases the ability of white blood cells to surround and destroy bacterial and viral invaders in the blood (**26a**). It stimulates the lymphatic system to clean up waste material and toxins, and it has definite antimicrobial activity (**27**). A russian scientist found that Echinacea stimulated wound healing and blood clotting (**26b**). *See Also BLOOD PURIFICATION/DETOXIFICATION; FEVERS & INFECTIONS*

**YELLOW DOCK ROOT** has been established clinically to be a good alterative, with especially good activity in conditions of chronic skin disorders (**28**). Among those conditions that have responded well to Yellow Dock treatment are eczema, ringworm and related diseases, leprosy, psoriasis, and cancer (**29**). In India it has even been used to toughen up weak gums, softened by malnutrition (**30**). As with other herbs in this blend, Yellow Dock possesses some antibiotic properties (**31**). *See Also BLOOD PURIFICATION/DETOXIFICATION; NERVES & GLANDS*

**KELP & CAYENNE** are present in this blend for their stimulant and anti-infectious properties. They also supply nutritional support required for proper tissue repair.

# OTHER NUTRIENTS

*The skin can be nourished, cleansed, moistened and otherwise maintained through the proper intake of vital nutrients. Individual needs may depart substantially from the following general recommendations.*

## VITAMINS

*(Daily requirements unless otherwise noted)*

Vitamin A *25,000-30,000 I.U.*
Vitamin B1 *25-50 mg*
Vitamin B2 *25-50 mg*
Vitamin B6 *25-100 mg*
Vitamin B Complex
Vitamin C *1,000-3,000 mg*
Vitamin D *1,000 I.U.*
Vitamin E *600-1,600 I.U.*
Niacinamide *100 mg*
Pantothenic Acid *200-300 mg*
PABA up to *1,000 mg*
Biotin *150 mg*
Choline *1,000 mg*
Inositol *1,000 mg*
Folic Acid *up to 5 mg*

## MINERALS

Zinc
Calcium/Magnesium
Potassium

## MISCELLANEOUS

Essential Fatty Acids
HCl
Lecithin
Brewer's Yeast

# REFERENCES

1. Smart, C.R., Hogle, H.H., Robins, R.K., Broom, A.D., & Bartholomew, D. "An interesting observation on nordihydroguaiaretic acid (NSC-4291; NDGA) and a patient with malignant melanoma—a preliminary report." **Cancer Chemotherapy Reports, Part 1,** 53, 147-151, 1969.
2. Mowrey, D.B. "Questions and Answers," **The Herbalist,** 28-29.
3. Burk, D. & Woods, N. "Hydrogen peroxide catalase, glutathione peroxidase, quinones, nordihydroguaiaretic acid, and phosphopyridine nucleotides in relation to X-ray action on cancer cells." **Radiation Research Supplement,** 3, 212-226, 1963.
4. Kaufman, H.P. & Ahmad, A.K.S., **Fette, Seifen, und Anstrichmittel,** 68, 837, 1967.
5. Sporn, A. & Schobesch, O. "Toxicity of nordihydroguaiaretic acid." **Igiena** (Bucharest), 15(12), 725-726, 1966.
6. Buu-Hoi, N.P. & Ratsimamanga, A.R., "Retarding action of nordihydroguaiaretic acid on aging in rats." **Comptes Rendus des Seances de la Societe de Biologie et de Ses Filiales,** 153, 1180-1182, 1959.
7. Baba, K., Abe, S., Mizuno, D. "Antitumor activity of hot water extract of dandelion, Taraxacum officinale—correlation between antitumor activity and timing of administration." **Yakugaku Zasshi,** 101(6), 538-543, 1981.
8. Millspaugh, C.F. **American Medicinal Plants.** Dover Publications, New York, 1974 (1st published in 1892).
9. **Martindale: The Extra Pharmacopoeia.** 1977. The Pharmaceutical Press. London.
10. Kiangsu Insititute of Modern Medicine. 1977. **Encyclopedia of Chinese Drugs.** 2 vols. Shanghai Scientific and Technical Publications. Shanghai, People's Republic of China.
11. Ellingwood, F. **American Materia Medica, Therapeutics and Pharmacognosy.** Eclectic Medical Publications, Portland, Oregon, 1983.
12. Scully, V. **A Treasury of American Indian Herbs.** Bonanza Books, New York, 1960.
13. Li Shih-Chen (Translated by Smith, F.P. & Stuart, G.A.) **Chinese Medicinal Herbs.** Georgetown Press, San Francisco, 1973.
14. Shvarev, I.F., Konovalova, N.K. & Putilova, G.I. "Effect of triterpenoid compounds from glycyrrhiza glabra on experimental tumors." **Voprosy Izuch. Ispol'z. Solodki SSSR. Akad. Nauk SSSR,** 167-170, 1966.

15. Mitsher, L.A., Park, Y.H., Clark, D. & Beal, J.C. "Antimicrobial agents from higher plants. Antimicrobial isoflavanoids and related substances from Glycyrrhiza glabra L. var. typica." **Journal of Natural Products,** 43(2), 259-264, 1980.

16. Abe, N., Ebina, T., & Ishida, N. "Interferon induction by glycyrrhizin and glycyrrhetinic acid in mice." **Microbiology and Immunology,** 26(6), 535-539, 1982.

17. Atherden, L.M. "Glycyrrhetinic acid inhibition of metabolism of steroids in vitro." **Biochemistry Journal,** 69, 75-80, 1958.

18. Adamson, A.C. & Tillman, W.G. "Hydrocortisone." **British Medical Journal,** 2, 1501, 1955.

19. Annan, W.G. "Hydrocortisone and glycyrrhetic acid." **British Medical Journal,** 1, 1242, 1957.

20. Colin-Jones, E. "Glycyrrhetinic acid." **British Medical Journal,** 1, 161, 1957.

21. Somerville, J. "Glycyrrhetinic acid." **Britsih Medical Journal,** 1, 282-283, 1957.

22. Anonymous. "Glycyrrhetinic acid ointment." **British Medical Journal,** 1, 914, 1959.

23. Chakravorti, S. "Glycyrrhetinic acid." **British Medical Journal,** 1, 161-162, 1957.

24. Evans, Q. "Glycyrrhetinic acid." **British Medical Journal,** 2, 1239, 1956.

25. Colin-Jones, E. "Some aspects of dermatological clinical trials." **Postgraduate Medical Journal,** 36, 678-682, 1960.

26. Colin-Jones, E. & Somers, G.F. "Glycyrrhetinic acid, a non-steroidal anti-inflammatory agent in dermatology." **Presse Medicales (Paris),** 238, 206, 1957.

26. (a) Chone, B. "Geziete steuerung der leukozytentinetik durch echinacin." **Arzneimittel-Forshung,** 11, 611-615, 1965.

26. (b) Nikol'skaya, B.B., "The blood clotting and wound-healing properties of perparations of plant origin." **Trudy Vsesoyuz. Obshchestva Fiziologov, Biokhimikov i Farmakologove Akademi Nauk, S.S.S.R.,** 2, 194-197 1954.

27. Samochowiez, E., Urbanska, L., Manka, W. & Stolarska, E. "Evaluation of the effect of Calendula officinalis and Echinacea augustifolia extracts on Trichomonus vaginalis in vitro." **Wiadomosci Parazytologiczne,** 25(1), 77-81, 1979.

28. Felter, H.W. **The Eclectic Materia Medica, Pharmacology and Therapeutics.** Eclectic Medical Publications, Portland, Oregon, 1983 (first published, 1922).

29. Gessner, O. **Die Gift.—Arzneipflanzen von Mitteleuropa.** Heidelburg, Germany, 1931.

30. Nadkarni, K.M. **The Indian Materia Medica. Bombay,** 1927.
31. Nishikawa, H. "Screening tests for antibiotic action of plant extracts." **Japanese Journal of Experimental Medicine,** 20(3), 337-349, 1949.

# STOMACH/INTESTINAL

## HERBS

**Form:** Capsule, Tea

**CONTENTS: GOLDENSEAL** root *(Hydrastis canadensis),* **LICORICE** root *(Glycryrrhiza glabra),* **Gentian root** *(Gentiana lutea),* **Papaya leaf** *(Carica papaya),* **Myrhh gum,** *(Commiphora myrrha),* **Irish Moss** *(Chondrus crispus),* **Fenugreek seeds** *(Trigonella foenum-graecum),* & **Ginger root** *(Zingiber officinale).*

**PURPOSE: To soothe and heal gastrointestinal tract disorders, such as upset stomach, gas, heartburn, ulcers (peptic and gastric), diverticulitis, irritable bowel syndrome, ulcerative colitis, Crohn's disease.**

**Other Applications:** Inflammations, Diarrhea, Giardiasis, Indigestion, Nausea.

**USE:** 1. Gas, Upset Stomach: 2-4 capsules as needed.
2. Chronic Heartburn: 2 capsules after each meal.
3. Ulcers: 2 capsules before each meal.
4. Other Applications: 2-3 capsules as needed.
5. Digestion: 2 capsules before meals with 2 capsules of DIGESTION blend.
6. Inflammatory diseases: 2 capsules with each meal.

**Contraindications:** Pregnant women should avoid Papaya-containing blends until possible effects of papain on the placenta are more fully understood. Use the NAUSEA blend instead. For a discussion of Licorice root see Appendix A.

**Note:** Ingest capsules with 1/2 glass of water since Myrrh and Irish Moss tend to swell.

There are not many diseases of the gastrointestinal tract that cannot be prevented by proper dietary habits. There was a time, before the advent of industrialized food processing and refining, when careful people could quite easily obtain adequate and balanced nutrition. Now, the abundance of available foods, both good and bad, makes getting just the right foods like looking for the proverbial needle in a haystack. Lack of nutritional education compounds the problem. So people make mistakes and suffer the consequences. Two of the biggest mistakes are eating too much red meat and too little dietary fiber. Other serious errors are eating too much refined carbohydrate (sugar), eating too much fat, and abusing substances such as alcohol and drugs. A diet weak in essential minerals, vitamins and fatty acids, without supplementation, is another common but potentially hazardous condition. Consider that thousands of people make several of the above mistakes all at the same time, and you have a pretty grim but realistic picture of the nation's current gastrointestinal health. The judicious use of herbs will probably not single-handedly restore the country's gastrointestinal health, but it may prove to be a significant aid in an overall program toward that end.

This is a multi-purpose blend designed to prevent and remedy several more or less related problems of the stomach and intestinal tract. It is also a specific remedy for all kinds of ulcers. Ulcers are one of the main medical problems of modern man. Over 200 million dollars are spent each year on antacid therapy alone, more than half of which is earmarked directly for ulcer treatment. And yet traditional treatments, antacid and anticholinergic drugs, are not very effective and they carry with them the very real threat of severe side effects. The herbs in this blend should provide a good treatment without side effects. This blend can also be used along with the DIGESTION blend for a broader spectrum of action, or used alone as a general treatment. It should also be used whenever the PARASITES & WORMS blend is being used to supplement the action of that blend. Prevention of G.I. tract disease can be substantially facilitated by using the CHOLESTEROL REGULATION Blend. In this blend, digestion is promoted by Papaya, Gentian, Licorice root, Fenugreek, Ginger root and Goldenseal. Ulcers are prevented by Ginger root, Irish Moss and Fenugreek. Ulcers are remedied by Licorice root, Irish Moss, Myrrh gum, Ginger root and Goldenseal. Upset stomach, gas and heartburn are treated with Gentian, Papaya, Ginger root, Goldenseal, and Licorice root.

**GOLDENSEAL ROOT.** Physicians of the 19th century, proficient in the use of natural remedies, were practically unanimous in the opinion that Goldenseal root, by itself, would cure indigestion, nausea, gas and heartburn. Twentieth century users of herbs, though concurring with that opinion, would rather use blends of herbs for gastrointestinal tract problems, such as indigestion and ulcers. This product was competently fashioned to meet that desire. The berberine alkaloids (hydrastine, berberine, berberastine) in Goldenseal not only stimulate bile production and secretion (**1**), but destroy noxious bacteria in the G.I. tract (**2**). Berberine increases the tone and movement of the gastrointestinal tract (**3**), and has been effectively used to treat gastroenteritis (**4**) and diarrhea in adults (**5**) and children (**6**).

Of concern to health officials around the world is the increasing threat of drinking water contamination by giardia. This pathogen exists in almost all surface waters, including lakes, reservoirs and mountain streams. And it is not destroyed by normal water treatment procedures, including chlorination. The symptoms of giardiasis can be broadly classified as severe G.I. distress. While eighty per cent (80%) of all cases yield to treatment, about 10-15% of the cases are incurable, even lethal. Berberine has been found to specifically remedy this ailment (**7**). Administered orally in a dose of 10 mg/kg/day for 10 days, it has cured patients at rates equal to, if not better than, established antigiardial drugs. The berberine in many studies is non-specific, i.e., it could have come from anywhere. In one important Japanese study, however, berberine and other alkaloids taken directly from Goldenseal were compared with alkaloids from related plants. The Goldenseal extract proved to be the most potent in terms of intestinal antibacterial activity (**8**). In terms of activity, berberine and hydrastine have been shown to be very similar (**9**). It is no wonder that Goldenseal is often called the "wonder herb." *See Also INFLUENZA; VAGINAL YEAST INFECTION; NERVES & GLANDS; EYES; FEVERS & INFECTIONS; HEMORRHOIDS*

**LICORICE ROOT** promotes the healing of peptic, gastric and duodenal ulcers. The earliest account of using Licorice root for ulcers is probably that recorded by Hippokrates in 400 B.C. Pliny & Gerard were other early authors with knowledge of this property, as were the ancient Chinese herbalists. The modern era of research on the anti-ulcer property of Licorice root began officially with the clinical use of the extract in 1946 (**10**). In 1962, research on Licorice root was advanced considerably when an English scientist turned the spotlight from Licorice root extract to its separate constituents (**11**). The primary constituent, glycyrrhetinic acid, eventually became known as carbenoxolone sodium (CS). This substance worked faster than Licorice root extract, but had more potent side effects. By 1965, CS had proved itself to be the #1 drug in treating ulcers **(12-15)**. In 1974, an editorial in **The Medical Journal of Australia** stated that only three therapeutic treatments had ever been conclusively shown to accelerate the healing of gastric ulcers: hospital admission; the cessation of smoking; and carbenoxolone sodium. Throughout the '60s, doctors in Britain hailed CS as the first effective cure for ulcers, ever. Meanwhile, side effects were being played down, researchers from other countries were carrying out their own studies, and the United States was more or less ignoring the entire phenomenon. In terms of side effects, Licorice root extract had produced sodium and water retention with subsequent loss of potassium in a small percentage of patients. CS was more potent, i.e., its side effects appeared in a greater percentage of people and were more pronounced. All side effects disappeared without permanent harm when the treatment was halted.

A startling event occurred when a group of researchers, seeking a substitute Licorice root derivative without side effects, discovered that Licorice root, from which 97% of the glycyrrhetinic acid (GLA) had been removed, was still capable of healing ulcers, but without side effects. This substance, known as deglycyrrhizinated licorice (DGL), was an unlikely candidate for an anti-ulcer drug because it had been assumed that GLA was the only active principle in Licorice root. In subsequent years, DGL was proven to have good healing effects **(16-22)**. In most studies DGL produced a 75-80% reduction in ulcerative indexes. One study found that CS was only a little more effective than DGL, and the difference was not statistically significant **(23)**. Whole Licorice root must, then, possess at least two anti-ulcer principles. The first, GLA, has been shown effective in literally hundreds, of animal and human studies. This component also contains the principles with aldosterone-like activity (see ARTHRITIS & Appendix A). The second, DGL, became the focus of serious research attention when it was discovered that it healed ulcers without the aldosterone side effects of the GLA. Whole Licorice root, of course, combines both active principles, but has not been experimentally studied at all. Such research is expensive and whatever monetary gain could be realized from marketing an unregulated, non-patentable herb would not begin to repay the costs of the research. The use of Licorice root extract is also not a profitable venture for pharmaceutical companies. From a research point of view, one important question should be answered as soon as possible: How does whole (powdered, encapsulated) Licorice root compare with DGL for speed of action, effectiveness and side effects. I suspect, as explained in Appendix A, that whole Licorice root is also devoid of side effects, but it is impossible to say beforehand whether or not it would be faster acting or as effective. The mode of action of these Licorice compounds has not been conclusively demonstrated, but the most probable theory is that they primarily reinforce the defenses of the stomach wall against the damaging effect of back diffusion of hydrogen ions and against excesses of duodenal bile. Licorice root also has an important anti-inflammatory effect on stomach mucous membranes. This effect may be due to the adrenocortical property of the herb which inhibits the secretory activity of the stomach and lowers the level of stomach juices without influencing enzymatic activity or hydrochloric acid levels (**24**). *See Also INFERTILITY; ARTHRITIS; RESPIRATORY AILMENTS; SKIN; FEMALE TONIC; BLOOD PURIFICATION/DETOXIFICATION; CIRCULATION; FATIGUE; WEIGHT LOSS; ENVIRONMENTAL POLLUTION; FEVERS & INFECTIONS; THYROID; WHOLE BODY; DETOXIFY/NURTURE; MENTAL ALERTNESS/SENILITY*

**GENTIAN ROOT** is a potent bitter from the Old World that is a remarkable aid to digestion, eliminating along the way, gas, heartburn and flatulence. In a classic study from Germany, it was discovered that this herb, in conjunction with lesser amounts of Ginger root (see below), Wormwood and Cayenne, was remarkably effective in curing indigestion and heartburn in human patients (**25**). Other studies have provided dramatic proof that Gentian root stimulates the gallbladder and pancreas (e.g., **26-27**). It also causes strong stimulation of the appetite, increases saliva and digestive juice secretion, and accelerates the emptying of the stomach (**28**). Administration of Gentian root should precede mealtimes by about one half hour for maximum benefit. But its activity begins about five minutes after reaching the stomach, as digestive juices begin to flow and bile secretion increases. Whatever level of digestive liquid is achieved during the first 30 minutes will be maintained for 2-3 hours without increasing further. This simply means that digestion, especially of fat and protein, will take place more quickly and thoroughly with the herb than without it (**29**). Experts in Gentian research are convinced that it acts on the mucous membranes of the stomach and mouth and directly on the gallbladder to stimulate its emptying (**30**). Gentian works in this manner more potently than almost every other bitter. *See Also CIRCULATION; NERVES & GLANDS; THYROID; DIGESTION*

**PAPAYA LEAF** is known primarily for its digestive properties. However, it does have other effects on the gastro-intestinal tract. The most important of these is an anti-ulcer action. Knowledge of this activity comes to us by way of Taiwan, where Papaya was used as a folk medicine to treat G.I. disorders. Recently, a Taiwanese research team determined the relative veracity of the foklore claims. In their study, ulcers were induced in rats by aspirin and stress and corticosteroids. Rats that had ingested Papaya for a period of 6 days prior to the stress period were significantly more resistant than untreated animals (**31**). This study, and a previous one that found similar effects, may stimulate more research along these lines. The mode of action could involve either one, or both of the known properties of Papaya. The first is based on the herb's tendency to coagulate blood (**32**). This property could protect the stomach mucosa from damage and ulcer formation. The second involves the finding that Papaya reduces acid secretion (**34**); less acid, less damage. *See Also DIGESTION; MENSTRUATION*

**MYRRH GUM** is a disinfectant, astringent and deodorant for air passages and the urinary tract. It acts primarily on mucous membranes of the respiratory tract. It acts directly and rapidly on the peptic glands to increase activity, in this way increasing digestion. In cases of dyspepsia accompanied with excess mucous formation, Myrrh is highly recommended by herbablists. *See Also FEVERS & INFECTIONS; VAGINAL YEAST INFECTION*

**IRISH MOSS** contains an abundance of mucilaginous essence that soothes inflamed and ulcerated surfaces. Being an unassimilated hydrocolloid, Irish Moss is a very effective bulk laxative, but is used throughout the food industry to impart stability (ice creams, sherbets, whipped creams, etc.), texture, and body (creamed soups and chowder, etc.). Among the proven effects of Irish Moss are the abilities to reduce gastric secretions, reduce high blood pressure, and alleviate peptic and duodenal ulcers (**34**). Ulcers appear to be susceptible to the medicinal properties of various marine plants. A recent U.S. Patent describes an Iceland Moss preparation for treating gastric and duodenal ulcers (**35**). Kelp, another marine plant, has been used for decades to effectively treat ulcers. Irish Moss also possesses anticoagulant, hypotensive and immunosuppressive properties (**34**). *See Also LAXATIVE*

**FENUGREEK SEED** has been used in folk medicine as a digestive aid, to allay stomach pains, and to stimulate liver function. In recent years, these uses have received some amount of experimental verification. For example, in a successful attempt to verify the ability of

Fenugreek seeds to improve severe diabetes in humans, a group of French scientists discovered that the seeds stimulate general pancreatic secretion which, as a by-product, would improve digestion (**36**). In a second study, these authors verified the blood cholesterol and blood glucose lowering actions of Fenugreek seeds (**37**). These effects were not due to the essential oil of the seeds, as was predicted, but to the defatted portion of the seeds, which is high in fiber, cellulose and lignin. Fenugreek seeds are also high in protein, with large amounts of amino acids: lysine, tryptophan, leucine, histidine and arginine. These chemicals could also contribute to better digestion and assimilation of nutrients. In addition, the mucilaginous nature of Fenugreek would act in a like fashion to Irish Moss in relieving the pain and irritation of ulcers. Other research shows that the seeds have galactagogue effects due to lactation factors in the fatty acids. Measurable improvement in general health, an increase in body weight, better protein utilization, inhibition of phosphorous secretion, and notable increases in erythrocyte count can be expected through ingestion of the seeds (**27**). *See Also CHOLESTEROL REGULATION; FEMALE TONIC*

**GINGER ROOT** is present in several blends in this book because of its many beneficial properties. Of these, none is so well known as its carminative or very soothing and mildly stimulating effects on the stomach. I try to influence everybody I know to use it for almost every kind of stomach discomfort, from nausea to indigestion, from simple stomachache to ulcers. Laboratories of modern science provide much interesting data. A German study has shown that Ginger root increases the flow of saliva, increases the amylase concentration in saliva, activates peristalsis, and increases tonus of the intestinal muscles (**38**). Another German study confirmed that a combination of Ginger root and Gentian root (with some Cayenne and Wormwood) is very effective in remedying indigestion and heartburn (**39**). An English study determined that Ginger root contains a proteolytic enzyme, zingibain, that is more effective than papain (from Papaya) or ficin (**40**). An American pair of investigators demonstrated that Ginger root is more effective than Dramamine in preventing motion sickness (**41**). Finally, Ginger root has been clincially proven to decrease signficantly, nausea and diarrhea associated with the common three-day, or 24-hour type flus (**42**). *See Also DIGESTION; NAUSEA; LOW BLOOD SUGAR; LAXATIVE; CIRCULATION; NERVOUS TENSION; FATIGUE*

## OTHER NUTRIENTS

*A healthy gastro-intestinal mucosa depends upon nutritional support from you. If you have problems in this area, the nutrients in the following table may help to restore and maintain health to your G.I. tract. Individual requirements may depart significantly from the following general recommendations.*

### VITAMIN & MINERALS

*(Daily requirements unless otherwise noted)*

Vitamin A *25,000 I.U.*
Vitamin B1 *25-100 mg*
Vitamin B2 *25-100 mg*
Vitamin B6 *25-100 mg*
Vitamin C *500-1000 mg*
Vitamin D *4,000 I.U.*
Vitamin E *400 I.U.*
Niacinamide *100 mg*
Folic Acid *400 mcg*
Pantothenic Acid *100-200 mg*
Inositol
Bioflavanoids

### MINERALS

Calcium/Magnesium
Potassium

### MISCELLANEOUS

Lecithin
Yogurt/Acidophilus
Digestive Enzymes
Brewer's Yeast
GLA

## REFERENCES

1. Kulkarni, S.K., Dandiya, P.C., Varandani, N.L. "Pharmacological investigations of berberine sulphate." **Japanese Journal of Pharmacology,** 22, 11-16, 1972.

2. Subbaiah, T.V. & Amin, A.H. "Effect of berberine sulphate on entamoeba histolytica." **Nature,** 215, 527-528, 1967.
3. Chopra, R.N., Dikshit, B.B., Chowhan, J.S. "Pharmacological action of berberine." **Indian Journal of Medical Research,** 19(4), 1193-1203, 1932.
4. Kamat, S.A. **Journal of the Association of Physicians of India,** 15, 525, 1967.
5. Lahiri, S.C. & Dutta, N.K. "Berberine and chloramphenicol in the treatment of cholera and severe diarrhea." **Journal of Indian Medical Association,** 48(1), 1-11, 1967.
6. Sharda, D.C. "Berberine in the treatment of diarrhea of infancy and childhood." **Journal of the Indian Medical Association,** 54(1), 22-24, 1970.
7. Gupte, S. "Use of berberine in the treatment of giardiasis." **American Journal of Diseases of Childhood,** 129, 866, 1975.
8. Haginiwa, J. & Harada, M. "Pharmacological studies on crude drugs. V. Comparison of the pharmacological actions of berberine type alkaloid-containing plants and their components." **Yakugaku Zasshi,** 82, 726-731, 1962, and 81, 1387, 1961.
9. Preininger, V. in **The Alkaloids,** Vol. 15, R.H.F. Manske, Ed., Academic Press, New York, 1975, 207.
10. Revers, R.E. "Heeft succus liquiritae een genezende weking op de maagzeer?" **Nederlands Tijdschrift voor Geneeskunde,** 90, 135-137, 1946. (The original study)
11. Doll, R., Hill, I.D., Hutton, C. & Underwood, D.J. "Clinical trial of a triterpenoid liquorice compound in gastric and duodenal ulcer." **Lancet,** 2, 793-796, 1962.
12. Sircus, W. "Progress report on carbenoxolone sodium." **Gut,** 13, 816-824, 1972.
13. Nagy, G.S. "Evaluation of carbenoxolone sodium in the treatment of duodenal ulcer." **Gastroenterology,** 74, 7-10, 1978.
14. Cliff, J.M. & Milton Thompson, G.J. "A double blind trial of carbenoxolone capsules in the treatment of duodenal ulcer." **Gut,** 11, 167-170, 1970.
15. Amure, B.O. "Clinical studies of duogastrone in the treatment of duodenal ulcers." **Gut,** 11, 171-175, 1970.
16. Turpie, A.G.G., Runcie, J. & Thompson, T.J. "Clinical trial of deglycyrrhizinized liquorice in gastric ulcer." **Gut,** 10, 299-302, 1969.
17. Anderson, S., Brany, F., Caboda, J.L.F. & Mizuno, T. "Protective action of deglycyrrhizinated licorice on the occurrence of stomach ulcers in pylorous-ligated rats." **Scandanavian Journal of Gastroenterology,** 6, 683-686, 1971.

18. Cooke, W.M. & Baron, J.H. "Metabolic studies on deglycyrrhizinated licorice in two patients with gastric ulcer." **Digestion,** 4, 264-268, 1971.
19. Tewari, S.N. & Wilson, A.K. "Deglycyrrhizinated licorice in duodenal ulcer." **The Practitioner,** 210, 820-823, 1973.
20. Mills, D.H. & Damrau, R. "Dedglycyrrhizinized glycyrrhiza in treatment of peptic ulcer." **International Medical Digest,** 4, 36-44, 1969.
21. Gassman, R. & Forster, G. "Experience with the liquorice juice preparation Caved-(S) in the treatment of ulcers of the alimentary tract." **Therapeutische Umschau,** 20, 306, 312, 1963.
22. Russell, R.I. & Dickie, J.E.N. "Clinical trial of a deglycyrrhizinated liquorice preparation in peptic ulcer." **Journal of Therapeutics and Clincial Research,** 1, 2-5, 1968.
23. Wison, J.A.C. "A comparison of carbenoxolone sodium and deglycyrrhizinated liquorice in treatment of gastric ulcer in the ambulant patient." **The British Journal of Clinical Practice,** 26, 563-566, 1972.
24. Lutomski, J. "Chemistry and therapeutic uses of licorice root." **Pharmazie in Unserer Zeit,** 12(2), 49-54, 1983.
25. Glatzel, H. "Treatment of dyspeptic disorders with spice extracts." **Hippokrates,** 40(23), 916-919, 1969.
26. Deininger, R. "Amarum-bitter herbs: common bitter principle remedies and their action." **Krankenpflege,** 29(3), 99-100, 1975.
27. List, P.H. & Hoerhammer, L. **Hagers Handbuch der Pharmazeutischen Praxis.** Volumes 2-5, Springer-Verlag, Berlin.
28. Glatzel, H. & Hackenberg, K. "Roentgenological studies of the effect of bitters on digestive organs." **Planta Medica,** 15(3), 223-232, 1967.
29. Ivancevic, J. & Kadrnka, S. **Archiv fuer Pharmakologie und Experimentelle Pathologie,** 189, 557-567. 1938.
30. Yamamoto, A. in **Enzymes in Food Processing,** 2nd Ed., G. Reed, Ed., Academic Press, New York, 1975, p. 123.
31. Chen, C., Chen, S., Chow, S. & Han, P.W. "Protective effects of carica papaya Linn on the exogenous gastric ulcer in rats." **American Journal of Chinese Medicine,** 9(3), 205-212, 1981.
32. Su, C.Y., Hus, S.Y. & Wang, Y.T. "Prevention of the experimental gastric ulcer in the rate by some folk medicinal plants in Taiwan." **Journal of the Formosan Medical Association,** 69(10), 507, 1970.

33. Prousset, J.L. "Antihemolytic action of an extract of carica papaya bark. Possibilities of use in glucose-6-phosphate dehydrogenase deficiencies." **Dakar Medical,** 24(3), 255-262, 1979.
34. Leung, A.Y. **Encyclopedia of Common Natural Ingredients.** New York, 1980.
35. Szturma, W. "Method for treating gastro-intestinal ulcers with extract of herb cetaria." U.S. Patent 4150123, issued April 17, 1979.
36. Ribes, G., Sauvaire, Y., Baccou, J.C., Valette, G., Chenon, D., Trimble, E.R. & Mariani, M.M.L. "Effects of fenugreek seeds on endocrine pancreatic secretions in dogs." **Annals of Nutrition and Metabolism,** 28, 37-43, 1984.
37. Valette, G., Sauvaire, Y., Baccou, J.C. &Ribes, G. "Hypocholesterolemic effect of fenugreek seeds in dogs." **Atherosclerosis,** 50, 105-111, 1984.
38. Glatzel, H. **Deutsche Apotheker Zeitung,** 110, 5, 1970.
39. Glatzel, H. "Treatment of dyspetic disorders with spice extracts." **Hippokrates,** 40(23), 916-919, 1969.
40. Thompson, E.H., Wolf, I.D. & Aleen, C.E. "Ginger rhizome: a new source of proteolytic enzyme." **Journal of Food Science,** 38(4), 652-655, 1973.
41. Mowrey, D.B. & Clayson, D.E. "Motion Sickness, ginger, and psychophysics." **Lancet,** 1(8273), 655-657, 1982.
42. Mowrey, D.B. "The effects of ginger root on the symptoms of the common flu." Paper presented at the Rocky Mountain Psychological Association, May, 1978.

# THYROID

## HERBS

**Form:**  Capsule, tablet

**CONTENTS:  KELP** *(Laminaria, Macrocystis, Ascophyllum),* **Gentian root** *(Gentiana lutea),* **Saw Palmetto berries** *(Serenoa repens-sabal),* **Cayenne** *(Capsicum annum),* & **Irish Moss** *(Chondrus crispus).*

**PURPOSE:  A gentle tonic to heal, strengthen and maintain the Thyroid gland.**

**Other Applications:**  For the adrenal, pineal, pituitary, lymph and other glands.

**USE:**  1. Thyroid tonic: 2-6 capsules per day as needed or desired.
2. During dieting: 1-2 capsules per day.
3. For added thyroid help while using the WHOLE BODY TONIC: 1-2 capsules per day.
4. To supplement the SKIN DISORDERS blend: 2-3 capsules per day.

**Contraindications:**  None. For discussion of Cayenne, see Appendix A.

An active, healthy thyroid produces hormones that are vital in maintaining normal growth and metabolism. Too much thyroid activity produces nervousness, heart palpitations and insomnia. Too little activity produces drowsiness, fatigue, impaired mental functioning, atherosclerosis, irritability, and lethargy. Severe inactivity produces obesity and coarsened features. An enlarged thyroid (usually with hyperthyroidism) is called goiter. The main thyroid hormones stimulate the activity of organs, tissues and cells, control skeletal growth and sexual development, influence the texture of skin and luster of hair, and are responsible for a person's energy or lack of it. Quite a responsibility for one gland. It is also the main repository of iodine in the body, and requires dietary iodine for proper development and functioning.

**KELP,** in supplying the thyroid with all the iodine it needs, increases the chances that this gland will not develop goiter, helps regulate the texture of the skin, and helps prevent dull hair. Iodine is essential for the proper regulation of energy through its effect on metabolism, i.e., by helping the body burn off excess fat (it may therefore prevent atherosclerosis that is due to disturbances in fat metabolism) (**1**). Thyroxine, the major thyroid hormone aids in protein synthesis, carbohydrate absorption and the conversion of carotene to vitamin A. Kelp not only absorbs iodine from seawater but sponges up an enormous supply of essential nutrients, and delivers them to the thyroid gland and the rest of the body. These nutrients include protein, essential fatty acid, carbohydrates, fiber, trace elements, sodium and potassium salts, and a variety of other chemicals, such as alginic acid (**2**). Iron, copper, magnesium, calcium, potassium, barium, boron, chromium, lithium, nickel, silicon, silver, strontium, titanium, vanadium and zinc are found in biologically important amounts in Kelp (**3**). Among the Japanese, who consume up to 25% of their diet in Kelp, thyroid disease is practically unknown, but among the Japanese who are becoming more Westernized, thyroid disease is on the rise (**4**). *See Also FEVERS & INFECTIONS; WEIGHT LOSS; FATIGUE; HEART; BLOOD PURIFICATION/DETOXIFICATION; INFERTILITY; PAIN; MENTAL ALERTNESS/SENILITY; CIRCULATION; DIABETES; PROSTATE*

**GENTIAN ROOT** provides bitter principles that are known to normalize the functioning of the thyroid, probably through an indirect means. More directly, the herb stimulates the powers and organs of appetite, digestion, and assimilation. These principles are fully explained under STOMACH/INTESTINAL. *See Also DIABETES; NERVES & GLANDS; CIRCULATION*

**SAW PALMETTO BERRY** assists the thyroid in regulating sexual development and in normalizing the activity of those glands and organs. These berries have been used by several cultures, but mainly Americans, as a nutritive tonic. The reputation of this herb is beginning to become known internationally, but research interest in other countries has not yet encompassed it. Clinical evidence, of which there is an abundance, from physicians in the modern United States is positive and enthusiastic. However, good controlled studies are presently lacking. In my own mind, the clinical evidence is convincing enough just as it stands. For example, one physician of my acquaintance, as a small part of a much larger study, gives half of his patients suffering from thyroid deficiency a supplement containing Saw Palmetto berries, and gives the other half the same supplement minus the berries. At this writing, the data for the past 11 months (total of 4 patients) shows a more rapid recovery, a stronger sense of well-being, and increased sexual activity in patients receiving the Saw Palmetto Berries. *See Also INFERTILITY; RESPIRATORY AILMENTS; DIABETES; FEMALE TONIC; PROSTATE; NERVES & GLANDS; DIGESTION*

**CAYENNE** operates by distributing nutrients, catalyzing reactions, stimulating glandular activity, and providing its own important vitamins and minerals.

**IRISH MOSS,** a close relative of Kelp, supplies its own quantities of iodine, trace elements and tissue salts.

## OTHER NUTRIENTS

*The thyroid requires good nutritional support in addition to adequate iodine. Individual needs may depart substantially from the following general recommendations.*

### VITAMINS

(Daily requirements unless otherwise noted)

Vitamin A *25,000 I.U.*
Vitamin C *3,000-5,000 mg*
Vitamin B Complex
Vitamin E *400 I.U.*
Vitamin D *1,000 I.U.*
Pantothenic Acid *200 mg*

## MINERALS

Iodine
Calcium/magnesium
Phosphorous
Potassium
Iron

## MISCELLANEOUS

Water


# REFERENCES

1. Guyton, A.C. **A Textbook of Medical Physiology,** 4th Ed., W.B.Saunders Co., Philadelphia, 1971.
2. Johnston, H.W. "Composition of edible seaweeds." in **Proceedings of the Seventh International Seaweed Syposium,** Wiley & Sons, New York, 1972, pp. 429-435.
3. Yamamoto, T. & Ishibashi, M. "The content of trace elements in seaweeds." in **Proceedings of the Seventh International Seaweed Symposium,** Wiley & Sons, New York, 1972, pp. 511-514.
4. Kagawa, Y. "Impact of westernization on the Japanese. Changes in physique, cancer, longevity and centenarians." **Preventative Medicine,** 205-217, 1978.

# VAGINAL YEAST INFECTION

## HERBS

**Form:** Capsule, Sitz bath

**CONTENTS:** **GOLDENSEAL** root *(Hydrastis canadensis)*, **BUCHU** leaves *(Barosma crenata)*, **Witch Hazel leaves** *(Hamamelis virginiana)*, **Plantain** *(Plantago ovata)*, **Myrrh Gum** *(Commiphora myrrha)*, **Juniper berries** *(Juniperis communis)*, & **Squaw vine** *(Mitchella repens)*.

**PURPOSE:** **To treat Vaginal Yeast Infection (Vaginitis); As a tonic for other female problems including cervical infection and urinary tract infection.**

**Other Applications:** Unusual bleeding (Menses, Nosebleeds, etc.), Hemorrhoids, Varicose Veins, Difficult Urination, Tonic.

**USE:** 1. Vaginal yeast infection: 2 capsules, 4 times daily. For best results, supplement with 4-6 capsules of Garlic per day and 3-5 capsules of the FEVERS & INFECTIONS blend.
2. Urinary Tract Infection: 4-6 capsules per day.
3. Cervical Infections: 6 capsules per day.
4. To supplement the DIURETIC Blend: 3-4 capsules per day.

**Contraindications:** Persons with known potassium insufficiency should exercise caution and consider using supplemental potassium when using products containing diuretics.

271

Vaginal infections (vaginitis) may be caused by several means, the most common being yeast (candida albicans); others are bacteria, vitamin B and A deficiencies, intestinal worms and improper hygiene. Every herb in this blend, by some means, has been shown to be effective in reducing symptoms of leukorrhea and related vaginal, cervical and uterine problems. The combined mode of action of these herbs is to soothe inflamed and infected mucous membranes and inhibit discharges, while disinfecting the area in the interest of good health.

**GOLDENSEAL ROOT** and its major constituent, hydrastine, have been repeatedly proven through global research first, to reduce inflammation of mucous membranes (vaginal and uterine) (**1-2**), second, to control uterine hemorrhaging (**3**), and third, to destroy harmful bacteria and other germs (**4-5**). It has been suggested that berberine (a primary constituent of Goldenseal, along with hydrastine) acts on mucosal surfaces by coagulating proteins and thus decreasing the inflammatory congestion (**6**). This mechanism was also suggested for the herb's remarkable success in treating patients during successive cholera epidemics in Calcutta, India, in 1965 and 1966. During those sieges, berberine proved more effective, with fewer side effects, than antibiotics (**7**). Another possible explanation of Goldenseal's anti-hemorrhoidal property, as demonstrated in pharmacological tests, is that it possesses a potent peripheral vessel constricting property (**8-10**). These modern research findings confirm the experience of past generations (**5**). Primary related material on Goldenseal root can be found in the following chapters: INFLUENZA; STOMACH/INTESTINAL; NERVES & GLANDS. *See Also FEVERS & INFECTIONS; EYES; HEMORRHOIDS/ASTRINGENT.*

**WITCH HAZEL LEAF** possesses a unique kind of astringency whose main locus of action is on the venous system, acting to restore tone, health and vigor throughout that system. It also has a powerful hemostatic property. Hemorrhoids and varicose veins are even benefited by this plant. In fact, almost any sort of minor bleeding such as nosebleed, scratches, etc., can be quickly mended with the application of Witch Hazel tincture or poultice. But the primary usefulness of Witch Hazel leaves is for treating congestive conditions of the uterus, cervix, and vagina, including vaginitis, prolapsus, and the aching sensation of weight or fullness. The plant's effectiveness is normally ascribed to the strong astringency of tannic acid, present in large amounts in Witch Hazel. But the common "Witch Hazel" water has all tannin removed, yet is nevertheless astringent. The plant's effectiveness is probably also due to proven bacteriostatic activity, and the presence of two or three important volatile oils, such as eugenol and carvacol. (General references on Witch Hazel: **10-12**). *See Also HEMORRHOIDS/ASTRINGENT*

**PLANTAIN** imparts a necessary soothing mucilage to products designed for internal symptomatic relief of the irritated urinary tract and for external relief of inflamed and painful mucous membranes. The Plantain provides the necessary cooling balm that takes the harsh astringent edge away from the blend. By itself, Plantain has often been used to treat female disorders that are accompanied by fluent discharges (**13**). It was used by American Indians, early physicians, and is still used by modern herbalists, to treat hemorrhoids (as well as snakebite, coughs, venereal disease, and countless other ailments) (**14**). *See Also BONE-FLESH-CARTILAGE; WEIGHT LOSS; RESPIRATORY AILMENTS; CHOLESTEROL REGULATION*

**BUCHU LEAF** is a recognized urinary antiseptic (**15**) that acts to eliminate mucous, acid urine and irritation, and is given to combat many forms of inflammation and infection, including cystitis, pyelitis, urethritis, and prostatitis (**16**). *See Also DIURETIC; PROSTATE*

**MYRRH GUM**'s three great actions are on digestion, infection and vaginitis, the first two of which are discussed in the chapters on STOMACH/INTESTINAL and FEVERS & INFECTIONS. The third effect was observed and recorded several centuries ago in China (**17**) from which date forward the Chinese have used the herb to treat menstrual difficulties, leukorrhea and other forms of bleeding, including hemorrhoids and ulcerated sores. But several centuries before the Chinese learned about Myrrh gum, other Asians were using it. The herb was introduced to the West from Asia and Africa, and has become an important source of botanical medicine. It is antiseptic to mucous membranes, and, curiously, both inhibits oversecretion as well as disinhibits undersecretion of these tissues; thus, it *normalizes* mucous membrane activity (**13**). The anti-infectious nature of Myrrh also plays an active role in this blend. The bacteriostatic and antiseptic properties of the herb have been experimentally verified in both America and China (**18-19**), in which studies Myrrh was shown to inhibit gram positive bacteria such as *stapholococcus aureus*. *See Also STOMACH/INTESTINAL; FEVERS & INFECTIONS*

**JUNIPER BERRY** has been used in America for a couple of hundred years as a urinary antiseptic, and, by some physicians, to treat vaginitis (**20**). It was recommended for several years in the U.S.P. and N.F. as an emmenagogue (an agent that promotes menstrual flow). Its primary application is as a diuretic. *See Also DIURETIC*

**SQUAW VINE** acquired its name because it was popular among many American Indian tribes as an aid to parturition, being used in large quantities during the last few weeks of pregnancy (**15**). The plant was also used extensively to treat several uterine difficulties, including painful menstruation and threat of miscarriage. Some early American physicians used the plant quite successfully (**21**), but it wasn't until 1926 that it gained official recognition and was allowed into the National Formulary. *See Also FEMALE TONIC*

## OTHER NUTRIENTS

*Vaginitis and related infections and irritations of the vagina and cervix can be prevented and remedied with the aid of various nutritional substances. Individual needs may depart substantially from the following general recommendations.*

### VITAMINS
*(Daily requirements unless otherwise noted)*

Vitamin A *25,000-50,000 I.U.*
Vitamin B Complex—High potency
Vitamin B1 *25-50 mg*
Vitamin B2 *25-50 mg*
Vitamin B6 *25-100 mg*
Vitamin D *400 I.U.*
Vitamin E
Vitamin C *1,000-2,000 mg*
Pantothenic Acid *100 mg*

### MINERALS

Zinc
Calcium/Magnesium

## MISCELLANEOUS

Nizoral
Digestive enzymes
Essential Fatty Acids
Nystatin
Protein

# REFERENCES

1. **U.S. Dispensatory** (26th ed), Lippencott. Philadelphia, PA, p. 576.
2. Chopra, R.N., Dikshit, B.B. & Chowhan, J.S. "Pharmacological action of berberine." **Indian Journal of Medical Research,** 1932, 19(4), 1193-1203.
3. Gibbs, O.S. "On the curious pharmacology of hydrastis." **Federation of American Societies for Experimental Biology Federation Proceedings,** 1947, 6(1), 332.
4. Johnson, C.C., Johnson, G. & Poe, C.F. "Toxicity of alkaloids to certain bacteria. II. Berberine, physostigmine and sanguine." **Acta Pharmacologica et Toxicologica,** 1952, 8(1), 71-78.
5. Welch, A.D. & Henderson, V.E. "A comparative study of hydrastine, bicuculline, and adlumine." **Journal of Pharmacology and Experimental Therapeutics,** 1934, 51(4), 482-491.
6. Sharda, D.C. "Berberine in the treatment of diarrhea of infancy and childhood." **Journal of the Indian Medical Association,** 54(1), 22-24, 1970.
7. Lahiri, S.C. & Dutta, N.K. "Berberine and chloramphenicol in the treatment of cholera and severe diarrhea." **Journal of the Indian Medical Association,** 48(1), 1-11, 1967.
8. Genest, K. & Hughes, D.W. "Natural products in canadian pharmaceuticals." **Candadian Journal of Pharmaceutical Sciences,** 4(2), 41-45, 1969.
9. Ikram, M. "A review of the chemical and pharmacological aspects of genus berberis." **Planta Medica,** 28, 353-358, 1975.
10. List, P.H. & Hoerhammer, L. **Hagers Handbuch der Phaermazeutishen Praxis.** Vols 2-5. Springer-Verlag. Berlin. 1969-1976.
11. **Martindale: The Extra Pharmacopoeia.** The Pharmaceutical Press. London. 1977.
12. Trease, G.E., & Evans, W.C. **Pharmacognosy.** 11th ed. Bailliere Tindall. London. 1978.

13. Ellingwood, F. **American Materia Medica, Therapeutics and Pharmacognosy.** Eclectic Medical Pubs, Portland, Oregon, 1983.
14. Hutchens, A.R. **Indian Herbalogy of North America.** Merco, Ontario, Canada, 1969.
15. Claus, E.P. **Pharmacognosy.** 4th ed. Lea & Febiger, Philadelphia, 1961.
16. Youngken, H.W. **Textbook of Pharmacognosy.** 5th ed. Blakiston. Philadelphia. 1943.
17. Hartwell, J.L. "Plants used against cancer. A survey." **Lloydia.** 31(2), 71-170, 1968.
18. Kiangsu Institute of Modern Medicine. **Encyclopedia of Chinese Drugs.** 1977. 2 vols. Shanghai Scientific and Technical Publications. Shanghae. People's Republic of China.
19. Majno, G. **The Healing Hand—Man and Wound in the Ancient World.** Harvard University Press, Cambridge, Mass. 1975. 217-218.
20. Gunn, J.C. & Johnson, **J.H. Gunn's Newest Family Physician.** Philadelphia, 1878.
21. Skinner, H.B. **The Family Doctor, Or Guide to Health...** Boston, published for author, 1844.

# WEIGHT LOSS

## HERBS

**Form:** Capsule

CONTENTS: **PLANTAIN** *(Plantago ovata)*, **Fennel seed** *(Foeniculum vulgare)*, **Burdock root** *(Arctium lappa)*, **Hawthorn berries** *(Crataegus oxyacantha)*, **Kelp** *(Laminaria, Macrocystis, Ascophyllum)*, & **Bladderwrack** *(Fucus vesiculosus)*.

**PURPOSE: To lose weight safely, naturally and effectively.**

**Other Applications:** Arthritis, gout, edema, high cholesterol levels, psoriasis, appetite suppressant.

**USE:** 1. While Dieting: 3-4 capsules immediately before each meal with a glass of water. May also wish to use 1-2 capsules of the DIURETIC blend and 1-2 capsules of the HEART blend.
2. While not Dieting: 2-3 capsules per meal.
3. For nutritional supplementation during fasts: 4-6 capsules per day.

**Contraindications:** None. If used in conjunction with a diuretic, care should be exercised to avoid serum potassium depletion as may occur when using diuretics.

   An herbal supplement to a weight reducing program should supply necessary nutrients, including vitamins, minerals and salts to sustain and nurture vital body systems, including the nerves, glands, skin, blood and organs. In addition, one should expect some help from the product in actually losing pounds. These two purposes are fulfilled by this blend full of Seeds and Seaweed, Berries and Burs. However, if you just sit around, you will not obtain any benefit from the increased metabolic capacity these herbs provide.

**NOTE:**  I have never been satisfied with the use of Chickweed to promote weight loss. No experiment, either with animals or with humans, has ever convinced me, or, indeed, shown the slightest indication that Chickweed is active in this respect. So why include it in a reduction plan when there are so many other herbs with proven effectiveness? I have recommended for years that Plantain be used in the place of Chickweed. Plantain, an herb whose contribution to weight loss is receiving more scientific substantiation all the time, successfully does what Chickweed is supposed to do.

**PLANTAIN** mucilage in the diet dramatically reduces serum cholesterol levels. An effective agent will reduce total serum cholesterol as well as low and very low density lipoprotein (LDL) while not affecting (or raising) high density lipoprotein (HDL) levels. Dietary fiber has been shown to have positive effects on serum lipid levels. Most fiber is composed of lignin and different kinds of nonabsorbable carbohydrates like cellulose. Pectin, mucilage and algae gums are also carbohydrates, that of Plantain being mainly D-xylose, L-arabinose and aldobiouronic acid (**1**). Different metabolic effects are achieved with different types of fibers (see CHOLESTEROL REGULATION for more details). Plantain before meals causes a definite decrease in triglycerides and beta cholesterol (the bad guys) with a proportional increase of serum levels of alpha cholesterol (the good guy) (**2**). Since deficiency in the latter substance has been implicated in obesity (**3**), type II diabetes and atherosclerosis (**4**), it is likely that Plantain mucilage provides some protection against those diseases. In Italy, a study on the effects of Plantain in a reducing diet for women who averaged about 60% overweight resulted in weight loss greater than that obtained by the diet alone (**5**). Three grams of Plantain was administered half an hour before meals, twice daily with half a glass of water. The diet was a standard hypocaloric, hypoglucidic (800 calories/day, 45% protein, 20% lipid, 35% carbohydrates). The effect of Plantain on weight loss was dramatic. Plantain works probably because it satiates the appetite (**6**) and reduces the absorption of lipids (**7**). In Russia, the cholesterol reducing property of Plantain and its relationship to weight loss have been shown to depend not only on the mucilage but on certain polyphenol compounds found in the leaves

**(8)**. In summary, it appears that Plantain produces weight loss by limiting caloric intake, due to its appetite-satiating effect, and by reduced intestinal absorption of lipids. *See Also VAGINAL YEAST INFECTION; BONE-FLESH-CARTILAGE; RESPIRATORY PROBLEMS; CHOLESTEROL REGULATION*

**FENNEL SEED** was used as a dietary aid as far back as the first century **(9)**. It is still successfully used today. Though the plant has received much experimental attention as an estrogenic agent **(10)**, the basis for many of its other properties has not been determined. Fennel does not directly affect weight, rather it has soothing, mildly stimulating properties, which are probably due to its essential oil. Oil of this kind is of immense importance to a gastro-intestinal system undergoing a weight loss regimen for it maintains tone and stasis, sterilizes, stimulates, and suppresses some anti-social consequences of dietary changes (if you get my drift); it also reduces any tendency toward colic that may arise **(11)**. *See Also DIGESTION*

**BURDOCK ROOT** is the herb of which the American Medical Botanist Millspaugh wrote, ". . . is so rank that man, the jackass, and caterpillar are the only animals that will eat of it." But it is included here to help cleanse the blood of toxins during the weight loss regimen. It markedly enhances liver and gall/bile functions as shown clinically **(12)** and experimentally **(13)**. Though the ingestion of Burdock root probably will not lead to weight loss, any good weight loss program should incorporate an herb to strengthen and purify the blood. *See Also DETOXIFY/NURTURE; SKIN PROBLEMS; BONE-FLESH-CARTILAGE; BLOOD PURIFICATION/DETOXIFICATION*

**HAWTHORN BERRY** is added to the blend to offset the increased demands made on the heart by the condition of being overweight. It also helps recondition and tone up the heart muscle while reducing, especially if the reducing plan includes, as it should, some form of exercise. In that case, it is very important that the heart be able to supply sufficient oxygen to the tissues. Hawthorn berries have been shown to have an oxygen-saving effect on the myocardium under stress **(14)**, as measured with an EKG during exercise. A Hungarian study showed that Hawthorn has a very strong vasodilatory action, and it lowers peripheral resistance to blood flow **(15)**. An Austrian team of investigators studied the effect of Hawthorn in human patients after 14 hours of food abstinence. They found that the herb led to a significant decrease in free fatty acids and in lactic acid. Also decreased, though not as much, were glucose and pyruvic acid. Triglyceride levels were increased (16). These findings indicate that Hawthorn has an anabolic, or building up, effect on the metabolic processes. That effect is probably achieved by an influence on the enzymatic system, leading to a decrease in oxygen and energy demands. The above experiments show that Hawthorn helps reduce coronary stress induced by over-weight and by exercise. *See Also HEART; CHOLESTEROL REGULATION*

**KELP** and **BLADDERWRACK** are two of the best weight-reduction plants available. Iodine in Kelp maintains a healthy thyroid, thereby significantly reducing one major cause of obesity. In addition, sea-weeds, through a healthy supply of nutrients and oxygen, increase the body's ability to burn off fat through exercise (17). Stamina is boosted, allowing cells to consume energy more efficiently. Kelp also lowers blood cholesterol levels (18). The mechanism of action of this latter effect may be related to the presence of fiber, and its ability to bind bile acid and bile salts (19). In support of this hypothesis, it has been found that Kelp increases concentrations and daily excretion of fecal cholesterol, deoxycholic acid, lithocholic acid, and total bile acids (20). An interesting industrial innovation for improving lipid metabolism, preventing hyperlipemia and treating diabetes recently appeared (21). It involves feeding Kelp to chickens who biologically incorporate the iodine in the eggs they lay. These iodine rich eggs can then be used for the above stated purposes.

## OTHER NUTRIENTS

*Everyone agrees that diet plays a major role in gaining and losing weight. The trick is to get all the nutrients and calories you need without overdoing it in the calorie department. Sometimes the use of dietary supplements can help. Individual requirements may differ significantly from the following recommendations.*

### VITAMINS & MINERALS

(Daily requirements unless otherwise noted)

Vitamin B-1 *25-100 mg*
Vitamin B-2 25-100 mg
Vitamin B-6 *25-100 mg*

Vitamin B-12 *4 mcg*
Vitamin C *500-1,000 mg*
Vitamin E *100-600 I.U.*
Inositol *1,000 mg*
Choline *1,000 mg*

**MINERALS**

Calcium/Magnesium

**MISCELLANEOUS**

Lecithin

# REFERENCES

1. Leung, A.Y. **Encyclopedia of Common Natural Ingredients.** New York, 1980.
2. Frati-Munari, A., Fernandez, H.J.A, Becerril, M., Chavez, N.A., Banales, H.M. "Decrease in serum lipids, glycemia and body weight by plantago in obese and diabetic patients." **Archivos de Investigacion Medica (Mexico),** 14(3), 259-268, 1983.
3. Krauss, R.M. "Regulation of high density lipoprotein levels." **Medical Clinics of North America,** 66, 403, 1982.
4. Eder, H.A., Gidez, L.I. "the clinical significance of the plasma high density lipoproteins." **Medical Clinics of North America,** 66, 431, 1982.
5. Enzi, G, Inelmen, E.M. & Crepaldi, G. "Effect of hydrophilic mucilage in the treatment of obese patients." **Pharmatherapeutica,** 2(7), 420-428, 1980.
6. Gugielmi, G, Spagnoletto, P. & Messina, B. "Risultati clinici e comportamento di alcuni parametri biologici in corso di trattamento con mucillagine idrofila." **Clinica Terapeutica,** 87, 27, 1978.
7. Forman, D.T., Garvin, G.E., Forestner, J.E., & Taylor, C.B. "Increased excretion of fecal bile acids by an oral hydrophillic colloid." **Proceedings of the Society for Experimental and Biological Medicine,** 127, 1060, 1968.
8. Maksiutina, N.P., Nikitina, N.I., Lipkan, G.N., Gorin, A.G. & Voitenko, I.N. "Chemical composition and hypocholesterolmic action of some drugs from plantago major leaves." **Farmatsevtychnyi Zhurnal,** 4, 56-61, 1978.

9. Guenther, R.T. **The Greek Herbal of Dioscorides.** Book 3:81, Hafner Publishing Company, London and New York, 1968, pp. 229 & 314.
10. Albert-Puleo, M. "Fennel and anise as estrogenic agents." **Journal of Ethnopharmacology,** 2, 337-344, 1980.
11. Shipochliev, T. "Pharmacological study of several essential oils. I. effect on smooth muscle." **Veterinarno-Meditsinski Nauki,** 5, 63, 1968 (Chem Abstracts 70, 86144e, 1969.
12. Felter, H. W. **The Eclectic Materia Medica, Pharmacology and Therapeutics.** Eclectic Medical Publications, Portland, Oregon, 1983 (first published 1922).
13. Charbrol, E. & Charonnat, R. "Therapeutic agents in bile secretion." **Ann. Med.,** 37, 131-42, 1935.
14. Kandziora, J. "The effects of Crataegus on perfusion disorders of the heart." **Muenchen Medizinische Wochenschrift,** 111(6), 295-298, 1969.
15. Kovach, A.G.B., Foedl, M. & Fedina, L. "Effects of extract obtained from Crataegus oxyacantha on Coronary blood flow in dogs." **Arzneimittelforschungen,** 9(6), 378-379, 1959.
16. Hammerl, H., Kranzl, C., Pichler, O., & Studlar, M. "Clinical and experimental investigations on metabolism using an extract of Crataegus." **Arztliche Forschung,** 21(7), 261-264, 1967.
17. Johnston, H.W. "Composition of edible seaweeds." **Proceedings of the Seventh International Seaweed Symposium.** Wiley and Sons, New York, 1972, pp. 429-435.
18. Kimura, A. & Kuramoto, M. "Influences of seaweeds of metabolism of cholesterol and anticoagulant actions of seaweed." **Tokushima Journal of Experimental Medicine,** 21, 79-88, 1974.
19. Story, J.A. & Kritchevsky, D. "Bile acid metabolism and fiber." **American Journal of Clinical Nutrition,** 31, s199-s202, 1978.
20. Reddy, B.S., Watanabe, K. & Sheinfil, A. "Effect of dietary wheat bran, alfalfa, pectin and carrageenan on plasma cholesterol and fecal bile acid and neutral sterol excretion in rats." **Journal of Nutrition,** 110, 1247-1254, 1980.

21. Kamimae, H. & Ishikawa, T. U.S. Patents 4410541, 4394376 & 4338304. "Composite for improving lipid metabolism." "Method for preventing hypertriglyceridemia." & "Composite for treating diabetes." 1983, 1983, 1982.

# TONIC—
# WHOLE BODY

## HERBS

**Form:** Capsule

**CONTENTS:** **SARSAPARILLA** **root** *(Smilax officinalis),* Siberian **GINSENG** *(Eleutherococcus senticosus),* **Fo-Ti** *(Polygonum multiflorum, ho-shou-wu),* **Gotu Kola** *(Hydrocotyle asiatica),* **Saw Palmetto berries** *(Serenoa repens-sabal),* **Licorice root** *(Glycyrrhiza glabra),* **Kelp** *(Laminaria, Macrocystis, Ascophyllum),* **Stillingia** *(Stillingia sylvatica),* **Alfalfa** *(Medicago sativa),* & **Cayenne** *(Capsicum annum).*

**PURPOSE:** **To supplement all other blends in this manual; to use daily as a regular dietary supplement; generally, to increase the vitality of the entire body, especially its resistance to disease and ability to rebound from illness or poor health.**

**Other Applications:** Longevity.

**USE:** 2-12 capsules per day as desired. Generally, use more during periods of convalescence, poor health and high stress.

**Contraindications:** None. For complete discussion of Licorice root and Cayenne, see Appendix A.

This blend is the ultimate tonic. It is like the finale of a Holiday fireworks display—you've seen the big sparklers individually and in small bursts, but now you get to see them all together. The blend

285

contains the true heavy-weights of the herbal kingdom. It's like an international all-star show: from the West you have **Sarsaparilla, Saw Palmetto, Stillingia,** and **Alfalfa;** and from the East you have **Ginseng, Fo-ti, Gotu Kola,** and **Kelp;** co-hosting the event is that favorite international pair, **Cayenne** and **Licorice root.** This blend is for those who are really serious about wholistic health, those who cherish the daily rejuvenation of the body's vital substances, the inexorable growth of stamina, strength and resistance to disease. For patient individuals, willing to forgo the quick pick-me-up in order to experience the subtle, sublime development and unfolding of their body's potential. For those willing to pay the price required to eventually achieve a more perfect inward unity and outward physical realization.

On the other hand, the blend is also great for those who just want to get on with life, mirthfully reveling in stress and risk, who live life to the max, who find developing optimum dietary routines both a waste of time and boring, but don't want to physically degenerate before their time. This blend will serve their purposes admirably. Use it with impunity. There is not a gland, nerve, muscle, vein, artery, organ, or bone in the body that will not experience significant benefits. The longer you maintain daily usage, the greater those benefits will be.

The medical profession does not normally recognize the term "tonic" as a viable drug class. The use of tonics was derived from folk usage. Tonics are not usually used to "treat" disease, and that is why their use was not picked up by the medical profession which specializes in the treatment, not the prevention of disease. Please read the introduction to the chapter entitled TONIC—NERVE & GLAND for more information about what makes an herb a tonic and how they are investigated. Refer to that chapter for information on **Kelp, Cayenne** and **Saw Palmetto,** the discussions of which were omitted here to prevent redundancy.

The specific medical information about the herbs in this blend can be found in the chapters listed for each one. In this chapter, continuing the method introduced in the NERVE & GLAND chapter, I will discuss the factors that have contributed to the elevation of these herbs to tonic status.

**SARSAPARILLA** belongs to a large family of related *Smilax* species, the members of which are used in countries around the world for fairly similar purposes. But nowhere except in the United States has this herb attained the status of tonic. Ironically, the best control-led studies on the herb come from China. In the U.S. and other countries, extracts of Sarsaparilla are routinely used for flavoring beverages, baked goods, candy and other foods. Toxicity tests are negative, but few people have ever sought to determine medicinal value in laboratory tests. Americans learned about the uses of Sarsaparilla from the Indians. The Indians used several species of the plant for numerous purposes. Medically speaking, it was used internally for coughs, hypertension, pleurisy, as a diuretic and alterative, and most importantly as a general tonic. Externally, it was used for wounds, sore eyes, burns and so on. Further knowledge about this herb was obtained from the medical and clinical experience of naturopathic physicians. These professionals were often divided about its specific activity, but agreed that it was an excellent tonic. I have occasionally read and heard some rather outlandish claims being made for Sarsaparilla without a shred of evidence to back them up. Such errant claims notwithstanding, the herb has proven itself to be a refreshing herbal tonic for nerves, blood and glands, and deserves much more research attention than it has received. It is used as an alterative, tonic, diuretic, carminative, diaphoretic. *See Also INFERTILITY, ARTHRITIS, BLOOD PURIFIER/DETOXIFIER, DETOXIFY/NURTURE*

**SIBERIAN GINSENG** and related herbal species are among the most highly prized objects on earth. As early as 618 B.C., the T'ang Dynasty of China prized Panax Ginseng enough to give it as royal gifts and to drive up the price close to its weight in gold. At times it has been worth **more** than its weight in gold. The earliest important paper on Ginseng was written about 400 years ago by Li Wen-Yen, whose son spent 27 years writing the famed Chinese pharmacopoeia, *Pen Ts'ao kang-mu*. This book describes Ginseng in detail and is still considered a scholarly, precise and invaluable work on the traditions of China. Ginseng is the ultimate example of man's almost mystical interaction with nature. Because of its antiquity and shape, Ginseng plays the central role in a good deal of Chinese mythology. It represented the human form, the transformation of matter and energy, the essence of the earth, and possessed both spiritual as well as physical attributes. Western man's initial introduction to Ginseng is difficult to trace, but appears to have begun when Arabs familiar with China brought it to the attention of European physicians who then promptly forgot about it. Another failed attempt to introduce it to Europe was made by Marco Polo. Finally, after Vasco de Gama opened trade routes, everything made or grown in China became fashionable in Europe. For about a hundred years physicians sold Ginseng as fast as they could get it. It also became a cash crop for American growers and European merchants: these men were more interested in exporting it to China than importing it from China. Then, undermined by some negative clinical experiments, it rapidly fell into disrepute.

At any rate, for Western man, the economic value of Ginseng far outweighed its medicinal value until the past 15 years or so. In the last few years, research in the area has grown explosively. The Chinese recommend Ginseng for the following disorders: anemia, asthma, stomach aches, colds & fevers, colic, depression, dizziness, dropsy, exhaustion, headaches, heart failure, impotence, indigestion, insomnia, lack of appetite, menstrual disorders, nausea, nervous disorders, old age, rheumatism, vascular cramps, sexual dysfunction. They have used the plant for these purposes throughout the centuries with only minor changes in the list. On the American continent, Wild American Ginseng was used by the Indians for earache, fever, infertility, general tonic, headache, menstrual problems, cramps, shortness of breath, sore eyes, stomach pains, exhaustion, tonsillitis and vomiting. For white Americans, Ginseng was mainly a cash crop. As late as 1931, Grieve wrote this about Ginseng: "In Western medicine, it (Ginseng) is considered a mild stomachic, tonic and stimulant, useful in loss of appetite and in digestive affections that arise from mental and nervous exhaustion." Not much, compared to the volumes about the herb written in China, Russia, Korea and Japan. Modern research on Ginseng species has tended to verify and extend the medicinal claims, but in more precise terminology. This research can be summarized as follows: Ginseng species stimulate the central nervous system in small amounts and depress the central nervous system in large doses; they protect the body and nervous system from stress; they stimulate and increase metabolic function; increase physical and mental efficiency; lower blood pressure and glucose levels when high, and raise them when low; increase gastrointestinal movement and tone; increase iron metabolism; and cause changes in nucleic acid (RNA) biosynthesis. For research and references on Ginseng see INFERTILITY, FATIGUE, WHOLE BODY TONIC, MENTAL ALERTNESS/SENILITY, BLOOD SUGAR. (The preceding material on Ginseng was adapted from a forthcoming book on the subject coauthored by Dennis Clayson, Ph.D. and myself.)

**FO-TI** is used mostly as an aromatic, purgative and emetic. In India it is used against colic and enteritis; in Brazil, for hemorrhoids and gout; in China, for skin and stomach ulcerations and abscesses, and in geriatrics. In that country, Fo-ti (Ho-shou-wu) is one of the most popular herbal tonics among the elderly. Its use and value (but not properties) are comparable to Goldenseal in the United States and Chamomile in Europe. The properties of this herb are often justly compared to those of Ginseng, but it has not yet been subjected to rigorous experimental study. In Oriental philosophy, it is said to increase Yin, thereby improving physical and mental health. Research on the plant indicates that it does lower blood cholesterol levels, and prevents the formation of experimental atherosclerosis in animals (**1**). In studies with humans, Fo-Ti has been found to reduce hypertension, blood cholesterol levels and the incidence of coronary heart disease among individuals prone to these conditions (**2**). An important and reliable Chinese materia medica lists several classes of ailments and conditions for which Fo-Ti should be used: 1) neurasthenia, insomnia, sweating, dizziness; 2) elevated serum cholesterol, coronary disease; 3) weakness, pain, backache, etc.; and 4) tuberculous adenopathy (**3**). These uses conform to the traditional Chinese medical view that Fo-Ti has anti-toxic, anti-swelling and tranquilizing properties (**4**). In addition, according to a recent report by the American Herbal Pharmacology Delegation which brought a great deal of information back to us from China, Fo-Ti is used by the Chinese for "liver and spleen weakness," vertigo, scrofula, cancer, constipation, and insomnia (**5**). The report also verified that the plant is used outside of China for various reasons, including sedative and anti-cancer effects. Reviewing pertinent scientific literature, the report of the delegation revealed data showing sedative effects, anti-cancer properties, anti-fever, and beneficial effects on fertility and other female functions involving ovulation and corpus luteum formation. An intriguing hypothesis was offered by the delegation: since most *polygonum* species contain *leucoanthrocyanidins* (LAC), which have been shown to have anti-inflammatory activity, to decrease blood coagulability, and to have cardiotonic, hypotensive, and vasodilatory activity, much of Fo-Ti's activity would be explained if it also contained LAC. To my knowledge, that particular chemical has not yet been isolated from Fo-Ti. But if it is there (as it should be), then Fo-Ti should be effective in reducing inflammatory conditions such as ulcers and arthritis. It should also strengthen the heart and reduce hypertension. These effects are closely related to those ascribed to the herb in Chinese herbal pharmacology. (Technical information was included here because the herb does not appear in any other blend in the book.)

**GOTU KOLA** is a traditional blood purifier, tonic and diuretic, hailing from Pakistan, India, Malaysia and parts of Eastern Europe. It is commonly used for diseases of the skin, blood and nervous system.

In homeopathy, it is used for psoriasis, cervicitis, pruritis vaginitis, blisters and so forth. Gotu Kola contains asiaticoside which is being used in the Far East to treat leprosy and tuberculosis. Several years ago, while in graduate school, I accepted a small grant to investigate the anti-fatigue and stimulating effects of three of the herbs that are in this blend: Capsicum, Ginseng and Gotu Kola. I found that Capsicum had a pronounced, quick acting anti-fatigue property and that a *combination* of Ginseng and Gotu Kola was able to gradually increase the activity rate in laboratory animals over a period of several weeks. I did not investigate the activity of those two herbs individually due to the stipulations of the grant. For those of you who are into digging up obscure source material, that research was published, according to grant requirements, in the first two issues of an uncelebrated periodical, now defunct (**6-7**). One final note: As I have written elsewhere (**8**), Gotu Kola contains no caffeine at all. Kola nut contains caffeine. They are not the same plant, or even remotely related. *See Also FATIGUE; MENTAL ALERTNESS/SENILITY; BLOOD SUGAR*

**SAW PALMETTO BERRY** See TONIC—NERVE & GLAND for tonic information. *See Also INFERTILITY; RESPIRATORY AILMENTS; DIABETES; FEMALE TONIC; PROSTATE; NERVES & GLANDS; THYROID; DIGESTION*

**LICORICE ROOT,** for good reasons, is contained in many of the blends recommended in this book. Besides possessing numerous medicinal properties of its own, it modulates and strengthens the activity of other herbs. In both Western and Eastern medicine Licorice root has played a central role for hundreds, even thousands of years, and is used today in both cultures for almost exactly the same conditions. Licorice root is also one of the most studied of all plants, with literally hundreds of studies having been conducted during the last 30-40 years. The following is a list of serveral proven therapeutic effects: Activity against fevers, infections, coughs, ulcers, inflammations, edema, bacteria, viruses, cholesterol and nervousness. It has estrogenic, hypotensive and blood sugar raising properties as well. It's effect on the adrenal-pituitary system is well-documented. Licorice root's status as a tonic is undoubtedly due to the cumulative effect of all its medicinal properties. Unlike many other tonics, however, Licorice root is more specific and is recommended in *large* amounts only for very specific conditions. In small amounts, as occur in this blend, the herb can be used with impunity: its activity herein is not to act on any specific physiological substrate, but to temper and enhance qualities within the other herbs. For important information on the correct use of Licorice root, see Appendix A. For details on its specific actions *See Also INFERTILITY; ARTHRITIS; RESPIRATORY AILMENTS; SKIN; FEMALE TONIC; BLOOD PURIFIER/DETOXIFIER; LAXATIVE; LIVER DISORDERS; STOMACH/INTESTINAL; DETOXIFY/NURTURE; FEVERS & INFECTIONS; NAUSEA*

**KELP** See TONIC—NERVE & GLAND for information on its tonic activity. For details on specific activity see many other blends in this manual, but especially THYROID, ARTHRITIS, HEART, HIGH BLOOD PRESSURE, CIRCULATION, ENVIRONMENTAL POLLUTION, DETOXIFY/NURTURE, FEVERS & INFECTIONS, and WEIGHT LOSS.

**STILLINGIA** is discussed under DETOXIFIER/NUTRITIONAL SUPPLEMENT.

**ALFALFA** is included in this blend on the basis of its reputation as an appetite stimulant and vitality augmenter. Much of that reputation was gained during observations of its effect as a livestock feed. Subsequent additions to the diets of humans produced the same results. The idea of humans eating something generally grown for animals has never really caught on in a big way with the general public, yet is completely accepted by persons interested in natural health. As a spring tonic, Alfalfa has no equal. It is one the best sources for protein. In addition, it is very high in vitamins A, D, E, B-6, and K, calcium, magnesium, chlorophyll, phosphorous, iron, potassium, trace minerals and several digestive enzymes. The chapter on ARTHRITIS discusses Alfalfa's role further. *See Also ENVIRONMENTAL POLLUTION.*

**CAYENNE** See TONIC—NERVE & GLAND for information on its tonic value. *See Also CIRCULATION; HIGH BLOOD PRESSURE; FATIGUE; INFLUENZA; BLOOD PURIFICATION/DETOXIFICATION*

## OTHER NUTRIENTS

*A wide range of dietary nutrients is necessary for optimum health. The following recommendations will usually not apply in toto for any given individual. But you should be certain your daily intake is balanced.*

## VITAMINS

(Daily requirements unless otherwise noted)

Vitamin A *25,000 I.U.*
Vitamin B Complex
Vitamin B1 *25 mg*
Vitamin B2 *25 mg*
Vitamin B6 25 mg
Vitamin B12 *25 mcg*
Vitamin C *500 mg*
Vitamin D *400 I.U.*
Vitamin E *200 I.U.*
Biotin *150 mcg*
Niacinamide *50 mg*
PABA *30 mg*
Pantothenic Acid *100 mg*
Choline *1,000 mg*
Inositol *1,000 mg*
Bioflavonoids *100 mg*
Folic Acid *400 mcg*

## MINERALS

Calcium/Magnesium
Zinc
Selenium
Phosphorous
Manganese
Iron
Copper
Iodine
Chromium

## MISCELLANEOUS

GLA
Essential Fatty Acid
Lecithin
Protein
Brewer's Yeast
Yogurt
Wheat Germ
HCl

# REFERENCES

1. Zhuo, D., et.al. **Clinical Application of Traditional Chinese Drugs,** Guangzhou, Guangdong People's press, 1975, pp. 321-322, 376.
2. Zhuo, D. "Preventive geriatrics: an overview from traditional chinese medicine." **American Journal of Chinese Medicine,** 10(1-4), 32-39, 1982.
3. Cheung, S.C. & Li, N.H. (eds) "Polygonum multiflorum Thumb." In **Chinese Medicinal Herbs of Hong Kong,** 1980.
4. Kam, J.K. "Mutagenic activity of Ho Shao Wu (Polygonum multiflorum Thunb)". **American Journal of Chinese Medicine,** 9(3), 213-215, 1981.
5. **Atlas of Commonly Used Chinese Traditional Drugs,** Revolutionary Committee of the Institute of Materia Medica, Chinese Academy of Medical Sciences, 1970. Or Report of the American Herbal Pharmacology Delegation, National Academy of Sciences, 1975. Much of this material can also be found in **The Barefoot Doctor's Manual.**
6. Mowrey, D.B. "Capsicum, Ginseng and Gotu Kola in combination." **The Herbalist,** Premier issue, 22-28, 1975.
7. Mowrey, D.B. "The effects of Capsicum, Gotu Kola and Ginseng on activity: further evidence." **The Herbalist,** 1(1), 51-54, 1976.
8. Mowrey, D.B. "Questions & Answers." **The Herbalist,** June, 26, 1977.

# Appendix A

## Licorice Root

Nowhere has the interaction between pharmacognocists and peudo- or semi-professional herbalists produced more confusion than in the discussion of the relative merits and dangers of ingesting Licorice root. Pharmacognocists seem to take great academic pride in pointing out scores of recorded cases of supposed Licorice root toxicity to an audience that is typically unequipped to evaluate the situation objectively. But a lack of scientific expertise does not stop some members of that audience from publicizing, under the guise of privileged insiders, information on Licorice root that is out of context, inaccurate and misleading. Such complicity between pontificating professionals and bumbling, eager-beaver, got-tell-em-like-it-is herbalists and authors has created doubts in the minds of thousands of people about one of the most beneficial herbs known.

I cannot hope to rectify the damage that has been done, but at least I can set forth the facts as they stand. The major fact is that there are no reported cases of intoxication as a result of using whole Licorice root, neither in powdered nor stick nor tea form.

The culprits are derivatives and concentrated extracts of the herb. With very few exceptions, all recorded cases involve one of the following abuses:

1. Licorice Candy that contains real and highly concentrated Licorice extract: European varieties are like this. Most american kinds are not. (Licorice flavor is due to anise, not Licorice.) If large amounts of this potent candy are eaten every day, even normal persons can develop mild toxic symptoms. Sensitive persons can develop severe potassium depletion. In most cases of toxicity, victims report having ingested one half pound or more per day. Children can be sensitive to smaller quantities. Rarely, deaths have occurred, but if the condition is noticed anywhere up to that point, it is completely reversible; no long term damage occurs.

2. Licorice Extract-Containing Laxatives: There are reported cases of severe toxicity from using these kind of laxatives two or three times daily. Only hypersenstive persons experience problems. The potassium depletion caused by the laxative itself is further aggravated by the presence of concentrated Licorice extract. The symptoms are, again, completely reversible. The idea of using Licorice root in a laxative is sound, but it is stupid to do it this way.

3. Carbenoxolone Sodium-Containing Ulcer Medications: This is also a case of concentration. Since CS is a highly concentrated form of glycyrrhizinic acid, it is not surprising that abuse of this drug can have side effects in some portion of the population. I recommend whole deglycyrrhizinated Licorice root for it is effective in treating ulcers, but without side effects.

The use of whole Licorice root (powdered or otherwise prepared) has not posioned anyone. But the distinction between extract and whole herb is seldom made in the press. Often the form of the preparation is omitted from published reports altogether. I've spent weeks tracking down the real facts in some cases. The distillation of all I've discovered can be summarized in a few short statements, as follows:

1) There are some people in the population that are sensitive to Licorice root extracts and derivatives. These persons should avoid overuse of true Licorice candy, laxatives containing large amounts of Licorice extract, and antiulcer drugs that are nothing but concentrated Licorice derivatives.

2) DGL (deglycyrrhizinated Licorice) has never caused toxic symptoms, and would be an excellent product to use for treating ulcers.

3) Whole Licorice root has never caused toxicity.

4) Millions of people all over the world consider Licorice root to be one of the top two or three herbs found in nature; they use it daily without any signs of toxicity.

The bad press on Licorice root is exactly that. Inadequate familiarity with the research coupled with a characteristic susceptibility to scare tactics have led some writers, lecturers and other so-called health experts to be overly cautious about a situation that really needs very little caution at all.

Finally, Licorice root should generally be combined with other herbs whereby the effectiveness of all the herbs is enhanced. This principle has been known and practiced religiously and with great precision by Chinese physicians for thousands of years.

# Cayenne

The controversy surrounding the use of Cayenne concerns its effect on the mucous membranes of the gastro-intestinal tract. A hurried and often incompetent review of experimental data has convinced some people (usually the same ones that are down on Licorice root) that Cayenne can and will damage mucosal cells and even cause ulcers in anyone who uses it daily. That position typically ignores or dismisses the hundreds of purported Cayenne-induced ulcer cures.

The dominant research finding has been that *under certain conditions*, Cayenne ingestion can result in damage to cells in the mucous membranes. Such damage is observed when Cayenne extract, or capsaicin (the potent active principle of Cayenne) are applied directly to isolated tissue and when high doses of these substances are ingested either by themselves or in conjunction with a poor diet (high fat, low protein).

Administration of low doses of Cayenne or capsaicin, or high doses with adequate nutrition does not produce mucosal damage.

Over time, the gastric mucosa adapts to Cayenne stimulation, so that if use is increased gradually from an initial very small amount to an eventual very high level, damage to the mucosa can be avoided altogether.

*Capsaicin* has been found to stimulate the appetite of rats, but to inhibit weight gain. It is postulated by the investigators that damage to gastro-intestinal epithelial cells prevents the absorption of nutrients. On the other hand, several investigators have found that the addition of *Cayenne* to a basic diet increases the growth rate of rats by as much as 25%. In one study the addition of Cayenne led to a significant increase in food intake, weight gain and food efficiency ratio. Adding the equivalent amount of pure *capsaicin* had the reverse effect: it significantly lowered food intake, weight gain and food efficiency ratos. These latter findings invalidate all of the research that uses capsaicin to study the toxic effects of Cayenne.

The following guidelines for proper use of Cayenne are offered. Conforming to these principles should result in full benefit from the herb with no toxicity.

1. Non-Cayenne users, beginning Cayenne users, infrequent users, and people who routinely reject hot sauce for their tacos should not attempt to treat their ulcers with large doses of Cayenne. They must begin small and work up. Remember that the herb is caustic for a reason; just because you can take a handful of capsules and bypass the unpleasant effect on the tongue, doesn't mean Nature intended for you to do that. Even one capsule, once per day, is not too small of a starting point.

2. Moderate and heavy users will probably experience some benefit from moderate doses of Cayenne to treat ulcers. Properly, however, such people should never get ulcers. But never say never. If you have ulcers, and have been a heavy Cayenne user, back off; use less and you will run less chance of aggravating the condition and you will have a better chance of experiencing the good effects Cayenne can have on the body.

3. If beginning and infrequent users want to avoid getting ulcers or other gastrointestinal problems from using Cayenne they should ingest very small amounts at first and gradually work up from there. After a few months, they will be able to ingest several capsules per day without irritating the gastric mucosa. This is especially important if one has a predisposition toward ulcers or stomach problems of any kind.

4. A high protein, low fat diet will counteract almost all negative effects of Cayenne on the gastric mucosa. In countries where Cayenne use is high, but other aspects of the diet are terrible, especially in a low protein, high fat situation, gastro-intestinal ailments, including ulcers, are very high, and appear to be aggravated by the Cayenne.

# INDEX

abortion, *Black haw bark*, 111, 188; 185

abscesses, *Echinacea root*, 250; *Fo-ti*, 288

acetylcholine, *Shepherd's purse*, 187

acidosis, 1

acne, 17, 247

ACTH, 27

Addison's disease

adrenal failure, *Licorice root*, 26

adrenal glands, *Licorice root*, 4, 26, 172

adrenal-pituitary axis, *Ginseng, siberian*, 192

adrenalin, *Gentian root*, 49

adrenals, *Chaparral*, 3, 32, 249; see also 4, 19, 25, 267

adrenergic, *Ginger root*, 218

adrenocortical, *Ginseng, siberian*, 102; see also 4, 25

adsorption vs. absorption, *Clay*, 130

afterpains, *Wild yam root*, 112

aftertaste, *Ginger root*, 197

aging, 191

ajoene, *Garlic*, 11

alcohol, 178

aldosterone, *Licorice root*, 258

**ALFALFA**, anti-cancer, 91; anti-rheumatic, 2; antibacterial, 91; appetite stimulant, 291; arthritis, 1, 2; bile acids, 91; cholesterol lowering, 2, 91; detoxification, 2; environmental pollution, 87, 91; estrogenic, 2; fiber, 91; nutritive, 2, 91; protein, 291; radiotherapy, 91; saponins, 2, 91; steroidal properties, 2, 91; tonic—whole body, 285, 291; vitality, 291; vitamin k, 91

algenic acid, *Kelp*, 268

**ALGIN**, anti-cancer, 88; anti-oxidant, 88; bile, 88; breast cancer, 88; cholesterol lowering, 88; environmental pollution, 87, 88; fiber, 88; heavy metals, 88; immune system, 88; pollution, 88; radioactivity, 88; strontium-90, 88; toxins, 88

allergenic, *Wild yam root*, 177

allergens, 130

allergens, *Mullein leaf*, 131; *Wild cherry bark*, 131

allergies, *Clay*, 129-130; *Horehound*, 129, 131; *Mullein leaf*, 129, 131; *Wild cherry bark*, 129, 131; see also 239

allicin, *Garlic*, 10, 122, 230

allyl sulfide, *Garlic*, 230

aloe-emodin, *Buckthorn bark*, 60; *Cascara sagrada bark*, 58

alterative, *Burdock root*, 3, 57, 249, 279; *Kelp*, 20; *Licorice root*, 249; *Red clover*, 54; *Sarsaparilla root*, 19, 287; *Stillingia*, 57; *Yellow dock root*, 19, 250; see also 18, 20

**ALUM**, anus, 147; astringent, 145, 147; canker sores, 147; hematuria, 147; hemoptysis, 147; hemorrhoids, 145, 147; inflammation, 147; menorrhagia, 147; neuralgia, 147; piles, 147; pyorrhea, 147; sore gums, 147

amenorrhea, *Black haw bark*, 111

amoebic infection, 117

amylase, *Ginger root*, 261

analgesic, *Blue vervain*, 120, 206, 223, 226; *Chaparral*, 3; *Kelp*, 223, 226; *Passion flower*, 110, 216; *Raspberry leaf*, 186; *Rosemary leaf*, 138, 225; *Skullcap*, 223, 225; *White willow bark*, 223, 224; *Wood betony*, 223, 224

androgen, 26

anemia, *Blue vervain*, 206; *Yellow dock root*, 19, 207; see also 17

anesthetic, *Echinacea root*, 118; *Uva-ursi*, 187

angina, *White willow bark*, 224; 135

anorexia, *Gentian root*, 205; 203

antacid, 256

anthelminitic, *Black walnut*, 230; *Pumpkin seed*, 236; see also 229

anthraquinones, *Buckthorn bark*, 60; *Cascara sagrada bark*, 169; *Cascara sagrada bark*, 58

anti-aggressive, *Valerian root*, 12

anti-arthritic, *Licorice root*, 4

anti-cancer, *Alfalfa*, 91; *Algin*, 88; *Kelp*, 112; *Black walnut*, 230; *Chamomile*, 205; *Chaparral*, 3, 54-56, 248; *Fo-ti*, 289; *Kelp*, 60; *Rhubarb root*, 171; *Uva-ursi*, 187

anti-coagulant, *Irish moss*, 260

anti-convulsive, *Valerian root*, 12

anti-diarrheal, *Blue vervain*, 206 *Raspberry leaf*, 186; *Wood betony*, 224

anti-epileptic, *Skullcap*, 217

anti-fatigue, *Cayenne*, 102; *Ginseng, siberian*, 102; *Gotu kola*, 103, 290

anti-fever, *Fo-ti*, 289

anti-fungal, *Burdock root*, 58; *Garlic*, 122

anti-granulomatous, 4

anti-infectious, *Bayberry root bark*, 99; *Cayenne*, 250; *Kelp*, 250 anti-inflammatory, *Black cohosh root*, 42, 108; *Blue vervain*, 120, 206, 50; *Chamomile*, 110, 205; *Gentian root*, 68; *Licorice root*, 4, 109, 120, 242, 259; *Peppermint leaf*, 75; *Saw palmetto berry*, 242; see also 60.

anti-leukemia, *Cascara sagrada bark*, 58

anti-rheumatic, *Alfalfa*, 2; *Kelp*, 60; *Chaparral*, 3, 32; see also 6

anti-scorbutic, *Uva-ursi*, 67

anti-tumor, *Burdock root*, 58; *Licorice root*, 56; see also 37

anti-tussive, *Licorice root*, 242

anti-ulcer, *Chamomile*, 205; *Peppermint leaf*, 75

anti-viral, *Cinchona*, 121; *Licorice root*, 109, 119

antibacterial, *Alfalfa*, 91; *Chamomile*, 110, 205; *Chaparral*, 32; *Garlic*, 122; *Goldenseal root*, 257; *Kelp*, 123; *Licorice root*, 119; *Oregon grape root*, 57; *Parsley*, 33; *Rhubarb root*, 171; *Yellow dock root*, 19

antibiotic, *Bayberry root bark*, 157; *Burdock root*, 58; *Cascara sagrada bark*, 58; *Catnip*, 76; *Cayenne*, 159; *Chickweed*, 241; *Cleavers*, 83; *Garlic*, 122; *Goldenseal root*, 98, 119, 158, 204, 272; *Horsetail (shavegrass)*, 32; *Kelp*, 123; *Kelp*, 139; *Kelp*, 235; *Mullein leaf*, 241; *Red clover*, 54; *Sarsaparilla root*, 58; *Uva-ursi*, 187; *Yellow dock root*, 250

antibodies, 130

antigen-antibody reaction, 130

antihemolytic, *Papaya leaf*, 187; *Shepherd's purse*, 187

antimalarial, *Cinchona*, 121; *Rosemary leaf*, 226

antimicotic, *Chamomile*, 110, 205

antimicrobial, 67, 75

antimicrobial, *Chaparral*, 249; *Echinacea root*, 250; *Garlic*, 122; *Licorice root*, 120; *Licorice root*, 249; *Parsley*, 67; *Peppermint leaf*, 75; *Sarsaparilla root*, 19

antioxidant, *Algin*, 88; *Chaparral*, , 553; *Celery seed*, 180; *Kelp*, 88; see also 32, 55

antipyretic (antifever), *Goldenseal root*, 158

antipyretic, *Bayberry root bark*, 159; *Cinchona*, 121; White willow bark, 224

antiseptic, *Buchu leaf*, 235; *Echinacea root*, 118; *Goldenseal root*, 98, 119, 158; *Juniper berry*, 274; *Myrrh gum*, 273; *Uva-ursi*, 67, 83, 187; *White willow bark*, 224

anti-spasmodic, *Black haw bark*, 111; *Chamomile*, 110, 205; *Hops*, 218; *Motherwort*, 138; *Passion flower*, 165; *Skullcap*, 217; *Wild yam root*, 181

antistress, *Ginseng, siberian*, 152

antitoxic, *Fo-ti*, 289; *Kelp*, 88

anus, *Alum*, 147

anxiety, *Rosemary leaf*, 139; *Valerian root*, 12, 164; see also 9- 10, 191, 203, 213, 223

aperient, *Licorice root*, 172

aphrodisiac, *Damiana*, 152; *Ginseng, siberian*, 152

apiol, *Parsley*, 234

appetite stimulant, *Alfalfa*, 291; *Catnip*, 76; *Cinchona*, 121; *Gentian root*, 205, 259; *Saw palmetto berry*, 77, 209

appetite suppressant, *Plantain*, 41-42, 277-278

**APPLE PECTIN**, bile acids, 39, 90; blood sugar, 40; cholesterol regulation, 37, 39, 89-90; coronary heart disease, 89; diabetes, 40, 89; effects on intestine, 89-90; environmental pollution, 87, 89; fiber, types of, 89; food additives, 91; gallstones, 40, 90; heavy metals, 91; insulin, 40; lipids, 39; mucilage, 90; obesity, 89; toxins, 89; vegetarians, 89

arbutin, *Uva-ursi*, 83, 187

aromatic, *Buchu leaf*, 68; *Fo-ti*, 288; *Peppermint leaf*, 103

arsenic, *Kelp*, 20

arteriosclerosis, 10, 135

arthritis, *Alfalfa*, 1, 2; *Burdock root*, 1, 3; *Cayenne*, 1, 4; *Celery seed*, 1-3,; *Chaparral*, 1, 3; *Fo-ti*, 289; *Kelp*, 1, 4, 53, 208, 226; *Licorice root*, 1, 4; *Queen-of-the-meadow*, 1, 4; *Sarsaparilla root*, 1, 3, 58; *White willow bark*, 224; see also 17, 31, 81, 151, 277

arythmia, 136

ascorbic acid levels, *Chaparral*, 3, 32, 249

asculetin, *Black haw bark*, 111

asiaticoside, *Gotu kola*, 290

aspirin, *White willow bark*, 224

asthma, *Black haw bark*, 188; *Marshmallow*, 33; *Mullein leaf*, 241; *Parsley*, 83; *Passion flower*, 165; *Wood betony*, 224; see also 129

astringent tannins, *Rhubarb root*, 171

astringent, *Alum*, 145, 147; *Bayberry root bark*, 99; *Cranesbill root*, 186; *Goldenseal root*, 145, 148; *Mullein leaf*, 145, 147; *Myrrh gum*, 260; *Queen-of-the-meadow*, 84; *Raspberry leaf*, 99, 186; *Shepherd's purse*,

nurture, 53, 58; gallstones, 179; immunosuppressant, 58; in elderly patients, 170; intestinaltonus, 170; jaundice, 179; laxative, 167, 179, 58; liver disorders, 177, 179; liver, 58; non-griping, 170; non-habituating, 170; non-toxic, 170; rhein, 58
cataracts, 97
catarrh, *Saw palmetto berry*, 242; *Wood betony*, 224
cathartic, 168
**CATNIP**, antibiotic, 76; appetite stimulant, 76; bronchial infections, 76; carminative, 76; colds, 76; colic, 76; digestion, 73, 76; tonic, 76
**CAYENNE**, anti-fatigue, 102; anti-infectious, 250; antibiotic, 159; arthritis, 1, 4; atherosclerosis, 40; bile acids, 40; blood detoxification, 17, 19; blood pressure, 9, 12; blood purification, 17, 19; capsaicin, 12, 40; cardiac stimulant, 19, 139; carminative, 208; cholesterol lowering, 12, 37, 40; cholesterol regulation, 40; circulation, 47, 48, 102, 139, 208, 242; colds, 159; diaphoretic, 19; diuretic, 81, 84; expectorant, 242; eyes, 97, 99; fatigue, 101, 102; gastric secretion, 48; gastro-intestinal stimulant, 208; glands, 203, 208; heart, 135, 139, 208; hypertension, 40; infections, 157, 159; influenza, 157, 159; laxative, 167, 172; lipids, 40; liver disorders, 177, 180; liver, 12; metabolism, 209; mucous, 242; nausea, 197; nerves, 203, 208; nutritive, 4, 84, 99, 139, 242; oxygen, 242; prostate, 233, 235; respiration, cellular, 209; respiratory ailments, 209; respiratory reflex, 102; skin disorders, 247; sore throat, 159; stimulant, 4, 19, 48, 102, 139, 198, 208, 235, 250; stress, 102; thyroid, 267, 269; tonic, 203, 208
**CELERY SEED**, antioxidative, 180; arthritis, 1-3,; blood cleanser, 2; blood pressure lowering, 3, 180; diuretic, 2, 180; gout, 3; hyperglycemia, 180; insulin, 180; liver disorders, 177, 180; rheumatism, 2; sedative, 180
cellulitis, *Peppermint leaf*, 75
central nervous system depressant, *Ginseng, siberian*, 288
central nervous system stimulant, *Ginseng, siberian*, 192, 288
cervical infection, 271
cervicitis, *Gotu kola*, 193, 290

cervix, *Black cohosh root*, 108
chamazulen, *Chamomile*, 206
**CHAMOMILE**, anti-cancer, 205; anti-inflammatory, 110, 205; anti-ulcer, 205; antibacterial, 110, 205; anti-micotic, 110, 205; antispasmodic, 110, 205; bisabolol, 206; bitter, 205; carminative, 110; chamazulen, 206; dermatological ailments, 110, 205; female tonic, 107, 110; glands, 203, 205; liver, 205; nerves, 203, 205; nontoxic, 110; pain, 205; panacea, 205; sclerosis, 205; sedative, 110, 205; teeth, 205; tonic, 203, 205
**CHAPARRAL**, adrenals, 3, 32, 249; analgesic, 3; anti-rheumatoid, 3, 32; antibacterial, 32; anticancer, 3, 54-56, 248; antimicrobial, 249; antioxidant, , 553; arthritis, 1, 3; ascorbic acid levels, 3, 32, 249; bone-flesh-cartilage, 31, 32; dental carries, 32; detoxify/nurture, 53-56; glycolysis, 248; inflammation, 32; mitochondrial respiration, 3; NDGA, 3, 32, 55, 248; pain relief, 3; rheumatism, 3, 32; skin cancer, 32, 56; skin disorders, 247, 248; vasodepressant, 3
chelating agent, *Cascara sagrada bark*, 58
chickweed, 278
**CHICKWEED**, antibiotic, 241; blood disease, 241; bronchitis, 241; colds, 241; eye inflammation, 241; flu, 241; gout, 241; hemorrhoids, 241; joint disease, 241; nutritive, 241; panacea, 241; respiratory ailments, 239, 241; rheumatism, 241; sore throat, 241; tuberculosis, 241; whooping cough, 241
childbirth, *Wild yam root*, 12; *Slippery elm bark*, 241
childhood behavior disorders, *Valerian root*, 12, 215
children, hyperactive, 191
children, suitability of *Rhubarb root* for, 171
cholekinetic, *Dandelion root*, 179
cholera, *Garlic*, 122; *Goldenseal root*,
cholera, *Garlic*, 122; *Goldenseal root*, 158, 272; *Marshmallow*, 33; *Prickly ash bark*, 59; *Slippery elm bark*, 146.
choleretic, *Dandelion root*, 179; *Peppermint leaf*, 75
cholesterol lowering, *Alfalfa*, 2, 91; *Algin*, 88; *Bladderwrack*, 280; *Cayenne*, 12, 37, 40; *Garlic*, 10; *Ginger root*, 48, 200; *Kelp*, 193; *Kelp*, 280; *Kelp*, 88; *Plantain*, 41, 277; *Skullcap*, 225; *Wild yam root*,

ne, 203, 208; *Chamomile*, 203, 205; *Dandelion root*, 203, 206; *Gentian root*, 203, 205, ; *Goldenseal root*, 203, 204; *Kelp*, 203, 208; *Saw palmetto berry*, 203, 209; *Skullcap*, 203, 207; *Wood betony*, 203, 208; *Yellow dock root*, 203, 207; see also 267
glucocorticoids, *Licorice root*, 26
glucose metabolism, 25, 28, 66
glucose, *Hawthorn berry*, 280
glycolysis, *Chaparral*, 248
glycosides, *Buckthorn bark*, 60; *Passion flower*, 216
glycyrrhetic acid, *Licorice root*, 4
glycyrrhizin, *Licorice root*, 4, 153, 180, 257
goiter, *Kelp*, 268
**GOLDENSEAL ROOT**, antibacterial, 257; antibiotic, 98, 119, 158, 204, 272; antipyretic (antifever), 158; antiseptic, 98, 119, 158; astringent, 145, 148; berberine, 158, 204, 257, 272; bile, 257; blood, coagulation of, 272; cholera, 158, 272; cinchona, comparison to, 158; colds, 158; congestion, 158; conunctivitis, 98; diarrhea, 257; eyes, 97, 98; fevers, 117, 119, 158; gas, 257; gastroenteritis, 257; giardia, 257; giardiasis, 158; glands, 203, 204; heartburn, 257; hemorrhage, uterine, 272; hemorrhoids, 145, 148; hydrastine, 158, 204, 257, 272; indigestion, 257; infections, 117, 119, 157, 158; inflammation, 148; influenza, 157, 158; laxative, 167, 171-172; mucous membranes, 158; nausea, 257; nerves, 203, 204; panacea, 204; sore throat, 158; stomach/intestinal, 255, 257; tonic, 203, 204; tuberculosis, 158; ulcers, 257; uterine tonic, 204; vaginal yeast infection, 271, 272; vasoconstrictor, 204
gonorrhea, *Marshmallow*, 33; *Prickly ash bark*, 59; *Saw palmetto berry*, 153
**GOTU KOLA**, antifatigue, 103, 290; asiaticoside, 290; blood purifier, 193; cervicitis, 193, 290; diuretic, 193, 289; fatigue, 101, 103; leprosy, 193, 290; longevity,, 193; low blood sugar, 25, 27; memory, 193; mental alertness, 191, 193; pruritis, 290; psoriasis, 193, 290; senility, 191, 193; skin disorders, 193, 289-290; stamina, mental, 193; stimulant, 290; stress, 103; syphilis, 193; tonic, 193, 290; tonic—whole body, 285, 289; tuberculosis, 290; vaginitis, 193, 290
gout, *Celery seed*, 3; *Chickweed*, 241; *Fo-ti*, 288; *Queen-of-the- meadow*,

4; *Red clover*, 54; *White willow bark*, 224; *Wood betony*, 224; see also 1, 17, 81, 223, 277
granulomatous, *Echinacea root*, 119
gum disease, 18

hair, *Kelp*, 268
harman, *Passion flower*, 216
**HAWTHORN BERRY**, atherosclerosis, 40; cardiac insufficiency, 137; cholesterol regulation, 37, 40; coronary stress, 280; digitalis, 137; exercise, 137; free fatty acids, 279; glucose, 280; heart, 135-137, 279; hepatitis, 137; hypertension, 40; lipids, 40; nutritive, 40; obesity, 277, 279; oxygen, 137, 279; pyruvic acid, 280; stress, 279; triglycerides, 280; vasodilation, 137; weight loss, 277, 279
hayfever, *Clay*, 129-130; *Horehound*, 129, 131; *Mullein leaf*, 129, 131; *Wild cherry bark*, 129, 131
headache, *Cinchona*, 121; *Ginger root*, 104, 200; *Hops*, 164*Rosemary leaf*, 226; *Skullcap*, 225; *Valerian root*, 164; *White willow bark*, 224; *Wood betony*, 216; see also 197, 223
heart disease, *Bladderwrack*, 69; *Fo-ti*, 289; *Garlic*, 11; *Kelp*, 208; see also 3, 37, 82, 89, 135
heart murmur, 136
heart stimulant, 136
heart, *Black cohosh root*, 42; *Cayenne*, 135, 139, 208; *Hawthorn berry*, 135-137, 279; *Kelp*, 103; *Kelp*, 135, 139; *Motherwort*, 135, 138; *Rosemary leaf*, 135, 138
heartburn, *Gentian root*, 68, 259; *Ginger root*, 261; *Goldenseal root*, 257; *Peppermint leaf*, 75; *Wood betony*, 21, 224; see also 47, 73-75, 177, 255
heavy metals, *Algin*, 88; *Apple pectin*, 91; *Bran*, 91; *Kelp*, 88
hematuria, *Alum*, 147
hemolysis, 19, 32
hemolytic (blood clotting), *Horsetail (shavegrass)*, 32
hemoptysis, *Alum*, 147
hemorrhage, *Goldenseal root*, uterine, 272; *Papaya leaf*, 187; see also 182
hemorrhoids, *Alum*, 145, 147; *Chickweed*, 241; *Cranesbill root*, 186; *Fo-ti*, 288; *Goldenseal root*, 145, 148; *Mullein leaf*, 145, 147; *Myrrh gum*, 273; *Plantain*, 273; *Rhubarb root*, 171; *Slippery elm bark*, 145, 146; *Witch hazel leaf*, 145-147, 272
hemostatic, *Witch hazel leaf*, 272
Hepatichol, *Dandelion root*, 179
hepatitis, *Bayberry root bark*, 159; *Corn*

oil, unsaturated, 38
oligouria, *Corn silk*, 235
**OREGON GRAPE ROOT**, antibacterial, 57; berberine, 57; detoxify/nurture, 53, 56-57; hydrastine, 57; skin problems, 57
otitis media, *Peppermint leaf*, 75
ovarian troubles, *Kelp*, 154; *Saw palmetto berry*, 111; *Wild yam root*, 112, 181
ovulation, *Fo-ti*, 289; *Licorice root*, 109, 153
oxygen, *Bladderwrack*, 280; *Cayenne*, 242; *Hawthorn berry*, 137, 279; *Kelp*, 242, 280

pain killer, *Burdock root*, 3; *Uva-ursi*, 187; *Wood betony*, 223, 224
pain relief, *Blue vervain*, 223, 226, 206; *Chaparral*, 3; *Kelp*, 223; *Raspberry leaf*, 186; *Rosemary leaf*, 138, 223; *Skullcap*, 223, 225; *White willow bark*, 223, 224; see also 107, 118, 163
pain, *Chamomile*, 205; *Fenugreek seed*, 261; *Fo-ti*, 289; *Plantain*, 34, 241; *Rosemary leaf*, 225; *Skullcap*, 165; *Wild yam root*, 181
palpitations, *Motherwort*, 135, 138
panacea, *Chamomile*, 205; *Chickweed*, 241; *Goldenseal root*, 204
pancreas, *Dandelion root*, 67; *Fenugreek seed*, 261; *Gentian root*, 68, 259; see also 65-66, 177
papain, *Papaya leaf*, 74, 255
**PAPAYA LEAF**, antihemolytic, 187; biological scalpel, 74; blood, coagulation of, 260; chymopapain, 74; digestion, 73, 74, 260; emmenagogue, 187; hemorrhage, 187; menorrhagia, 187; menstruation, 185, 187; papain, 74, 255; skin problems, 74-75; stomach/intestinal,255, 259; ulcers, 75, 260
paramecicidal, *Bayberry root bark*, 159
parasites, *Black walnut*, 229; *Butternut root bark*, 229, 231; *Garlic*, 229, 230; see also 117, 256
parasympathetic, *Blue vervain*, 226, 49
**PARSLEY**, antibacterial, 33; antimicrobial, 67; apiol, 234; asthma, 83; bone-flesh-cartilage, 31, 33; diabetes, 65, 67; digestion, 83; diuretic, 81, 234; essential oil, 33; expectorant, 82; gallstones, 67; hypotensive, 33, 67, 82, 83; jaundice, 67, 83; laxative, 67, 82; liver, 67; menstrual problems, 83; myristicin, 234; nutritive, 33, 234; prostate problems, 233, 234; uterine tonic, 67
parturition, *Passion flower*, 110; *Raspberry leaf*, 186; *Squaw vine*, 274

**PASSION FLOWER**, analgesic, 110, 216; anti-spasmodic, 165; asthma, 165; cardiovascular, 165; circulation, 165; concentration, mental, 165; convulsions, 165; female tonic, 107, 110; flavanoids, 216; geriatrics, 165; glycosides, 216; harman, 216; insomnia, 163, 165, 216; menopause, 110; menses, 110; mental acuity, 165; parturition, 110; relaxation, 165; restlessness, 165; sedative, 110, 165, 216; sleep, 165; tonic, 110; tranquilizing, 215
pectin, *Plantain*, 278
**PECTIN**, see APPLE PECTIN
penicillin, *Garlic*, 122
**PEPPERMINT LEAF**, anti-inflammatory, 75; anti-ulcer, 75; antimicrobial, 75; aromatic, 103; bile, 75; calmative, 192; cellulitis, 75; choleretic, 75; circulation, 192; colic, 75; concentration, mental, 192; constipation, 75; cramps, 75; cystitis, 75; diarrhea, 75; digestion, 73, 75, 103; energy, 103; enteritis, 75; essential oils, 192, 75; fatigue, 101, 103; gallbladder, 75; gastritis, 75; heartburn, 75; herpes, 75; indigestion, 75; influenza A virus, 75; mental alertness, 191, 192; mumps, 75; otitis media, 75; senility, 191, 192; stimulant, 103; test taking, 192; throat infections, 75; vaginal yeast infection, 75; viruses, 75; vitality, 103; volatile oils, 75, 192
peptic glands, *Myrrh gum*, 260
peristalsis, 168; *Ginger root*, 172; *Rhubarb root*, 171
phagocytic, 21
pharyngitis, *Bayberry root bark*, 159
phelbitis, *Witch hazel leaf*, 147
phenolic glycosides, *Uva-ursi*, 67
phlebitis, 145
phospholipids, *Garlic*, 11
piles, *Alum*, 147
pineal gland, 267
pituitary disease, *Licorice root*, 27
pituitary, 25, 267
**PLANTAIN**, appetite control, 41, 42; appetite suppressant, 278; atherosclerosis, 278; bile, 41; bone-flesh-cartilage, 31, 34; bronchitis, 241; cholesterol lowering, 41, 277; cholesterol regulation, 37, 41; colds, 241; constipation, 41; coughs, 241, 273; diabetes, 278; feet, pain and fatigue of, 34; fiber, 278; hemorrhoids, 273; inflammation, 34; itching, 34; lipids, 41, 278; lipoprotein, 278; mucilage, 34, 41, 241, 273, 277; obesity, 41, 277; pain, 34, 241; pectin, 278; poison ivy dermatitis, 34; respiratory ailments,

venereal disease, *Burdock root*, 249;
    *Sarsaparilla root*, 58, 153; *Stillingia*,
    57; see also 17
verbenalin, *Blue vervain*, 226
vermifuge, 229; *Butternut root bark*,
    231
vertigo, 197; *Black cohosh root*, 216;
    *Ginger root*, 199
viral warts, 17
viruses, *Peppermint leaf*, 75
vision, 97
vitality, *Alfalfa* 291; *Peppermint leaf*,
    103
vitamin A, *Dandelion root*, 207
vitamin C, 32
vitamin k, *Alfalfa*, 91
volatile oils, *Buchu leaf*, 83; *Fennel
    seeds*, 76; *Juniper berry*, 83; *Myrrh
    gum*, 119; *Peppermint leaf*, 75, 192
vulnerary, *Blue vervain*, 206; *Wood be-
    tony*, 216

warts, 17
wastes, body, 18, 21
weakness, 101
weight loss, *Bladderwrack*, 277, 280;
    *Burdock root*, 277, 279; *Fennel
    seeds*, 277, 279; *Hawthorn berry*,
    277, 279; *Kelp*, 277, 280; *Plantain*,
    278
white blood cells, *Myrrh gum* 119
**WHITE WILLOW BARK**, analgesic,
    223, 224; angina, 224; antipyretic,
    224; antiseptic, 224; arthritis, 224;
    aspirin, 224; disinfectant, 224; fever,
    224; gout, 224; headache, 224;
    malaria, 224; pain relief, 223, 224;
    rheumatic fever, 224; rheumatism,
    224; salicin, 224; salicylic acid, 224
whooping cough, *Chickweed*, 241; *Mul-
    lein leaf*, 241; see also 33, 54
**WILD CHERRY BARK**, allergens, 131;
    allergies, 129, 131; cough, 240;
    hayfever, 129, 131; respiratory ail-
    ments, 239, 240
**WILD YAM ROOT**, afterpains, 112;
    allergenic, 177; antispasmodic, 181;
    biliouscolic, 180; blood pressure,
    181; child birth, 12; cholesterol-
    lowering, 181; contraseptives, 112;
    cortisone, 112; cramps, 112;
    diosgenin, 112; dysmenorrhea, 112,
    181; estrogens, 112; female tonic,
    107, 111-112; gallstones, 181; in-
    digestion, 181; liver disorders, 177,

180-181; menses, 112; miscarriage,
    111; ovarian neuralgia, 112, 181;
    pain, 181; progesterone, 112; ster-
    oidal, 111; steroids, 180; stress,
    181
**WITCH HAZEL LEAF**, astringent, 145-
    147, 272, 187; bacteriostatic, 147,
    273; carvacol, 273; eugenol, 273;
    hemorrhoids, 145-147, 272;
    hemostatic, 272; menstruation, 185,
    187; phlebitis, 147; prolapsus, 272;
    tannin, 146, 272; vaginal yeast in-
    fection, 271, 272-273; varicose
    veins, 272; venal system, 146
**WOOD BETONY**, analgesic, 223, 224;
    antidiarrheic, 224; asthma, 224;
    astringent, 216, 224; bladder
    stones, 224; carminative, 224;
    catarrh, 224; fatigue, 224; glands,
    203, 208; gout, 224; headache,
    216; heartburn, 21, 224; hypoten-
    sive, 193, 208, 216, 223; insanity,
    216; kidney stones, 224; mental al-
    ertness, 191, 193; nerves, 203, 208;
    nervine, 193; nervous tension, 213,
    216; nervousness, 193, 224; neural-
    gia, 216; pain killer, 223, 224; re-
    laxant, 208, 216; sedative, 193,
    216, 224; senility, 191,193; tonic,
    203, 208, 216; tuberculosis, 225;
    vulnerary, 216
worms, *Black walnut*, 229; *Butternut
    root bark* 229, 231; *Garlic*, 229,
    230; see also 73, 256
wound healer, *Marshmallow*, 33
wounds, 32, 33
wounds, *Sarsaparilla root*, 287; *Slippery
    elm bark*, 34, 241; see also 32-33
yeast, 271
**YELLOW DOCK ROOT**, alterative, 19,
    250; anemia, 19, 207; antibacterial,
    19; antibiotic, 250; astringent, 207;
    blood detoxification/purification, 17,
    19; cancer, 250; cleanses, 207; de-
    toxification, 19, 207; eczema, 250;
    gall bladder problems, 207; glands,
    203, 207; inflammation, 207; iron,
    207; leprosy, 250; liver ailments,
    207; liver, 19; nerves, 203, 207;
    psoriasis, 250; ringworm, 250; scur-
    vy, 19; skin disease, 19, 207, 247,
    250 ; thiamine, 19; tonic, 203, 207
yin, *Fo-ti*, to increase, 289
zinc, 20
zingibain, *Ginger root*, 76, 261